Obesity and Diabetes

Second edition

Other titles in the Wiley Diabetes in Practice Series

Exercise and Sport in Diabetes Second Edition
Edited by Dinesh Nagi
978 0470 022061

Complementary Therapies and the Management of Diabetes and Vascular Disease
Edited by Patricia Dunning
978 0470 014585

Diabetes in Clinical Practice: Questions and Answers from Case Studies
Edited by N. Katsilambros, E. Diakoumopoulou, I. Ioannidis, S. Liatis, K. Makrilakis, N. Tentolouris and P. Tsapogas
978 0470 035221

Prevention of Type 2 Diabetes
Edited by Manfred Ganz
978 0470 857335

Diabetes – Chronic Complications Second Edition
Edited by Kenneth Shaw and Michael Cummings
978 0470 865798

The Metabolic Syndrome
Edited by Christopher Byrne and Sarah Wild
978 0470 025116

Psychology in Diabetes Care Second Edition
Edited by Frank J. Snoek and T. Chas Skinner
978 0470 015049

The Foot in Diabetes Fourth Edition
Edited by Andrew J. M. Boulton, Peter R. Cavanagh and Gerry Rayman
978 0470 015049

Gastrointestinal Function in Diabetes Mellitus
Edited by Michael Horowitz and Melvin Samson
978 0471 899167

Diabetic Nephropathy
Edited by Christopher Hasslacher
978 0471 589924

Nutritional Management of Diabetis Mellitus
Edited by Gary Frost, Anne Dornhorst and David R. Hadden
978 0471 962045

Hypoglycaemia in Clinical Diabetes Second Edition
Edited by Brian M. Frier and Miles Fisher
978 0470 018446

Diabetic Cardiology
Edited by Miles Fisher and John McMurray
978 0470 862049

Diabetes in Old Age
Edited by Alan Sinclair
9780470065624

Obesity and Diabetes

Second Edition

Editors

Anthony H. Barnett

Department of Medicine, University of Birmingham and Birmingham Heartlands and Solihull NHS Trust, UK

Sudhesh Kumar

Warwick Medical School, University of Warwick, UK

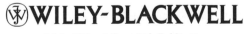

WILEY-BLACKWELL

A John Wiley & Sons, Ltd., Publication

Library of Congress Cataloging-in-Publication Data

Obesity and diabetes / editors, Anthony H. Barnett, Sudhesh Kumar. – 2nd ed.
   p. ; cm.
  Includes bibliographical references and index.
  ISBN 978-0-470-51981-3 (cloth)
 1. Obesity. 2. Non-insulin-dependent diabetes. I. Barnett, A. H. (Anthony H.), 1951– II. Kumar, Sudhesh.
  [DNLM: 1. Diabetes Mellitus, Type 2–etiology. 2. Obesity–complications. 3. Diabetes Mellitus,
Type 2–epidemiology. 4. Diabetes Mellitus, Type 2–therapy. 5. Obesity–therapy. WK 840 O12 2009]
  RC628.O2263 2009
  616.3'98–dc22
                2008047104

ISBN: 978-0470-51981-3(H/B)

A catalogue record for this book is available from the British Library.

Set in 10.5/12.5 pt Times by Thomson Digital, New Delhi
Printed in Great Britain by CPI Antony Rowe, Chippenham, Wiltshire

Contents

Foreword

Diabetes and obesity are amongst the biggest scourges of the twenty-first century – the twin horsemen of the apocalypse. Until 50 years ago diabetes was considered to be a disease of developed countries and commonest in Europids. In the 1960s it became clear that diabetes was very common in certain other groups – Pima Indians and Nauruans in the Pacific. In both these groups it was associated with rapid improvement in economic status. Since that time there has been an inexorable increase in the number of people with diabetes world-wide. In some areas this rise started later than others, for example rural sub-Saharan Africa, but now there are few parts of the world which are spared. By far the majority of this rise has been in type 2 diabetes, although for unknown reasons there has been an increase in type 1 diabetes as well. In 1990 there were approximately 100 million people with diabetes. This had risen to almost 250 million by 2007 and is predicted, conservatively, to increase further to 350 million by 2030. In addition, there are about the same number of people with impaired glucose tolerance, many of whom will develop diabetes in the future.

Several factors have contributed to this epidemic rise in prevalence. These are largely related to lifestyle changes. Ethnicity and family history contribute – thus people of South Asian origin and Afro-Caribbeans have a much greater susceptibility than Europids – but only if their lifestyle changes. The latter encompasses obesity as well as decreased physical activity and increasing urbanization.

The major problem is, of course, obesity. This has shown a parallel rise world-wide with that found for diabetes. In the United States a recent survey showed that 26% of adults were obese (body mass index, BMI $> 30\,\mathrm{kg/m2}$) with highest rates in the 50–59 year age group and in non-Hispanic black women (39%). Other countries are showing similar rates, with the United Kingdom and Australia rapidly catching up. This is not however restricted to the economically advantaged world. Obesity rates are rising in all countries and there is now a U-curve for BMI in many countries, with malnutrition and underweight still rife at the same time as obesity rates are rising. Of even greater concern are obesity rates in children, which have also risen dramatically – up to 20% in many countries – and are now associated with the appearance of type 2 diabetes in children and adolescents, a previously unknown phenomenon. The costs are crippling – both economically and to the individual. The National Health Service already spends £4.2 million a year on the direct effects of obesity and £15.8 million on the wider costs.

This is predicted to rise to £50 million by 2050. It has also been calculated that 58% of the rise in type 2 diabetes can be attributed to obesity.

Obesity is linked to diabetes through insulin resistance, which is directly related to weight. Susceptible people may have sufficient insulin secretion to maintain normoglycaemia if they retain sensitivity to insulin. However, when they become less insulin sensitive through increased weight and decreased activity then hyperglycaemia develops and eventually diabetes supervenes. The distribution of weight is also important with central adiposity more damaging than peripheral fat deposition.

The editors of the current book have recognized the importance of the link between obesity and diabetes – this indeed is the second edition. They have assembled an international team of experts to discuss many of the key aspects of type 2 diabetes, obesity and their treatment. The discussions range from basic pathophysiology and genetics to behavioural change, the role of bariatric surgery and childhood obesity to the impact of ethnicity and obesity and employment. I recommend the volume to you strongly.

Sir George Alberti

Contributors

Anthony Barnett

Birmingham Heartlands Hospital
Undergraduate Centre
Bordesley Green East
Birmingham
B9 5SS UK

Iain Broom

The Robert Gordon University
School of Life Sciences
St. Andrew Street
Aberdeen
AB25 1HG UK

Ian Campbell

Park House Medical Centre
61 Burton Road
Carlton
Nottingham
NG4 3DQ UK

Tahseen Chowdhury

Department of Metabolic Medicine
The Royal London Hospital
Whitechapel Road
London
E1 1BB UK

Carlton Cooke

Carnegie Research Institute
Leeds Metropolitan University
Headingley Campus
Leeds
LS6 3QS UK

Paul Gateley

Carnegie Research Institute
Leeds Metropolitan University
Headingley Campus
Leeds
LS6 3QS UK

Susan A Jebb

MRC Human Nutrition Research
Elsie Widdowson Laboratory
Fulbourn Road
Cambridge
CV1 9NL UK

Laura Johnson

Health Behaviour Unit
Department of Epidemiology and Public
Health
University College London
2–16 Torrington Place
London
WC1E 6BT UK

David Kerrigan

Gravitas
Murrayfield Hospital
Holmwood Drive
Wirral
CH63 1AU UK

Sudesh Kumar

Warwick Medical School
University of Warwick
Coventry
CV4 7AL UK

Victor Lawrence

Department of Diabetes and Endocrinology
St Mary's Hospital
Parkhurst Road
Newport, Isle of Wight
PO30 5TG UK

Joana Lindstrom

Department of Public Health
Diabetes and Genetic Epidemiology Unit
University of Helsinki
Helsinki
Finland

Konstantinos Lois

Clinical Sciences Research Institute
Clinical Sciences Building
University Hospitals of Coventry
and Warwickshire
Clifford Bridge Road
Coventry
CV2 2DX UK

Krys Matyka

Clinical Sciences Research Institute
Clinical Sciences Building
Walsgrave Hospital
Clifford Bridge Road
Coventry
CV2 2DX UK

John Pinkney

Gravitas
Murrayfield Hospital
Holmwood Drive
Wirral
CH63 1AU UK

Diana Raskauskiene

Department of Endocrinology
School of Medicine
Keele University
Thornburrow Drive
Hartshill
Stoke-on-Trent
ST4 7QB UK

Catherine Rolland

School of Life Sciences
St. Andrew Street
Aberdeen
AB25 1HG UK

Ponnusamy Saravanan

Clinical Sciences Research Institute
Warwick Medical School
University of Warwick
Coventry
CV4 7AL UK

Jayadave Shakher

Diabetes and Endocrinology
Birmingham Heartlands Hospital
Bordesley Green East
Birmingham
B9 5SS UK

Karri Silventoinen

Department of Public Health
Diabetes and Genetic
Epidemiology Unit
University of Helsinki
Helsinki
Finland

Jaakko Tuomilehto

Department of Public Health
Diabetes and Genetic Epidemiology Unit
University of Helsinki
Helsinki
Finland

Brent Van Dorsten

Department of Rehabilitation Medicine
University of Colorado Health Science
Center
Box 1650 MS F-713
Anschutz Outpatient Pavilion
Aurora
CO 80010 USA

Jonathan Webber

Diabetes Centre
Selly Oak Hospital
Raddlebarn Road
Birmingham
B29 6JD UK

John Wilding

University Hospital Aintree
Longmoor Lane
Liverpool
L9 7AL UK

Nerys Williams

12 Brueton Avenue
Solihull
West Midlands
B91 3EN UK

1

Changing epidemiology of obesity – implications for diabetes

Jonathan Webber

University Hospital Birmingham NHS Foundation Trust, Birmingham, UK

1.1 Introduction

There is a global epidemic of obesity [1] and the enormous implications for diabetes of this epidemic are now clear [2,3]. A large number of co-morbidities are associated with obesity, but it is type 2 diabetes that is most closely linked with increasing adiposity [4] and even within the normal weight range diabetes prevalence begins to rise with increasing adiposity [5,6]. There are currently about 110 million patients with diabetes on a worldwide basis, with this number projected to increase to 180 million by 2010 [7]. This will clearly have major economic implications with diabetes consuming ever higher proportions of healthcare budgets [8]. Being overweight or obese with an abdominal fat distribution probably accounts for 80–90% of all patients with type 2 diabetes [9].

1.2 Assessment of obesity in epidemiological studies

Most current epidemiological studies of body weight use body mass index (BMI) to define degrees of obesity. BMI is calculated as the subject's weight in kilograms divided by the square of their height in metres (kg/m^2). Cut-offs for underweight, normal weight, overweight and obesity are shown in Table 1.1.

BMI correlates well with total adiposity [10] and with morbidity and mortality from many diseases [4], although for a number of co-morbidities, including type 2 diabetes,

Obesity and Diabetes, Second Edition   Edited by Anthony H. Barnett and Sudhesh Kumar
© 2009 John Wiley & Sons, Ltd

Table 1.1 World Health Organization classification of obesity

WHO classification	BMI (kg/m^2)
Underweight	Less than 18.5
Healthy weight	18.5–24.9
Overweight (grade 1 obesity)	25–29.9
Obese (grade 2 obesity)	30–39.9
Morbid/severe obesity (grade 3 obesity)	Greater than 40

the relationship is closer with abdominal body fat distribution than total body fat [11]. In epidemiological studies intra-abdominal fat is most commonly estimated using measurements of waist and hip circumference and these can be used to identify increased risk of diabetes and other cardiovascular risk factors [12]. Worryingly, one recent study suggests there has been an increase in the prevalence of abdominal obesity in overweight subjects [13]. This would further drive up the risk of subsequent type 2 diabetes.

1.3 Prevalence of obesity

The prevalence of obesity is increasing throughout the world at an unprecedented rate. To be a healthy BMI, as defined by the World Health Organization (WHO), is now to be in a minority in much of western Europe as well as the United States. Indeed, in many developing countries overweight and obesity are now so common that they are replacing more traditional problems such as undernutrition and infectious diseases as the most significant causes of ill-health. In 1995, there were an estimated 200 million obese adults worldwide and another 18 million under-five children classified as overweight. As of 2000, the number of obese adults has increased to over 300 million. This obesity epidemic is not restricted to industrialized societies; in developing countries, it is estimated that over 115 million people suffer from obesity-related problems [1]. As the proportion of the population with a low BMI decreases, there is an almost symmetrical increase in the proportion with a BMI above 25.

The WHO Monitoring Trends and Determinants in Cardiovascular Disease (MONICA) project compares obesity rates in 48 populations spread throughout the world [14]. In the period 1983 to 1986 these rates varied from less than 5% in Beijing in China to about 20% in Malta. Recent data suggests that the BMI distribution is moving upwards in China as in the rest of the world. From 1989 to 1997 overweight (BMI $25–29.9 \, kg/m^2$) doubled in females (from 10.4 to 20.8%) and almost tripled in males (from 5.0 to 14.1%) [15]. Some of the highest prevalence figures come from the Pacific region where in urban Samoans obesity has increased from 38.8% in men in 1978 to 58.4% in 1991 [1].

Within the developed world the United States has led the obesity epidemic. In the adult population in the United States the prevalence of obesity, as determined from the National Health and Nutrition Examination Survey (NHANES), has increased from 22.9% in the period 1988–1994 to 30.5% in 1999–2000 [16]. Corresponding increases

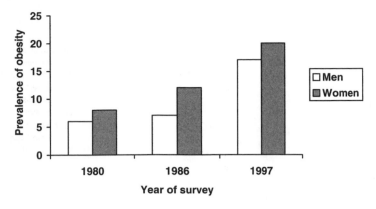

Figure 1.1   Prevalence of obesity in the UK from 1980 to 1997 from Joint Health Surveys Unit on behalf of the Department of Health 1999

have also occurred in overweight and in morbid obesity. Self-reported data (Behavioural Risk Factor Surveillance System) from much larger numbers of subjects confirm these worrying trends in the United States [2]. Indeed, if weight gain continues at the current rate in the United States by 2008 39% of the population will be obese [17]. The overall data on obesity prevalence masks other differences, including higher rates of overweight and obesity in non-Hispanic black women and in a number of minority ethnic groups. In the United Kingdom a number of surveys have documented the changes in obesity from 1980 to the current day [18] (Figure 1.1). There has been a tripling in obesity prevalence even in this relatively short period of time, with the likelihood that the UK rates will continue to rise to attain those already existing in the United States.

The age of onset of obesity is getting progressively younger [19]. This is reflected in the trends in overweight and obesity in children. In the United States the prevalence of overweight (defined as at or above the 95th centile of BMI for age) increased from 10.5 to 15.5% of 12 to 19-year olds between 1994 and 2000 and in the 2–5-year age group period the increase was from 7.2 to 10.4% in this 6 year time-span [20]; in England 9.0% of boys aged between 4 and 11 years were overweight in 1994 compared with 5.4% in 1984 [21]. The corresponding figures for girls were 13.5% (1994) and 9.3% (1984). Further recent increases were described in a recent Department of Health publication [22].

Though not all obese children become obese adults, a considerable proportion will do so [23]. The continuing rise in childhood obesity is likely to lead to a massive increase in the prevalence of those co-morbidities linked to obesity.

1.4   The epidemiological link between obesity and diabetes

The link between obesity prevalence and rates of diabetes in different populations was demonstrated by West with an increase in the prevalence of type 2 diabetes as the

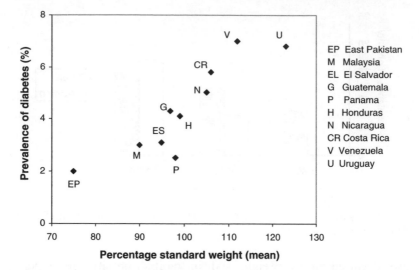

Figure 1.2 Diagram showing the relationship between the prevalence of diabetes (predominantly type 2 diabetes) and body weight in 10 representative populations. Body weight is expressed as the population mean, relative to a 'standard' weight that is given an arbitrary score of 100. Reproduced from West 1978 by permission of Elsevier Science

population becomes more obese [24] (Figure 1.2). Whilst there are changes in the incidence of type 1 diabetes, it is type 2 diabetes that is largely responsible for the global epidemic of diabetes.

Within populations there is clear evidence of a strongly positive relationship between obesity and the risk of diabetes. Data in the United States from the Health Professionals' Follow-up Study in men [5] and the Nurses' Health Study in women [6] graphically illustrates the increasing risk of diabetes that obesity brings (Figure 1.3). Compared with those of a BMI less than 21, women with a BMI greater than 35 had a 93-fold excess risk of developing diabetes. The risk of developing type 2 diabetes rises progressively with increasing adiposity (whether assessed by BMI, or percentage of ideal body weight). Data from NHANES shows that for each kilogram increase in weight of the population the risk of diabetes increases by 4.5% [25]. More recent examination of diabetes trends in the United States showed an even steeper increment of diabetes risk with weight gain, with a 9% increased risk of diabetes for each kilogram of body weight gain [26]. Whether this large difference is a real phenomenon, or is explained by increased public awareness of diabetes is not clear, as the later study depended on telephone surveys.

Where populations have changed their lifestyle and become more obese (e.g. Pima Indians of Arizona, Micronesian Nauruan Islanders) an epidemic of type 2 diabetes has followed on. Groups that were previously lean and had a low incidence of diabetes have become obese diabetics. Eighty per cent of adult Pima Indians are now obese and 40% of this population now has type 2 diabetes [27]. In comparison, a genetically almost identical Pima Indian population in Mexico has been described who are lean and

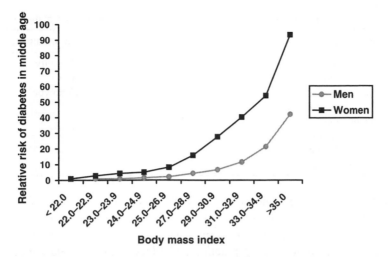

Figure 1.3   Relative risk of type 2 diabetes with increasing BMI. Drawn from data in [5] (reproduced by permission of American Diabetes Association) and [6] (reproduced by permission of American College of Physicians)

whose incidence of type 2 diabetes is virtually zero [28]. The importance of obesity in the development of diabetes is clearly demonstrated.

Amongst patients with type 2 diabetes excess adiposity is almost the rule. In the Diabetic Clinic in Dundee about 80% of patients attending are either overweight or obese [29]. Increasing obesity in the general population is now reflected in patients with diabetes. Of those patients newly presenting with diabetes in a clinic in Minnesota in the 1970s 33% were obese, whereas 49% of those diagnosed in the late 1980s were obese [30]. Thus, not only are we likely to see more patients with diabetes, but also to see more obese patients amongst our diabetic patients with the additional difficulties that accompany their clinical management.

In tandem with the rise in childhood obesity there is now a marked rise in type 2 diabetes in children and adolescents. There has been a 10-fold increase in type 2 diabetes amongst children between 1982 and 1994 in the United States [31]. Diabetes in this age group is clearly linked with obesity, although genetic and environmental factors also play a role with many such subjects having a family history of type 2 diabetes and belonging to minority populations [32]. In place of type 1 diabetes type 2 diabetes may soon become the more common form of childhood diabetes [33].

1.5 Factors modifying the relationship between obesity and diabetes

A large number of factors influence the relationship between obesity and diabetes and many of them are closely inter-related (Table 1.2). That obesity on its own is not sufficient to cause diabetes is apparent from the observation that 20% of patients with

Table 1.2 Factors mediating the relationship between obesity and diabetes

Modifiable	Not modifiable
Physical activity	Ethnicity
Infant feeding practices	Age
Duration of obesity	Genotype
Dietary composition	
Weight gain	
In utero environment	
Childhood stunting	
Social network	

type 2 diabetes are not obese and even in the highest risk group with high BMI and high waist–hip ratio over 80% will escape type 2 diabetes [6]. Other factors include body fat distribution, duration of obesity, weight gain, age, physical activity, diet, the in utero environment, infant feeding practices, childhood stunting and genetic factors. Methodological issues are also important in examining the relationship between obesity and diabetes. Some of the observed increase in diabetes prevalence attributed to obesity could be related to more awareness and detection of type 2 diabetes, rather than a true increase in numbers (previous Diabetes UK estimates are that 50% of patients do not know they have type 2 diabetes). The change in the diagnostic criteria for diabetes introduced by the American Diabetes Association in 1997, with less use of the oral glucose tolerance test and more emphasis on the fasting glucose, appear to underestimate the prevalence of diabetes in obese subjects who may have a relatively normal fasting blood glucose in the presence of a high post-load glucose [34].

Abdominal obesity may be an even better predictor of the development of type 2 diabetes than BMI [11]. The predictive value of high waist–hip ratios and high waist circumferences in mediating the risk of diabetes appears to be of most importance in those in the highest quintile of these measures [5] and perhaps in leaner subjects. For a given BMI many Asian populations have a much higher risk of type 2 diabetes, even at a BMI well within the normal range [35]. WHO is currently studying the use of a more limited range of normal BMI ($18.5–22.9 \, \text{kg m}^{-2}$) in these groups together with use of waist circumference [36].

The duration of exposure to obesity is an important modulator of the risk of diabetes. In Pima Indians, subjects' whose BMI was greater than $30 \, \text{kg/m}^2$ for more than 10 years had over twice the risk of type 2 diabetes compared with those who had been obese for less than 5 years [37]. The epidemic of childhood obesity allied with the influence of obesity duration suggests both increasing frequency of diabetes and its earlier onset.

Weight gain during adult life acts in addition to BMI per se to modify the risk of diabetes. In the Health Professionals' Follow-up Study men who gained more than 13.5 kg over the 5 years of the study had a 4.5-fold increased risk of diabetes in comparison with those men who remained within 4.5 kg of their weight at entry to the study [5]. Similar findings apply to women as described in the Nurses' Health Study where the relative risk of diabetes was 2.7 in those who gained 8–10.9 kg compared with those who were weight stable over a 14-year period [6].

Alongside the epidemic of childhood obesity and diabetes there is also an epidemic of diabetes related to the ageing population. The prevalence of type 2 diabetes increases progressively with age peaking at 16.5% in men and 12.8% in women at age 75–84 years [38]. Obesity rates plateau about 20 years earlier [18], but the age-related increases in total body fat and visceral adiposity make BMI a less good marker of adiposity in older age groups. Indeed, many normal weight elderly men and women are at high risk of type 2 diabetes due to increased visceral abdominal fat [39]. In the United Kingdom it is projected that due to population ageing by 2036 there will be 20% more cases of type 2 diabetes than in 2000 [8].

Decreasing levels of physical activity are undoubtedly implicated in the epidemic of obesity, but physical activity also has independent protective effects on the risk of diabetes. In the British Regional Heart Study, whilst BMI was the dominant risk factor for diabetes, men who engaged in moderate levels of physical activity had a substantially reduced risk of diabetes, relative to the physically inactive men, even after adjustment for age and BMI [40]. Similar data in women demonstrate a relative risk of type 2 diabetes of 0.67 in those who engaged in vigorous exercise at least once a week compared with women who did not exercise weekly [41]. At least in terms of reducing the risk of type 2 diabetes it is probably better to be overweight and physically active, than to be normal weight and inactive [42].

Dietary factors appear to have effects independent of those of obesity on the development of type 2 diabetes. Increasing fat in the diet is associated with both obesity and the development of diabetes [24], but much of this link is explained simply by the high energy intake that accompanies high fat diets. However, some populations with high fat diets (e.g. Eskimos and the Japanese) have a relatively low prevalence of diabetes compared with that expected from their obesity rates and this may be explained by a high intake of omega-3 polyunsaturated fatty acids [43]. A large prospective study of diet in women aged 34–59 years without diabetes at baseline and followed for 14-years found that total fat intake was not associated with risk of type 2 diabetes, but for a 5% increase in energy from polyunsaturated fat, the relative risk was 0.63 and for a 2% increase in energy from trans fatty acids the relative risk was 1.39 [44]. The authors estimated that replacing energy derived from trans fatty acids with polyunsaturated fat would lead to a 40% lower risk of type 2 diabetes. Alongside concerns about dietary fat, there is also evidence that the ready availability of sugar-sweetened drinks may contribute to obesity and diabetes [45]. In this study weight gain and greatest risk of diabetes were seen in those subjects with the highest consumption of sugar-sweetened soft drinks per day.

Whilst the vast majority of studies either show diabetes rates rising as obesity prevalence climbs, or project such a rise in diabetes from the observed obesity prevalence, one Swedish population survey has not demonstrated this [46]. From 1986 to 1999 the mean BMI in adults in northern Sweden increased from 25.3 to 26.2 kg/m^2 and the prevalence of obesity rose from 11 to 15%. However, in spite of the marked increase in obesity there was no increase in the prevalence of known diabetes. Dietary factors may account for some of this discrepant finding, with the diet over this period containing less saturated fat and having a lower glycaemic index. One additional observation was a decrease in waist–hip ratio (representing reduced visceral adiposity), perhaps also contributing to the absence of a BMI effect on diabetes. Findings such as these may mean that the gloomy picture of the diabetes epidemic painted by many authors is not quite as inevitable an outcome as projected.

In contrast, data from Australia show a dramatic increase in diabetes over the last 20 years, with a doubling of diabetes prevalence to its current value of 7.4% [47]. An additional 16.4% had abnormal glucose tolerance. Whilst obesity rates in this population have increased, neither obesity nor changes in the age profile of the population fully explain the extent of the diabetes epidemic. It is likely that some of the other factors discussed above, including body fat distribution, duration of obesity, dietary composition and physical activity account for this adverse pattern.

Currently there is much interest in the concept of social networks and the local neighbourhood as factors influencing the susceptibility to obesity and diabetes. Amongst participants of the Framingham Heart Study obesity appeared clustered in communities and in groups of friends [48]. One of the many factors that social networks share is their local environment. This environment includes resources for physical activity and for healthy eating. Exercise-friendly neighbourhoods are those with safe, walkable streets, parks and public gym facilities. In terms of healthy eating, examples of positive factors include ready availability of fruits and vegetables. A study looking at the relationship between local area facilities and insulin resistance (as measured by fasting insulin concentrations in those not known to have diabetes) found that greater physical activity resources were associated with lower insulin resistance with a similar inverse relationship for healthy food [49]. There are great opportunities to target obesity and diabetes prevention by more recognition of and investment in the local environment [50].

Whilst obesity is clearly important, other factors appear to influence the susceptibility both to weight gain and to the development of diabetes. The 'thrifty' gene hypothesis [51] suggests that the obese-type 2 diabetes mellitus genotype may have had some survival advantage, perhaps by favouring fat storage at times when food was abundant, so leading to improved survival during famines. However, this hypothesis remains an epidemiological explanation, with the exact genetic factors remaining unclear and no prospective data showing a survival advantage in subjects felt to have a thrifty genotype.

1.6 Early life influences on obesity and diabetes

Until relatively recently it was not felt that the in utero environment would be of any great significance in the later causation of obesity and type 2 diabetes. However, long-term follow-up of cohorts of small for gestational age babies, demonstrated an increased risk of later life type 2 diabetes and heart disease [52]. The 'thrifty' phenotype hypothesis generated from this and similar data, proposes that the epidemiological associations between poor fetal growth and the subsequent development of type 2 diabetes results from the effects of poor nutrition in early life, which produces permanent changes in glucose and insulin metabolism. These changes lead to reduced insulin secretion and increased insulin resistance and hence predispose to later type 2 diabetes.

Whether the critical factor for the development of childhood obesity and insulin resistance is in utero growth restriction *per se* is not clear. Rapid infancy weight gain, which may follow fetal growth restriction, also appears to be an important risk factor for the development of childhood obesity and insulin resistance [53]. Thus, rapid catch-up weight gain can lead to the development of insulin resistance, as early as 1 year of age, in association with increasing accumulation of central abdominal fat mass. Childhood stunting is another adverse early life phenomenon that affects later susceptibility to obesity and probably also to diabetes. Stunting remains common in lower income countries. Surveys in a number of countries show a significant association between stunting and overweight status in children in many countries [54]. With the transition from a lower income developing country to a more affluent developed one it is likely that the increased early stunting-mediated susceptibility to obesity will be compounded by later economic and social changes driving up obesity and diabetes rates.

At present there is more concern about large for gestational age babies and the later health consequences of this. One well-described group is those babies born to mothers with gestational diabetes. Maternal hyperglycaemia is proposed to influence not only fetal metabolism, but have more enduring effects throughout infancy and childhood leading to an increased risk of obesity and diabetes. This hypothesis has been supported by a large study demonstrating that increasing hyperglycaemia in pregnancy is linked with an enhanced risk of childhood obesity [55]. In this study it appeared that treatment of gestational diabetes attenuated the later risk of obesity. Longer-term follow up will be needed to show whether the type 2 diabetes risk is also reduced and how important this early metabolic imprinting is for long-term health.

1.7 Conclusions

There is no doubt that obesity is at present the major player in the increasing prevalence of type 2 diabetes. The current epidemic of obesity shows little sign of abating in most parts of the world and in contrast is still accelerating, particularly in children. Global predictions of the diabetes epidemic with 300 million patients with type 2 diabetes by 2025 are well on course [7]. Many of the factors that modify the relationship between obesity and diabetes, such as duration of obesity and physical activity levels are also changing adversely and are exacerbating the diabetes epidemic. The challenge for society is to reverse the ever-increasing prevalence of obesity.

References

1. World Health Organization (2000) Obesity: preventing and managing the global epidemic. Report of a WHO consultation. World Health Organization Technical Report Series, Vol. **894**, pp. i–xii, 1–253.

2. Mokdad, A.H., Ford, E.S., Bowman, B.A. *et al.* (2003) Prevalence of obesity, diabetes, and obesity-related health risk factors. *Journal of the American Medical Association*, **289**, 76–9.
3. Morabia, A. and Costanza, M.C. (2005) The obesity epidemic as harbinger of a metabolic disorder epidemic: trends in overweight, hypercholesterolemia, and diabetes treatment in Geneva, Switzerland, 1993–2003. *American Journal of Public Health*, **95**, 632–5.
4. Willett, W.C., Dietz, W.H. and Colditz, G.A. (1999) Guidelines for healthy weight. *New England Journal of Medicine*, **341**, 427–34.
5. Chan, J.M., Rimm, E.B., Colditz, G.A. *et al.* (1994) Obesity, fat distribution, and weight gain as risk factors for clinical diabetes in men. *Diabetes Care*, **17**, 961–9.
6. Chan, J.M., Rimm, E.B., Colditz, G.A. *et al.* (1994) Weight gain as a risk factor for clinical diabetes mellitus in women. *Diabetes Care*, **17**, 961–9.
7. King, H., Aubert, R.E. and Herman, W.H. (1998) Global burden of diabetes, 1995–2025: prevalence, numerical estimates, and projections. *Diabetes Care*, **21**, 1414–31.
8. Bagust, A., Hopkinson, P.K., Maslove, L. and Currie, C.J. (2002) The projected health care burden of Type 2 diabetes in the UK from 2000 to 2060. *Diabetic Medicine*, **19** (Suppl 4), 1–5.
9. Astrup, A. and Finer, N. (2000) Redefining type 2 diabetes: 'diabesity' or 'obesity dependent diabetes mellitus'? *Obesity Reviews*, **1**, 57–9.
10. Webster, J.D., Hesp, R. and Garrow, J.S. (1984) The composition of excess weight in obese women estimated by body density, total body water and total body potassium. *Human Nutrition and Clinical Nutrition*, **38**, 299–306.
11. Ohlson, L.O., Larsson, B., Svardsudd, K. *et al.* (1985) The influence of body fat distribution on the incidence of diabetes mellitus. 13.5 years of follow-up of the participants in the study of men born in 1913. *Diabetes*, **34**, 1055–8.
12. Han, T.S., van Leer, E.M., Seidell, J.C. and Lean, M.E.J. (1995) Waist circumference action levels in the identification of cardiovascular risk factors: prevalence study in a random sample. *British Medical Journal*, **311**, 1401–1405.
13. Li, C., Ford, E.S., McGuire, L.C. and Mokdad, A.H. (2007) Increasing trends in waist circumference and abdominal obesity among US adults. *Obesity (Silver Spring)*, **15**, 216–24.
14. Berrios, X., Koponen, T., Huiguang, T. *et al.* (1997) Distribution and prevalence of major risk factors of non-communicable diseases in selected countries: the WHO Inter-Health Programme. *Bulletin of the World Health Organization*, **75**, 99–108.
15. Bell, A.C., Ge, K. and Popkin, B.M. (2001) Weight gain and its predictors in Chinese adults. *International Journal of Obesity*, **25**, 1079–86.
16. Flegal, K.M., Carroll, M.D., Ogden, C.L. and Johnson, C.L. (2002) Prevalence and trends in obesity among US adults, 1999–2000. *Journal of the American Medical Association*, **288**, 1723–7.
17. Hill, J.O., Wyatt, H.R., Reed, G.W. and Peters, J.C. (2003) Obesity and the environment: where do we go from here? *Science*, **299**, 853–5.
18. Prescott-Clarke, P. and Primatesta, P. (1999) Health Survey for England 1997. HMSO, London.
19. McTigue, K.M., Garrett, J.M. and Popkin, B.M. (2002) The natural history of the development of obesity in a cohort of young U.S. adults between 1981 and 1998. *Annals of Internal Medicine*, **136**, 857–64.
20. Ogden, C.L., Flegal, K.M., Carroll, M.D. and Johnson, C.L. (2002) Prevalence and trends in overweight among US children and adolescents, 1999–2000. *Journal of the American Medical Association*, **288**, 1728–32.
21. Chinn, S. and Rona, R.J. (2001) Prevalence and trends in overweight and obesity in three cross sectional studies of British children, 1974–94. *British Medical Journal*, **322**, 24–6.
22. Jotangia, D., Moody, A., Stamatakis, E. and Wardle, H. (2005) Obesity among children under 11. Joint Health Surveys Unit National Centre for Social Research. Department of Epidemiology and Public Health at the Royal Free and University College Medical School.

23. Kotani, K., Nishida, M., Yamashita, S. *et al.* (1997) Two decades of annual medical examinations in Japanese obese children: do obese children grow into obese adults? *International Journal of Obesity*, **21**, 912–21.

24. West, K. (1978) *Epidemiology of Diabetes and its Vascular Lesions*, Elsevier, New York.

25. Ford, E.S., Williamson, D.F. and Liu, S. (1997) Weight change and diabetes incidence: findings from a national cohort of US adults. *American Journal of Epidemiology*, **146**, 214–22.

26. Mokdad, A.H., Ford, E.S., Bowman, B.A. *et al.* (2000) Diabetes trends in the US: 1990–1998. *Diabetes Care*, **23**, 1278–83.

27. Zimmet, P. (1982) Type 2 (non-insulin-dependent) diabetes – an epidemiological overview. *Diabetologia*, **22**, 399–411.

28. Esparza, J., Fox, C., Harper, I.T. *et al.* (2000) Daily energy expenditure in Mexican and USA Pima Indians: low physical activity as a possible cause of obesity. *International Journal of Obesity*, **24**, 55–9.

29. Jung, R.T. (1997) Obesity and nutritional factors in the pathogenesis of non-insulin-dependent diabetes mellitus, in *Textbook of Diabetes* (ed. G. Williams), Blackwell Science Ltd, Oxford, pp. 19.4–19.5.

30. Leibson, C.L., Williamson, D.F., Melton, L.J., 3rd *et al.* (2001) Temporal trends in BMI among adults with diabetes. *Diabetes Care*, **24**, 1584–9.

31. Pinhas-Hamiel, O., Dolan, L.M., Daniels, S.R. *et al.* (1996) Increased incidence of non-insulin-dependent diabetes mellitus among adolescents. *Journal of Pediatrics*, **128**, 608–15.

32. Fagot-Campagna, A., Pettitt, D.J., Engelgau, M.M. *et al.* (2000) Type 2 diabetes among North American children and adolescents: an epidemiologic review and a public health perspective. *Journal of Pediatrics*, **136**, 664–72.

33. Zimmet, P., Alberti, K.G. and Shaw, J. (2001) Global and societal implications of the diabetes epidemic. *Nature*, **414**, 782–7.

34. Melchionda, N., Forlani, G., Marchesini, G. *et al.* (2002) WHO and ADA criteria for the diagnosis of diabetes mellitus in relation to body mass index. Insulin sensitivity and secretion in resulting subcategories of glucose tolerance. *International Journal of Obesity*, **26**, 90–6.

35. Mather, H.M. and Keen, H. (1985) The Southall Diabetes Survey: prevalence of known diabetes in Asians and Europeans. *British Medical Journal*, **291**, 1081–4.

36. James, P.T., Leach, R., Kalamara, E. and Shayeghi, M. (2001) The worldwide obesity epidemic. *Obesity Research*, **9**, 228S–33S.

37. Everhart, J.E., Pettitt, D.J., Bennett, P.H. and Knowler, W.C. (1992) Duration of obesity increases the incidence of NIDDM. *Diabetes*, **41**, 235–40.

38. Wilson, P.W. and Kannel, W.B. (2002) Obesity, diabetes, and risk of cardiovascular disease in the elderly. *American Journal of Geriatrics and Cardiology*, **11**, 119–25.

39. Goodpaster, B.H., Krishnaswami, S., Resnick, H. *et al.* (2003) Association between regional adipose tissue distribution and both type 2 diabetes and impaired glucose tolerance in elderly men and women. *Diabetes Care*, **26**, 372–9.

40. Perry, I.J., Wannamethee, S.G., Walker, M.K. *et al.* (1995) Prospective study of risk factors for development of non-insulin dependent diabetes in middle aged British men. *British Medical Journal*, **310**, 560–4.

41. Manson, J.E., Rimm, E.B., Stampfer, M.J. *et al.* (1991) Physical activity and incidence of non-insulin-dependent diabetes mellitus in women. *Lancet*, **338**, 774–8.

42. Wei, M., Gibbons, L.W., Mitchell, T.L. *et al.* (1999) The association between cardiorespiratory fitness and impaired fasting glucose and type 2 diabetes mellitus in men. *Annals of Internal Medicine*, **130**, 89–96.

43. Malasanos, T.H. and Stacpoole, P.W. (1991) Biological effects of omega-3 fatty acids in diabetes mellitus. *Diabetes Care*, **14**, 1160–79.

44. Salmeron, J., Hu, F.B., Manson, J.E. *et al.* (2001) Dietary fat intake and risk of type 2 diabetes in women. *American Journal of Clinical Nutrition*, **73**, 1019–26.

45. Schulze, M.B., Manson, J.E., Ludwig, D.S. *et al.* (2004) Sugar-sweetened beverages, weight gain, and incidence of type 2 diabetes in young and middle-aged women. *Journal of the American Medical Association*, **292**, 927–34.

46. Eliasson, M., Lindahl, B., Lundberg, V. and Stegmayr, B. (2002) No increase in the prevalence of known diabetes between 1986 and 1999 in subjects 25–64 years of age in northern Sweden. *Diabetic Medicine*, **19**, 874–80.

47. Dunstan, D.W., Zimmet, P.Z., Welborn, T.A. *et al.* (2002) The rising prevalence of diabetes and impaired glucose tolerance: the Australian Diabetes, Obesity and Lifestyle Study. *Diabetes Care*, **25**, 829–34.

48. Christakis, N.A. and Fowler, J.H. (2007) The spread of obesity in a large social network over 32 years. *New England Journal of Medicine*, **357**, 370–9.

49. Auchincloss, A.H., Diez Roux, A.V., Brown, D.G. *et al.* (2008) Neighborhood resources for physical activity and healthy foods and their association with insulin resistance. *Epidemiology*, **19**, 146–57.

50. Workplace Health Promotion: How to encourage employees to be physically active. National Institute for Health and Clinical Excellence (2008).

51. Neel, J. (1962) Diabetes mellitus: a thrifty genotype rendered detrimental by 'progress'? *American Journal of Human Genetics*, **14**, 353–62.

52. Hales, C.N. and Barker, D.J. (2001) The thrifty phenotype hypothesis. *British Medical Bulletin*, **60**, 5–20.

53. Dunger, D.B., Salgin, B. and Ong, K.K. (2007) Early nutrition and later health: early developmental pathways of obesity and diabetes risk. *Proceedings of the Nutrition Society*, **66**, 451–7.

54. Popkin, B.M., Richards, M.K. and Montiero, C.A. (1996) Stunting is associated with overweight in children of four nations that are undergoing the nutrition transition. *Journal of Nutrition*, **126**, 3009–16.

55. Hillier, T.A., Pedula, K.L., Schmidt, M.M. *et al.* (2007) Childhood obesity and metabolic imprinting: the ongoing effects of maternal hyperglycemia. *Diabetes Care*, **30**, 2287–92.

2

The genetics of human obesity

Victor J. Lawrence[1] and Tahseen A. Chowdhury[2]
[1]Consultant Physician, Department of Diabetes and Endocrinology, St Mary's Hospital, Isle of Wight, UK
[2]Consultant Physician, Department of Diabetes and Metabolism, The Royal London Hospital, London, UK

2.1   Introduction

Obesity tends to occur in families, is more common in twins and can arise as a result of single gene or syndromic disorders. It is now clear that genetic factors are important in the aetiology of obesity. However, common obesity is likely to be a polygenic disorder, with genetic expression significantly influenced by environmental factors. This chapter summarizes the principles by which the genetics of human obesity can be investigated and some of the recent results of such investigations.

In recent years there has been rapid progress in our understanding of single gene disorders. The genetic basis of the more important diseases of the twenty-first century, such as obesity and diabetes, however, remains elusive.

The rapidly changing field of obesity genetics renders any 'State of the Art' review obsolete even before publication. Fortunately, rapidly updated information on specific genes and syndromes is readily available by searching on-line databases (http://obesitygene.pbrc.edu/ or http://www.ncbi.nlm.nih.gov/sites/entrez?db=omim, both accessed 12 September 2008).

Over the last decade, significant advances in molecular biology have made genetic study of complex disease more feasible. In this chapter, we intend to illustrate some of the major challenges facing research in this area, to describe some of the methods and their limitations currently available and how, in principle, they may be used to advance our understanding of this heterogeneous condition.

Obesity and Diabetes, Second Edition   Edited by Anthony H. Barnett and Sudhesh Kumar
© 2009 John Wiley & Sons, Ltd

2.2   Why has the genetics of obesity been difficult to study?

Defining the phenotype

One of the first problems faced in attempting to define a genetic basis for obesity is deciding what kind of effect (phenotype) we seek to examine. Obesity is a heterogeneous clinical disorder. Whilst it can be conveniently defined and clinically measured in terms of elevated body mass index (BMI), this is a definition chosen to define people or populations thought to be most at risk from its complications. It is a composite measure of body mass in relation to height, and is dependant on fat mass, lean tissue, bone and fluid mass, all of which may be subject to independent genetic or environmental influence. As BMI is not based on any specific pathophysiological process, it is an inherently unsatisfactory endpoint when looking for the effects of single genes or gene clusters.

For this reason, some studies have investigated genetic influence on more specific measures of body composition such as percentage body fat, total fat mass, visceral fat mass, subcutaneous fat mass or waist-hip ratio. These variables can be measured by bioelectrical impedance, computed tomography (CT), magnetic resonance imaging (MRI), dual energy X-ray absorbimetry (DEXA) scanning or underwater weighing. Whilst there is often a reasonable correlation with BMI (e.g. 0.83 between BMI and fat mass in one recent study [1]), the strength of such relationships varies unpredictably according to sex and age. Furthermore, these variables are not easy to measure in the large populations required for genetic study and even then may result from complex individual interrelationships between factors such as energy intake, age, sex, resting, voluntary and diet-induced energy expenditure and environmental (e.g. dietary, psychological and socio-political) influences.

Some researchers have attempted to examine the effects of putative genes on basic 'intermediary' biological measures such as resting metabolic rate (RMR), which may be affected by 'candidate' genes such as those encoding mitochondrial uncoupling protein (UCPs) or elements of the sympathetic nervous system such as the β_3 adrenoceptor. This approach also has drawbacks; subjects with established obesity tend to have high rather than low resting metabolic rates, for example. Using more complex constructs such as the difference between predicted and measured metabolic rate is possible but moving away from the clinical phenotype may mean that people displaying abnormalities are not obese.

Gene interactions

Having chosen an appropriate phenotype upon which to build a specific hypothesis, it is then necessary to consider the potential for a range of temporal and other paragenetic factors to influence gene expression and effect. These include the potential for genes to act at critical periods during different developmental stages, the effect that age related fat accretion will have on phenotype and sexual dimorphism of lipid storage (e.g. 'gynoid vs. android' distributions and total body fat differences between males and females). Epistasis between genes, whereby the effect of one gene may be modified by other genes and interactions between genes and environment may further complicate the picture especially if they result in sequence abnormalities being present in the background (or control) population without necessarily causing disease. Conversely, 'phenocopies' of obesity may exist without possessing the genotype sought by any particular study hypothesis thus reducing the power to detect genetic influence.

Thus, despite the fascinating physiological (and pharmacological) insights into the pathways involved in body weight regulation provided by unravelling the aetiology of some forms of monogenic obesity, it is increasingly clear that ultimate genetic understanding of common forms of human obesity will rely upon dissection of many small effects of multiple genetic variants superimposed on a permissive environment.

Many of these principles are illustrated by recent progress in understanding the genetics of Bardet–Biedl syndrome (BBS). First, more accurate phenotyping has permitted this syndrome to be separated from the Lawrence–Moon syndrome, which appears to be a distinct entity. Second, it is apparent that more than one genetic abnormality may be responsible for the observed abnormalities in this condition – at the time of writing, at least eleven loci (BBS 1–11) have been identified with subtly different effects on phenotype such as stature, body weight or pattern of polydactyly [2]. Third, in at least some forms of the disease, it may be necessary to have up to three distinct mutations (tri-allelic inheritance) for full disease expression, illustrating the principle of epistasis between disease alleles [3].

2.3   How much of obesity is genetic?

Given that the explosion in obesity prevalence over the past 20 years is likely to have taken place against a background of relatively constant population genetic structure, the question of to what extent obesity is subject to genetic influence is one that merits careful consideration. Most studies have attempted to resolve the population variance of a specific obesity phenotype into genetic, environmental and unknown (or residual) effects. In principle, the total observed phenotypic variance, Vp may be considered to be due to the sum of genetic variance (Vg), shared environmental variance (Vc) and an unknown residual (unshared environmental) variance (Ve) such that $Vp = Vg + Vc + Ve$. The percentage genetic inheritability of the trait in question is represented by the term Vg/Vp. Modifications of this simple model to attempt detection of gene-gene and gene-environment interactions and the application of complex multivariate computational modelling in different study populations are reviewed in detail elsewhere [4].

Twin studies

Twin studies allow separation of genetic and environmental components of variance since monozygotic (MZ) twins share 100% of their genes whilst non-identical dizygotic

(DZ) twins share 50%. The fact that there is discordance in the prevalence of obesity between MZ and DZ twins raised together supports the concept of genetic heritability of obesity if it is assumed that twins share exactly the same environmental influences (although it has been suggested that MZ twins may share more environmental influences than DZ twins [5]). Total genetic variance may then be subdivided into 2 components; *additive variance* which results from the sum of contributions of many alleles at different loci and *non-additive* effects, which are principally determined by the dominance of one allele over another at the same locus. It follows that an additive model is suggested when intra-pair correlations of DZ twins are half that of MZ twins and a non-additive model is suggested when DZ twins have substantially less than half the intra-pair correlations of variance of MZ twins.

Comparison of MZ twins raised together with MZ twins raised apart probably represents the ideal study group. However, such study populations are difficult to find and, even then, twins will have shared the same intra-uterine environment (which may be important on the basis of the Barker hypothesis [6]). Furthermore, there may be indirect genetic effects in operation and the effect of environment may be under-estimated as certain environmental conditions are likely to be common to both twins (e.g. the general availability of fast foods).

One study [7] assessed BMI in a sample of 1974 MZ and 2097 DZ male twin pairs and found concordance in MZ twins to be around 0.8. This was twice as high as that in DZ twins both at age 20 and at 25 year follow up. Others [8], however, report an age specific effect such that only 40% of the genetic factors that influence body weight at the age of 20 continue to do so by the age of 48.

One of the best estimates of obesity heritability, accounting for 67% of variance, is derived from the Virginia cohort of 30 000 twins their parents, siblings, spouses and children [9]. Overall, weighted mean BMI correlations have been calculated to be 0.74 for MZ twins, 0.32 for DZ twins, 0.25 for siblings, 0.19 for parent–offspring pairs, 0.06 for adoptive relatives and 0.12 for spouses [10] and the overall relative risk of siblings lies within the approximate range 3–7 [11].

The heritability of gene-environment interactions thought capable of leading to obesity has also been demonstrated using MZ twin populations [4]. The principle of this approach lies in the variability of individual response to environmental perturbation (in this case, weight change in response to either overfeeding or to increasing exercise with energy intake held constant). Where the response differs more between than within pairs of MZ twins, it may be assumed that genetic factors are responsible. These studies have demonstrated considerably more variance (in some cases by up to a factor of 3–6 depending on the variable studied) between rather than within twin pairs for a number of measures of body fat accumulation, distribution and energy expenditure. This supports the hypothesis that individual responses to diet and exercise have a substantial genetic component and may go some way to explaining the observation of increasing obesity prevalence on the background of a relatively constant gene pool. To what extent there is a genetic basis for the fact that obese people of similar BMI may be variably subject to obesity-related complications such as type 2 diabetes (independent of other risk factors) is unclear.

Adoption studies

Adoption studies rely on the assumption that differences between adopted children and their adoptive parents/siblings are due to genetic differences and differences between them and their biological families are due to environmental influences. However, adoption studies are complicated by problems relating to ascertainment of the biological father (false paternity being found in some 8% of individuals in many studies), the effects of selective or late placement of the child and the inherent inability of such studies to assess gene–environment interactions.

Thus there has been considerable heterogeneity in published estimates of the heritability of obesity depending for the large part on the type of study and population used. Whereas twin studies are thought in general to overestimate the true heritability, adoption studies are thought to underestimate it. Thus, estimates for obesity heritability from adoption studies are lower than those from twin studies and range from around 0.2–0.6 with two very large family studies providing estimates of 0.3–0.4 [10].

2.4   Is there a major gene for obesity?

Several large population studies using segregation techniques predicted the existence of one or more 'major' recessive gene effects independent of the discovery of any specific obesity gene [12,13]. Studies based on candidate genes or obesity syndromes have reported concentration of mutations thought capable of contributing to the obese phenotype amongst the obese population at large.

Segregation studies

Segregation studies test the hypothesis that there exist one or more (uncharacterized) recessive genes with major effects on a specific obesity phenotype. Support for a putative large (recessively inherited) genetic component of obesity was initially suggested by observations that the obese proband in many studies often demonstrates a far greater degree of obesity than either their parents or siblings. If it is hypothesized that the parents carry heterozygous mutations, one would expect that the frequency of transmission of a recessive allele from a homozygous dominant, homozygous recessive or heterozygous parent would be close to 0, 100 and 50% respectively. Evidence for one or more major recessive genes accounting for some 45% of the variance in fat mass being so transmitted has been reported in 6% of individuals in one study population [14]. In addition, reports of major gene effects accounting for some 37–42% of the variance in regional fat distribution have raised the intriguing possibility of one major gene effect subtending total and visceral fat accumulation with another influencing subcutaneous fat topography elsewhere [4].

It has been suggested recently that 2.9% of the general obese population are heterozygotes for at least one of the eleven autosomal recessive genetic defects present in BBS [15] and mutations in the gene coding for the MC-4 receptor may be present in up to 4% of the obese [16]. However, it remains to be seen whether these mutations are biologically important in the sense of leading to alterations in protein function and their true significance is currently debated [17].

2.5   How to identify obesity genes

The ultimate goal of obesity genetics is to identify a gene defect found exclusively in obese patients producing a functional variant (for example with altered or absent protein function, the so-called 'smoking gun'). The approaches that may be used in the attempt to identify such mutations depend to a large extent on what is known a priori about the function of the normal protein product.

The candidate gene approach

If there is knowledge that an abnormal protein product is capable of causing obesity (or counteracting it), evidence for the presence of mutations in the responsible 'candidate gene' may be sought in the population at large and related to measures of adiposity. In general, a gene may be considered a candidate gene for obesity based either on knowledge of its physiological role or because it becomes implicated in one or more forms of experimental or naturally occurring animal or human obesity.

Candidate genes based on physiological function
The candidate gene approach has been applied directly to examine the role of a number of polymorphisms in genes known to encode proteins with a role in energy homeostasis including the trp64arg mutation of the β_3-adrenoceptor, mutations of the mitochondrial UCPs1-3 and lipoprotein lipase (LPL). Unfortunately, the results of this direct approach have often been confusing. Two meta-analyses published in the same year of the trp64arg β_3-adrenoceptor mutation, with data from over 40 studies of 7000 subjects, have concluded with rather different assessments of its significance [18,19]. A common reason for discordant results is that differences in polymorphism frequency in different populations may give rise to population stratification effects. Furthermore, the presence of a polymorphism may not necessarily lead to alterations in protein structure or function and even if the protein product is altered, this may not always lead to obesity (an effect seen with certain null mutations of the MC-4 receptor [20]). In addition, publication bias towards positive results may overestimate the strength of an association. Conversely, true candidate gene effects may be missed if they are modulated by the presence of gene-environment interactions (such as those reported to occur between exercise and polymorphisms in the β_2-adrenoceptor gene [21]) or have effects specific to certain ethnic groups or sexes.

   At the time of writing, there have been positive reports in human populations of significant association between over 240 candidate genes and various measures of body weight/body composition/energy expenditure/serum leptin and temporal changes in body weight although the evidence is somewhat conflicting for a number of these associations (e.g. leptin, leptin receptor, agouti-related peptide, dopamine D2 receptor, β_3-adrenoceptor, LPL, UCP1-3, pro-opiomelanocortin (POMC), tumour necrosis factor, peroxisome proliferator-activated receptor-γ, 5-hydroxytryptamine receptor 2C, G protein β_3 subunit, adiponectin, β_2-adrenoceptor, interleukin-6, low-density lipoprotein receptor, insulin and vitamin D receptor [22]).

The search for candidate genes amongst animal and human forms of monogenic or syndromic obesity has often been more illuminating.

Monogenic obesity

Following the identification of the leptin gene mutation in *ob/ob* mice, three highly obese children from two consanguineous but unrelated families who carried non-functioning mutations of the leptin gene were identified from a study population characterized by extreme obesity. The defect in both pedigrees was a homozygous deletion of a single guanine nucleotide at codon 133 of the leptin gene, which resulted in a frameshift mutation and truncated protein [23]. Although immunoreactive leptin concentrations are typically increased rather than decreased in obesity suggesting that this defect per se is certainly not a common cause of obesity in the general population, this discovery led to intensification of the search amongst other forms of both syndromic and non-syndromic forms of obesity for other candidate genes. Mutations of six genes have been characterized in human forms of monogenic obesity (Table 2.1). It is noteworthy that five of these genes code for proteins involved in the leptin pathway of appetite regulation (see Figure 2.2). Whether this is because this pathway is the dominant pathway of weight regulation, or whether it results from poor understanding of alternative regulatory pathways is not yet clear. It is also noteworthy that mutations in one gene – *MC4R* – may be responsible for tens of thousands of cases of obesity [24] (Figure 2.1).

Syndromic obesity

Prader–Willi syndrome (PWS).   Long known to result from the deletion of a paternally inherited 4–4.5 Mb segment of chromosome 15q11.2–q12, PWS exhibits the interesting phenomenon of 'genetic imprinting'; when the deletion is inherited from the mother, Angelman syndrome (which does not have obesity as a cardinal feature) results but when the deletion is inherited from the father, loss of expression of one or more of the many C/D box, snoRNAs encoded within the paternally expressed SNRPN locus permits the PWS phenotype to be expressed. Generalized disruptions to the normal paternal expression of genes in this region (such as maternal uniparental disomy (UPD) 15 and imprinting centre (IC) mutations and specific balanced translocations with breakpoints within the paternally expressed SNRPN locus have also been reported to lead to PWS phenotype expression [25]. The precise cellular function of snoRNAs has yet to be determined but they are thought to play a part in the cellular localization and processing of RNA transcripts. The only candidate gene that may have a role in human obesity and PWS is the ghrelin gene, although evidence for its link to PWS is tenuous [26]. To date, no link between common forms of human obesity and these abnormalities has been reported.

Table 2.1 Monogenic forms of human obesity

Gene product	Human phenotype	Linkage with common human obesity	Association with common human obesity
Leptin	1. Hypogonadotrophic hypogonadism 2. Immune dysfunction 3. Hypothalamic–pituitary–thyroid abnormalities 4. Hyperinsulinaemia (in proportion to fat mass in humans) 5. Possible peripheral effects of leptin (e.g. vascular) 6. Increased glucocorticoid production in animals but not in man	Yes	Yes
Leptin receptor	Similar to leptin above other than additional 1. Growth retardation 2. Secondary hypothyroidism	Yes	Conflicting results
POMC/CART	1. Adrenocortical insufficiency 2. Abnormal pigmentation	Yes	No
MC4 receptor	1. Non-syndromic obesity of widely varying extent 2. Hyperinsulinaemia	Yes	Conflicting results
PC1	1. Abnormal glucose homeostasis 2. Hypogonadotropic hypogonadism 3. Hypocortisolism 4. Elevated plasma proinsulin and POMC concentrations 5. Low insulin levels	No	No
SIM1	1. Massive overeating with normal energy expenditure 2. Likely to be due to developmental abnormalities of hypothalamic PVN	No	No
NTRK2	1. Severe childhood obesity 2. Developmental delay 3. Blunted pain response	No	No

CART, Cocaine and amphetamine related transcript; MC, melanocortin; NTRK2, neurotrophic tyrosine kinase receptor-2; PC, pro-hormone convertase-1; SIM1, single-minded 1.

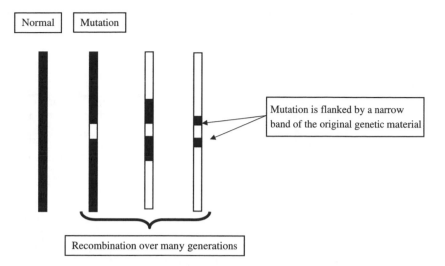

Figure 2.1 Linkage disequilibrium. A disease mutation initially arising on an ancestral haplotype becomes flanked by progressively smaller remnants of the original haplotype which are in LD with it and thus tend not to become separated from it by recombination events. These remnants may contain sequences which can be used to mark the position of the disease locus in a later generation. Although the detection of sequences derived from the ancestral haplotype may become more difficult after many generations, the precision of localization may be increased

BBS. This syndrome, until recently considered to be autosomal recessive in nature and frequently confused with the Lawrence–Moon syndrome, is diagnosed on the basis of the presence of a constellation of major and minor features of which obesity (in 72–96% of cases, preferentially distributed in the trunk and proximal limbs), retinal dystrophy, polydactyly, learning disabilities, male hypogonadism and renal abnormalities are most characteristic [27]. BBS prevalence varies widely, ranging from as little as 1 : 160 000 in ethnic Europeans to as much as 1 : 13 000 in populations such as Kuwait and Newfoundland where a founder effect has been postulated. Diagnostic difficulty has been compounded by a high degree of phenotypic variability, as much within as between families segregating the condition.

Since 1993, a combination of genome wide linkage scans in affected pedigrees and pooled sample homozygosity approaches have led to identification of the approximate position of eleven loci on chromosomes 11q13 (BBS1), 16 q21 (BBS2), 3p13 (BBS3), 15q22.3 (BBS4), 2q31 (BBS5), 20p12 (BBS6), 4q27 (BBS7), 14q32.11 (BBS8), 7p14 (BBS9), 12q21.2 (BBS10) and 9q33.1 (BBS11). BBS6 was first to be directly implicated in 2000 following its cloning as the gene responsible for a rather similar condition, the much rarer McKusick–Kaufman syndrome (MKKS) [28]. This knowledge, applied with increasingly detailed phenotyping, has permitted re-classification of some individuals previously thought to have MKKS as actually having BBS. Positional cloning of the BBS1, 2 and 4 loci has followed apace. Whereas BBS1 mutations appear sufficient for the development of classical BBS [29], it has been suggested that 3 specific mutations at the other loci may be necessary for disease expression, at least in

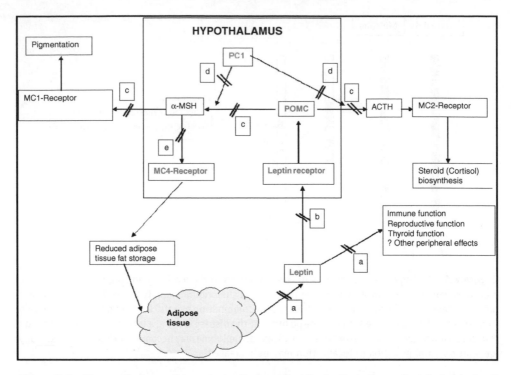

Figure 2.2   Monogenic forms of human obesity involving the leptin pathway. Protein products of genes known to be associated with human monogenic forms of obesity are shown in red (see also Table 2.1). POMC, pro-opiomelanocortin; α-MSH, α-melanocyte stimulating hormone; PC-1, pro-hormone convertase-1; MC-1, 2 and 4, melanocortin-1, 2 and 4 receptors. The *ob* gene mutation causing an absence of leptin is represented by (a) and leptin receptor mutations by (b). *POMC* mutations (c) disrupt cortisol biosynthesis and α-MSH-induced pigmentation as well as appetite regulation whereas *PC-1* mutations (d) do not appear to have a major effect on pigmentation but instead lead to hypogonadism and glucoregulatory abnormalities. *MC-4* mutations (e) are notable for causing little disturbance to regulatory pathways other than appetite and thus best represent common forms of non-syndromic obesity

some cases (tri-allelic inheritance). Six genes have been characterized in BBS, although their function is unclear. New candidate genes may be identified by detailed 'expression profiling' whereby expression is found to be qualitatively (e.g. in appropriate tissues) or quantitatively (e.g. variable gene expression under different nutrient or energy balance conditions) consistent with a role in body weight regulation. Alternatively, loci which become implicated in obesity by the use of 'positional' genetic approaches may then be further investigated using the candidate gene approach.

Positional approaches

Positional genetic techniques require no special previous knowledge of the function of an individual genomic region but implicate it in the causation of obesity purely on the grounds that identifiable markers in the region are found in obese phenotypes more frequently than would be expected by chance (i.e. they *segregate* in obesity and are identified in families by linkage or in populations by genetic association).

In practice, there is often a sequence of investigation using positional (described below) and then candidate approaches termed the 'positional candidate approach'. After identification of a region of interest using linkage studies in families, the genomic area of interest may be 'fine mapped' using techniques such as linkage disequilibrium (LD) to an area a few tens or hundred thousand base pairs in length. Subsequent association studies may attempt direct detection of an increased prevalence of a mutation (signalled either by a marker close to the mutation or a specific mutation itself) in affected individuals (probands) relative to unaffected population controls. Candidate studies then focus on genes with a plausible role in body weight regulation in the genomic region thus identified.

This 'positional candidate' approach may become more productive in its application to complex polygenic disease following publication of the human genome sequences. Functional annotation of the human genome sequence, now underway, may speed identification of possible candidate genes in stretches of genomic DNA identified by positional approaches. Furthermore, recent enhancements of single nucleotide poly-morphism (SNP) maps will provide many more identifiable genetic markers than have been available hitherto and may thus confer greater precision to gene mapping.

Once identified, further evidence for the potential role of a particular candidate gene in regulation of body weight may be sought from manipulation of the gene in animal models (e.g. transgenic or knockout models). Indeed, where the function of a locus revealed in association or LD studies is poorly understood, this may be vital in order to show that the proposed mutation is causative rather than simply being itself in linkage equilibrium with the real disease locus.

Linkage studies

Linkage is said to occur if two different alleles are passed to a subsequent generation in a proportion different to that expected by chance alone and is therefore a technique applied to family pedigrees rather than to cases and population controls. If two loci are completely linked (which usually means that they are very close together on the same chromosome), they will nearly always passed together via the gametes to the offspring. Thus no new combinations of these two alleles will be found to have occurred during meiosis in the transmitted chromosome. Where similar alleles at the two loci are completely un-linked, the alleles assort independently in meiosis and 50% of the offspring will have chromosomes with combinations not found in the parental strain. In practice, the proportion of new genotypes will be between 0 and 50% depending on the recombination percentage present (the number of gametes with a recombination that separates two particular parental alleles divided by the total number). Clearly, the closer the two gene loci (or a gene and a marker locus), the less likely it is for a recombination event to separate them. By convention, a 1% recombination frequency implies a distance of 1 centimorgan (cM) at least for differences less than 10 cM and this equates (depending on the region of the genome) to some 1 million base pairs in distance.

By detecting linkage with polymorphic markers whose location is known, it is possible to use this technique to infer the approximate location of a disease susceptibility gene.

In principle, genetic linkage may be sought between a particular marker variant and phenotype or throughout the entire genome, the latter requiring no assumptions to be made about gene function. However, the sheer scale of this endeavour must be appreciated. Typically, a genome scan might utilise some 300–400 polymorphic markers to localise linkage (with a given confidence interval, say 95%) to an area spanning approximately 10–20 cM (typically around 10–20 million base pairs). This genomic region may contain more than 200 genes, 60 000 common variants and many other rarer variants in intronic, exonic and regulatory sequences. It is clear from this that finer mapping techniques must then be used if there is to be any realistic prospect of cloning a specific gene.

The statistical significance of a linkage signal is denoted by the log odds likelihood ratio difference (LOD) score, which is the logarithm of the likelihood of the odds that two loci are linked compared with the likelihood of the odds for independent assortment. Correct interpretation of linkage signals relies critically on understanding the precise meaning of a LOD score to avoid inadvertent type 1 error. Whilst a LOD score of 3 for the effect of a single genotype on a single phenotype denotes a nominal p value of less than 0.0001, when repeated for multiple markers in a typical genome linkage scan, this equates to a true p value of around 0.09 and thus fails to reach classically defined statistical significance. It has been recommended that adopting LOD score thresholds of 3.3–3.8 to define definite linkage will result in less than 5% probability of type 1 error over a whole genome scan comprising 3–400 marker loci whilst linkage signals with LOD scores between 1.9 and 3.3 are best considered 'suggestive' and worthy of further investigation [30].

Limitations of traditional linkage analysis include its reliance on assumptions about disease transmission (genetic architecture) and the fact that linkage signals may be hard to detect when the gene in question contributes only marginally to the phenotype. The use of special relationships such as discordant sibling pairs has been used to circumvent these problems to some extent but, even with the advent of more complex study designs and elaborate computational methods (including models robust to assumptions about mode of inheritance such as non-parametric linkage analysis) it is still not possible to model the involvement of more than two disease loci and this is especially problematic in human obesity where disease susceptibility may depend more on particular con-figurations of more than one variant (as with calpain 10 in type 2 diabetes [31]) than on the presence or absence of a single variant.

Genome wide scans in various ethnic populations have uncovered a number of potential obesity loci [32]. Indeed, progress has been made in genome wide association studies into type 2 diabetes, which may have some relevance to obesity. Microchip technology has been developed that can analyse upto 500 000 SNPs in several thousand DNA samples. This technology has greatly facilitated genetic dissection of complex traits. Eleven common genetic variants have been confirmed to be involved in genetic risk for type 2 diabetes. Of these, the Fat Mass and Obesity associated (FTO) appears to have an important effect on obesity [33]. Examination of 30 000 adults has found that the 16% of Europeans that carry two copies of the diabetes associated allele were 2.3 kg heavier than the 35% of Europeans that had two copies of the non-risk allele. This finding has been replicated in a number of association studies subsequently.

Association studies

In contrast to linkage studies, association studies aim to detect co-segregation of a marker with a specific obesity phenotype in closely matched samples of affected and non-affected individuals who need not be related.

The simplest application of association is its use in testing the hypothesis that a specific polymorphism in a candidate gene is present in obese probands at a frequency greater than would be expected by chance (using χ^2 or similar tests) and is thus either causal or at least capable of conferring susceptibility to the development of obesity. It is clearly essential that controls and probands are from closely matched populations so that the overall population polymorphism frequency is similar otherwise a positive result may occur due to population stratification. Where there is no obvious candidate gene, controls and obese probands may be genotyped for the presence of one or more marker alleles and differences in respective frequencies are compared to determine whether particular markers are significantly associated with the phenotype of interest.

Association studies have traditionally been used further to evaluate signals detected by linkage methods and the greater a priori likelihood of a true association confers additional statistical confidence in a positive result. As they are usually more convenient to perform and can localize genes with only moderate or small effects on phenotype, association studies are increasingly being used as a first line of investigation, significant association suggesting that the allele either affects the phenotype of interest or at least is close enough to be in linkage disequilibrium with the allele that is actually responsible.

As with linkage studies, there are considerable inherent problems in determining the significance of an apparently positive finding and the literature is littered with uncorroborated reports of significant association, many of which are likely to prove spurious. Factors that have led to poor replication in association studies include latent population stratification, lack of detailed and accurate ascertainment of phenotype and lack of power to confirm or refute an association especially where there may be multiple SNPs in intronic, exonic, regulatory and upstream regions of the locus all of which require investigation in multiple populations before disease relevance may confidently be excluded [20].

Linkage disequilibrium

LD is defined as the non-random association between two alleles at two different loci on the same chromosome. Although similar to linkage and based on the same fundamental genetic principles, the method is population rather than pedigree based and has the distinct advantage of being able to localize a linkage signal with far greater precision than is possible with traditional linkage alone. When a gene mutation first occurs in an individual, it forms part of a unique haplotype, which tends to dissipate over many successive generations as recombination events dislodge alleles at loci on the same chromosome (Figure 2.2). As with linkage, loci situated furthest away from the disease gene are most subject to separation from it during meiosis. After many generations (assuming non-lethality and lack of effect on reproductive potential) all that is left of the original chromosome in descendents is the disease gene flanked by a few alleles from the original haplotype which can be used to mark its position. The ideal circumstances for fine LD mapping are encountered in founder communities (e.g. North American Hutterites, Amish, Finnish or French Canadian populations) because it is likely that the disease mutation was introduced by a single individual, producing the potential for a strong association between the disease and a specific haplotype in the current generation. Thus LD in such a population may be somewhat analogous to a family linkage study over many generations with an ancestral haplotype replacing a parental one. The ability to study many more 'offspring' (i.e. the present-day population) for linkage after many recombination events thus confers greater statistical power and much more precise localization than is possible with traditional linkage based methods.

The degree of LD depends on time elapsed since the mutation arose: in 'older' founder populations, the degree of LD often diminishes but, due to more recombination events elsewhere, the ability to fine map a mutation may often be greater. Important constraints of LD-based methods include the fact that they depend on the disease of interest existing in suitable founder populations in a way not obscured by marker mutation within the population, new disease mutations, genetic drift, locus heterogeneity, population admixture or the existence of multiple disease susceptibility loci. Problems related to population structure may also yield false positive results – that is, association without true linkage. Thus, assortive mating causing the eventual emergence of discrete genetic subpopulations (population stratification) and population admixture (where two genetically diverse populations have recently merged) may both lead to the association of unlinked loci.

Thus, additional studies are often required to determine whether a positive association is truly the result of genetic linkage between disease and marker loci. The transmission disequilibrium test (TDT) determines the transmission frequency of marker alleles from a heterozygous parent to an affected offspring. In the absence of true linkage, both alleles of a two allele marker locus will be transferred with equal frequency to an affected offspring. However, transmission of allele combinations with a frequency greater than that expected by chance is taken as evidence of true linkage.

Quantitative trait loci (QTLs)

QTLs are loci which individually have a small but measurable influence on a continuous phenotype such as body weight rather than giving rise to discrete disease present or absent phenotypes. The principal advantage of this methodology is that interactions between loci each having only a small phenotypic effect may be investigated particularly where the sum of more than one such effect is large. The principle of attempting to define QTLs as a tool for gene mapping relies on the fact that rodents may be selectively inbred to produce strains that differ widely in body weight and fat deposition under the influence of polygenic loci. Breeds with opposite poles of a phenotypic extreme may then be cross bred to produce F1 progeny whose phenotype will depend on the exact genotype inherited from each parental strain [34]. The resultant F1 generation may then be back-crossed to a parent or permitted to bred with siblings to generate a back-cross or sib-mated F2 population containing a number of allele combinations (and phenotypes) not encountered in either of the parental or F1 strains. Provided the two breeds differ in one or more molecular markers associated with each locus (e.g. restriction fragment length polymorphisms (RFLPs), microsatellites or SNPs), the F2 generation may be genotyped and phenotyped to associate genetic markers (and thus specific allele combinations) with the resulting phenotype.

Over 165 QTLs spanning the entire genome (except the Y chromosome) have been mapped in animals (mainly mice) to date [22]. Many appear to exert rather modest effects on phenotype (as may be expected in a complex polygenic disorder) although some do appear to have more major effects. Following identification of QTLs in mice, loci of interest may be mapped to the homologous (syntenic) region in man and the region further tested for association with obesity in a human population. Thus, the many benefits of performing genetic studies in mice may be reaped whilst maintaining relevance to human populations. These advantages include stable environmental conditions, pure breeding strains, the ability to perform sibling and back-cross mating, rapid breeding (generation) times and the ability to obtain accurate phenotypical data. The use of this method has identified QTLs having effects on intermediary phenotypes such as thermogenesis, serum leptin levels and insulin resistance, gene-environment interactions such as susceptibility to diet-induced obesity and with time of obesity onset and gender-specific susceptibility to obesity.

Because this technique examines the effects of many combinations of more than one allele, the opportunity to examine gene-gene interactions is presented. For example, the mouse strains *Mus spretus* and C57BL/6 are relatively lean as are the F1 progeny resulting from crossing these parental strains. However, backcrossed progeny (with allelic combinations not found in the parental or F1 strains) vary in percentage body fat content from about 1–60%. Significant association (LOD score >3.3) was found in the backcrossed F2 progeny between a number of intermediary phenotypes and 4 genomic regions (designated as mob1–4 on chromosomes 7, 6, 12 and 15 respectively). A further association with percentage body fat, accounting for some 7% of the observed variance of this trait, was considered 'suggestive' rather than statistically significant [35]. These loci include a number of plausible candidate genes including IGFR-1 (mob1), ob (mob2) and GH receptor (mob4). It is of interest that *M. spretus*-derived alleles appear to promote obesity at chromosomes 6, 7 and 12 whereas C57BL/6-derived alleles promote obesity only when present on chromosome 15 and then only when the loci at 6, 7 and 12 are heterozygous providing a clear demonstration of the complexities of epistasis in the aetiology of complex polygenic disorders such as obesity.

Animal models with altered genetic expression

Transgenic techniques involve introduction of genes (or regulatory sequences) into the germ line of mice so that target gene expression may be either introduced de novo or alternatively up or down-regulated whereas knockout techniques involve elimination of endogenous gene expression. These genetic manipulations have provided a powerful tool for the study of gene function in the intact animal but have led in some instances to the publication of confusing or unexpected results. Thus, animals lacking dopamine β hydroxylase are completely unable to synthesize catecholamines but do not develop obesity [36]. Also, animals carrying a knock-out version of the Y5 form of the NPY receptor are phenotypically normal until they develop a late onset form of obesity due to overfeeding rather than the underfeeding which might be expected from the known physiology of this receptor system [37,38]. Another problem is the fact that some germ line mutations are incompatible with foetal development and, with rare exceptions such as the intrauterine rescue of dopamine β-hydroxylase knockout mice with temporary provision of a downstream metabolite, it has not been possible to produce an adult animal model of such mutations.

It is likely that recent refinements of these techniques to permit both temporal activation/de-activation of the gene, and tissue specific modulation of gene activity will greatly enhance the usefulness of this research tool. Thus inserted or wild-type gene expression may be linked to a tissue specific promoter or to an inducible regulatory sequence (e.g. a tetracycline response element) so that, in this case, gene expression is either enabled or inhibited by the presence or absence of tetracycline in the animal's blood. However, even with advanced conditional (as opposed to classical germ line) gene expression targeting, there still remain problems of interpretation caused by factors such as the redundancy evident in the control of energy homeostasis leading to compensation for the failure of one regulatory component by up-regulation of another.

2.6   Summary and conclusions

In writing this chapter, we set out to illustrate some of the problems that have beset the study of obesity genetics, to evaluate some of the techniques currently available and to provide some examples of the progress made to date and future prospects for this rapidly moving field.

Progress in the past decade has been dizzying. The first definitive descriptions of genetic causes of obesity have been made, evidence that a monogenic form of obesity may be the commonest single gene disorder described, and increasing evidence that common genetic variants predispose to obesity in the wider population has been demonstrated. Further progress may lead to potential pharmacotherapeutic interventions which may reduce the burden of obesity, and its attendant complications.

References

1. Deng, H.W., Deng, H., Liu, Y.J. *et al.* (2002) A genomewide linkage scan for quantitative-trait loci for obesity phenotypes. *American Journal of Human Genetics*, **70**, 1138–51.
2. Iannello, S., Bosco, P., Cavaleri, A. *et al.* (2002) A review of the literature of Bardet–Biedl disease and report of three cases associated with metabolic syndrome and diagnosed after the age of fifty. *Obesity Reviews*, **3**, 123–35.

3. Katsanis, N., Ansley, S.J., Badano, J.L. *et al.* (2001) Triallelic inheritance in Bardet–Biedl syndrome, a Mendelian recessive disorder. *Science*, **293**, 2256–59.

4. Bouchard, C., Perusse, L., Rice, T. and Rao, D.C. (1998) The genetics of human obesity, in *Handbook of Obesity*, Marcel Dekker, New York, pp. 157–90.

5. Hebebrand, J., Sommerlad, C., Geller, F. *et al.* (2001) The genetics of obesity: practical implications. [Review] [70 refs]. *International Journal of Obesity & Related Metabolic Disorders*, **25** (Suppl 1), S10–S18.

6. Hales, C.N. and Barker, D.J. (1992) Type 2 (non-insulin-dependent) diabetes mellitus: the thrifty phenotype hypothesis. *Diabetologia*, **35**, 595–601.

7. Stunkard, A.J., Foch, T.T. and Hrubec, Z. (1986) A twin study of human obesity. *Journal of the American Medical Association*, **256**, 51–4.

8. Fabsitz, R.R., Carmelli, D. and Hewitt, J.K. (1992) Evidence for independent genetic influences on obesity in middle age. *International Journal of Obesity and Related Metabolic Disorders*, **16**, 657–66.

9. McLaughlin, J. (1991) The inheritance of body mass index in the Virginia 30,000. *Behavior Genetics*, **21**, 581, Abstract.

10. Maes, H.H., Neale, M.C. and Eaves, L.J. (1997) Genetic and environmental factors in relative body weight and human adiposity. *Behavior Genetics*, **27**, 325–51.

11. Allison, D.B., Faith, M.S. and Nathan, J.S. (1996) Risch's lambda values for human obesity. *International Journal of Obesity and Related Metabolic Disorders*, **20**, 990–9.

12. Borecki, I.B., Blangero, J., Rice, T. *et al.* (1998) Evidence for at least two major loci influencing human fatness. *American Journal of Human Genetics*, **63**, 831–38.

13. Rice, T., Tremblay, A., Dériaz, O. *et al.* (1996) A major gene for resting metabolic rate unassociated with body composition: results from the Quebec Family Study. *Obesity Research*, **4**, 441–9.

14. Rice, T., Borecki, I.B., Bouchard, C. and Rao, D.C. (1993) Segregation analysis of fat mass and other body composition measures derived from underwater weighing. *American Journal of Human Genetics*, **52**, 967–73.

15. Croft, J.B., Morrell, D., Chase, C.L. and Swift, M. (1995) Obesity in heterozygous carriers of the gene for the Bardet–Biedl syndrome. *American Journal of Medical Genetics*, **55**, 12–15.

16. Vaisse, C., Clement, K., Durand, E. *et al.* (2000) Melanocortin-4 receptor mutations are a frequent and heterogeneous cause of morbid obesity. *Journal of Clinical Investigation*, **106**, 253–62.

17. Jacobson, P., Ukkola, O., Rankinen, T. *et al.* (2002) Melanocortin 4 receptor sequence variations are seldom a cause of human obesity: the Swedish Obese Subjects, the HERITAGE Family Study, and a Memphis cohort. *Journal of Clinical Endocrinology and Metabolism*, **87**, 4442–6.

18. Allison, D.B., Heo, M., Faith, M.S. and Pietrobelli, A. (1998) Meta-analysis of the association of the Trp64Arg polymorphism in the beta3 adrenergic receptor with body mass index. *International Journal of Obesity and Related Metabolic Disorders*, **22**, 559–66.

19. Fujisawa, T., Ikegami, H., Kawaguchi, Y. and Ogihara, T. (1998) Meta-analysis of the association of Trp64Arg polymorphism of beta 3-adrenergic receptor gene with body mass index. *Journal of Clinical Endocrinology and Metabolism*, **83**, 2441–4.

20. Hirschhorn, J.N. and Altshuler, D. (2002) Once and again-issues surrounding replication in genetic association studies. *Journal of Clinical Endocrinology and Metabolism*, **87**, 4438–41.

21. Macho-Azcarate, T., Calabuig, J., Marti, A. and Martinez, J.A. (2002) A maximal effort trial in obese women carrying the beta2-adrenoceptor Gln27Glu polymorphism. *Journal of Physiology and Biochemistry*, **58**, 103–8.

22. Rankinen, T., Zuberi, A., Chagnon, Y.C. *et al.* (2006) The human obesity gene map: the 2005 update. *Obesity (Silver Spring)*, **14**, 529–44.

23. Montague, C.T., Farooqi, J.S., Whitehead, JP. *et al.* (1997) Congenital leptin deficiency is associated with severe early-onset obesity in humans. *Nature*, **387**, 903–8.

24. Alharbi, K.K., Spanakis, E., Tan, K. *et al.* (2007) Prevalence and functionality of paucimorphic and private MC4R mutations in a large, unselected European British population, scanned by meltMADGE. *Human Mutation*, **28**, 294–302.
25. Nicholls, R.D. and Knepper, J.L. (2001) Genome organization, function, and imprinting in Prader–Willi and Angelman syndromes. *Annual Review of Genomics and Human Genetics*, **2**, 153–75.
26. Goldstone, A.P. (2004) Prader–Willi syndrome: advances in genetics, pathophysiology and treatment. *Trends in Endocrinology and Metabolism*, **15**, 12–20.
27. Katsanis, N., Lupski, J.R. and Beales, P.L. (2001) Exploring the molecular basis of Bardet–Biedl syndrome. *Human Molecular Genetics*, **10**, 2293–9.
28. Slavotinek, A.M., Stone, E.M., Mykytyn, K. *et al.* (2000) Mutations in *MKKS* cause Bardet–Biedl syndrome. *Nature Genetics*, **26**, 15–16.
29. Mykytyn, K., Nishimura, D.Y., Searby, C.C. *et al.* (2002) Identification of the gene (*BBS1*) most commonly involved in Bardet–Biedl syndrome, a complex human obesity syndrome. *Nature Genetics*, **31**, 435–8.
30. Lander, E. and Kruglyak, L. (1995) Genetic dissection of complex traits: guidelines for interpreting and reporting linkage results. *Nature Genetics*, **11**, 241–7.
31. Altshuler, D., Daly, M. and Kruglyak, L. (2000) Guilt by association. *Nature Genetics*, **26**, 135–7.
32. Meyre, D., Bouatia-Maji, N., Tounian, A. *et al.* (2005) Variants of ENPPI are associated with childhoos and adult obesity and increase the risk of glucose intolerance and type 2 diabetes. *Nature Genetics*, **37**, 863–7.
33. Frayling, T.M., Timpson N.J., Weedon, M.N. *et al.* (2007) A common variant in the FTO gene is associated with body mass index and predisposes to childhood and adult obesity. *Science*, **316**, 889–94.
34. Brockmann, G.A. and Bevova, M.R. (2002) Using mouse models to dissect the genetics of obesity. *Trends in Genetics*, **18**, 367–76.
35. Warden, C.H., Fisler, J.S., Shoemaker S.M. *et al.* (1995) Identification of four chromosomal loci determining obesity in a multifactorial mouse model. *Journal of Clinical Investigation*, **95**, 1545–52.
36. Thomas, S.A. and Palmiter, R.D. (1997) Thermoregulatory and metabolic phenotypes of mice lacking noradrenaline and adrenaline. *Nature*, **387**, 94–7.
37. Erickson, J.C., Clegg, K.E. and Palmiter, R.D. (1996) Sensitivity to leptin and susceptibility to seizures of mice lacking neuropeptide Y. *Nature*, **381**, 415–21.
38. Palmiter, R.D., Erickson, J.C., Hollopeter, G. *et al.* (1998) Life without neuropeptide Y. *Recent Progress in Hormone Research*, **53**, 163–99.

3

Lifestyle determinants of obesity

Laura Johnson[1] and Susan A. Jebb[2]

[1]Health Behaviour Research Centre, Department of Epidemiology and Public Health, University College London, London, UK
[2]MRC Human Nutrition Research, Cambridge, UK

3.1 The importance of energy balance

Body weight is the integrated product of a lifetime's energy intake, offset by energy needs. Throughout the last century there has been a trend towards increased body weight and increases in body mass index, a measure of weight relative to height. Data from the annual Health Survey for England [1] shows that the average gain in weight of the adult population over the last 12 years has been approximately 0.3 kg/year, which is primarily adipose tissue, with modest concomitant increases in lean tissue. At an individual level, excess weight gain may occur gradually, almost imperceptibly, over many years or, in intermittent episodes of more pronounced positive energy imbalance, perhaps related to holidays or festive periods when usual diet and activity habits are distorted. However, spontaneous weight loss is rare, except in association with pathological processes. This asymmetry in energy balance is underpinning the rise in obesity.

Energy balance is the product of both innate and discretionary processes. Energy expenditure consists predominately of three components; resting energy expenditure (50–80%), thermogenesis (10%) and physical activity (10%) [2]. Resting energy expenditure is a product of an individual's body size and composition. Thermogenesis refers to energy expended by the digestion and processing of food, or thermoregulation. Only the energy used in physical activity is discretionary and thus modifiable.

The various mechanisms that control energy balance are the subject of intensive research. Although energy intake and physical activity are highly variable day-to-day [3], it is apparent that over the long term a complex physiological regulatory system exists to maintain body energy stores. Yet despite this innate capacity to cope with fluctuations in energy balance, imposed changes in lifestyle can have profound effects on body weight.

Obesity and Diabetes, Second Edition   Edited by Anthony H. Barnett and Sudhesh Kumar
© 2009 John Wiley & Sons, Ltd

Obesity is almost unknown in animals in the wild, but rapidly develops in captivity. Small animals housed in laboratories, fed standard chow are able to maintain a healthy body weight, yet when given access to highly palatable, refined diets, rich in fat and sugar, they rapidly gain excess weight and become obese. Modern lifestyles, characterized by access to abundant, diverse and palatable food, together with a low demand for physical exertion have created an environment in which individuals are very susceptible to weight gain, a situation described as 'passive obesity' [4].

3.2   Physical activity

A comparison of contemporary living with historical accounts quickly reveals that habitual physical activity has declined, but data on secular trends in activity using objective measures, is lacking. Physical activity is a complex, multidimensional behaviour that is difficult to quantify [5]. Physical activity questionnaires are notoriously unreliable, with inconsistent relationships between activity and fatness. Objective measures, which are unaffected by recall or over reporting biases, are increasingly being used. Recent cross-sectional analyses of objectively measured activity in children have reported an association between reduced fat mass with higher levels of physical activity [6,7]. However, the interpretation of cross-sectional analyses is limited due to difficulties in dissecting the directionality of the association. Physical activity may influence weight, but weight may equally influence the intensity or nature of physical activity.

Recent prospective studies more often provide supportive evidence that physical activity may attenuate weight gain, but overall the evidence is not consistent and suggests that activity only modestly attenuates age-associated increases in body weight [8]. For example, the UK Medical Research Council Ely Study followed up 739 healthy, middle-aged, white participants for 5.6 years. In multiple regression analysis each MJ/d of energy used in physical activity at baseline (measured by heart-rate monitoring) was associated with just 0.036 kg less fat mass at follow-up [9].

Randomized controlled interventions with prescribed increases in physical activity or exercise have yielded little evidence of effectiveness in halting the rise in excess weight [10]. The response to physical activity interventions is subject to considerable inter-individual variability, with some people much more likely to exhibit compensatory increases in appetite and energy intake, resulting in a smaller intervention effect on weight [11]. It is also acknowledged that compliance to such interventions is poor [12], and differences in motivation to commit to such lifestyle changes can affect the success of free-living trials. In many cases studies are limited by the lack of clear specification of a causal model, the absence of a theoretical basis for the design of an intervention and inadequate evaluation, which makes it impossible to disentangle exactly why an intervention was ineffective [8]. Much more research is needed, both to establish the true relationship between activity and weight gain and into how to establish and maintain changes in behaviour.

Physical activity has clear benefits for a range of chronic diseases and is potentially an important factor in preventing excess weight gain. The lack of quantitative information on exactly how much activity is needed to prevent obesity has resulted in a rather broad approach which includes recommendations to reduce sedentary pursuits, especially television viewing, increase activities of daily living and vigorous exercise sessions. Existing evidence suggests that the amount of activity required to prevent weight gain is probably large but any increased activity overall is likely to reduce obesity risk to some extent and make a positive contribution to public health.

3.3 Energy intake

Analysis of the dietary factors associated with obesity is confounded by difficulties in assessing food intake and eating behaviour [13]. Dietary surveys are increasingly beset by the problem of under-reporting, probably related to the increased awareness of nutrition issues and concern over body weight, which leads individuals to consciously mis-report their food intake. Under-reporting may also be subconscious as people may alter their dietary habits during periods of food recording, usually leading to a record of under-eating [14]. In 1986 Prentice *et al.* first demonstrated that obese women under-reported energy intake relative to energy needs by a mean of 3.5 MJ/d, while among lean women the two measures agreed to within 0.14 MJ/d [15]. This observation has been repeatedly reconfirmed, although it is now recognized that there is a spectrum of mis-reporting of food intake across the population, the nature of which is not easily predicted on the basis of individual phenotype or demographic statistics.

Analysis of the dietary determinants of obesity is also confounded by the problem of reverse causality, where increasing body weight may lead to changes in consumption. This makes it difficult to draw conclusions from cross-sectional studies of food intake and body weight. Relying on prospective studies that have reliable and accurate measures of diet and body composition severely limits the evidence base. Instead much of our understanding of the relationship between dietary factors and the risk of obesity comes from experimental studies in the laboratory or highly controlled intervention studies in the community. These may not truly mimic eating behaviour in a naturalistic setting, but they provide useful insights into the response to imposed dietary manipulations under standardized conditions.

Energy density

Energy density is a critical component in the regulation of human appetite and plays an important role in determining total energy intake. The results of many experiments where the energy density of foods have been covertly manipulated show that people tend to eat a standard volume of food regardless of it's energy content [16]. In one of the most robust experimental studies Stubbs *et al.* showed that lean, young healthy men, allowed to eat ad libitum, consumed significantly more energy as the fat content of the food was increased [17]. Over one week the men's body fat decreased by 0.86 ± 0.61 kg on the 20% fat diet, while increasing by 0.39 ± 0.59 kg and 2.24 ± 0.94 kg on the 40 and 60% fat diets respectively. Importantly, when the energy density of the food was

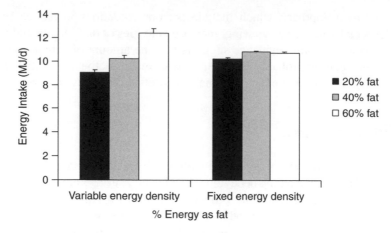

Figure 3.1 Impact of the proportion of dietary energy as fat on spontaneous energy intake of lean young men under conditions of variable or fixed energy density of food. Data from Stubbs *et al.* [18]

equalized, through careful experimental manipulation of the recipes, the high fat hyperphagia was abolished [18] (Figure 3.1). These studies provided no evidence of any physiological compensation for extra energy in food even after a week or more of sustained over-consumption. This process of 'passive over-consumption' implies that the bulk of food consumed is an important determinant of energy intake.

An energy dense diet frequently equates to a high fat diet, since fat (37 kJ/g) contains more than twice as much energy gram-for-gram as protein (17 kJ/g) or carbohydrate (16 kJ/g). Eating low-fat foods that contain substantially less energy than their full-fat equivalent can be one way to maintain the bulk of food in the diet while constraining energy intake. However, some food ranges that are low in fat have energy contents similar to their traditional equivalents, which is a result of the addition of large quantities of added sugars that help to maintain palatability. This emphasizes the importance of focusing on energy density and not just fat content as this type of low-fat, high-added-sugar food may lead to similar passive over-consumption as high-fat foods of similar energy density.

Water is also an important determinant of energy density and a paucity of fruits and vegetables is another feature of energy dense diets. Recent evidence has demonstrated that dietary advice encouraging a low energy-dense diet through a reduction of fat intake and increased consumption of fruits and vegetables resulted in similar weight loss but less hunger after 1 year compared to a reduction in fat intake alone (7.9 ± 0.9 kg vs. 6.4 ± 0.9 kg respectively); suggesting that reducing energy density and not just fat intake may be a more sustainable way of managing body weight [19].

Epidemiological studies of the effect of dietary energy density on body weight in free-living populations have reported mixed results to date. This is in part a result of an over-reliance on a cross-sectional study design (so reverse causality cannot be ruled out) but is also related to the method by which dietary energy density is calculated.

Excluding drinks from the calculation best represents the effect observed in experimental studies, which only manipulated food energy density. Studies of adults that calculated dietary energy density excluding drinks have consistently reported that a higher energy density is associated with increased body weight [20–22].

In children the effect of energy density may be more complex than that observed in adults. Energy density appears to interact with age-related changes in appetite control, such that younger, but not older, children are able to avoid excessive weight gain by responding to energy density and adjusting intake at subsequent meals. This is supported by prospective epidemiological studies that have identified a direct association between increased dietary energy density, in 7-year-old but not 3–5-year-old children, and higher subsequent obesity risk [23,24].

Sugar-rich drinks

It is important to recognize the energy density theory of appetite control cannot be equally applied across solid and liquid foods alike. Liquids have a lower energy density than solids because of their high water content, yet there is poorer energy compensation following isoenergetic liquids relative to solid food, perhaps due to differences in viscosity [25].

Highly controlled experimental studies provide evidence that soft drinks are an unhelpful addition to the diet of a nation prone to excess consumption since they tend to supplement rather than substitute for food. Two free-living studies have tested the effects on sugar-rich drinks on body weight. In the first, daily consumption of 1150 g soda sweetened with a high-fructose corn syrup (530 kcal/d) versus aspartame (3 kcal/d) or no beverage, over 3 weeks each, showed that the high-fructose corn syrup drink significantly increased energy intake and body weight relative to both the aspartame and control treatments (Figure 3.2) [26]. Second, a 10 week trial examined the impact of sugar-rich versus artificially-sweetened foods and drinks in which >80% of all intervention foods were beverages [27]. Over 10 weeks, weight increased by 1.6 kg in the high sugar group and decreased by −1.0 kg in the group in whom sugar rich foods and beverages were replaced by artificially sweetened varieties ($p < 0.001$). Overall, this data supports the hypothesis that consumption of sugar-rich drinks is a risk factor for obesity.

It is evident that increases in soft drink consumption have paralleled the rise in obesity. The increase has been marked, even among relatively young children. For example, in 4 year olds in Britain the consumption of soft drinks and juices has increased from only 13 g/week in 1950 to 446 g/week in 1992–1993 [28]. In adults, comparison of two nationally representative dietary surveys shows an increase from 669 to 1050 g/week in soft drinks (excluding diet varieties and juices) from 1986 to 2000–2001 [29,30]. Although this parallel increase does not prove causation a recent meta-analysis of prospective epidemiological studies provides some evidence of a detrimental effect [31]. Overall the results of three studies in adults and seven studies of children reported a small but positive correlation ($r = 0.14$ and $r = 0.03$ respectively)

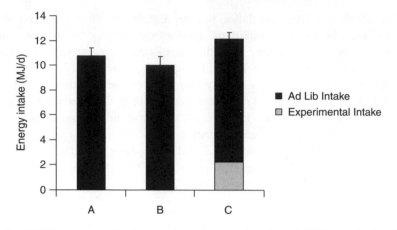

Figure 3.2 Ad libitum energy intake over three three-week periods (solid bars) plus intake from a prescribed beverage (hatched bars): A = no beverage, B = artificially sweetened, C = sweetened with high fructose corn syrup. Data from [26]

between sugar-rich drinks and body weight, which suggests that limiting the consumption of these drinks could benefit public health.

Portion size

The size of portions of food commonly served is increasing [32]. This trend, originally only in the United States, has rapidly swept across restaurants throughout the world as part of the process of globalization. It has been exploited by marketers and now also affects impulse snack purchases, household food and out of home eating occasions.

A series of studies in both laboratory and free-living settings have demonstrated that large portions foster increased consumption in both adults and children of both genders and irrespective of adiposity [33]. For example, when faced with increasing portions of amorphous foods such as pasta individuals consumed 30% more when the portion of food served was doubled [71] (Figure 3.3). There were no differences in reported hunger or satiety post-ingestion and less than half the participants recognized that the portion size varied on each occasion. High intakes at a single meal may be compensated for at subsequent meals or over the following days intake but recent studies have shown that this effect on energy intake is maintained over many days, suggesting that individual appetite regulation adjusts to accommodate the larger portion [35,36].

Of greater concern is when energy dense foods are served in large portions. Experimental studies in adults and children have shown that high energy density and portion size have additive and sustained effects on raising energy intake, with no concomitant effect on hunger and fullness, leading to an even greater over-consumption of energy [37,38].

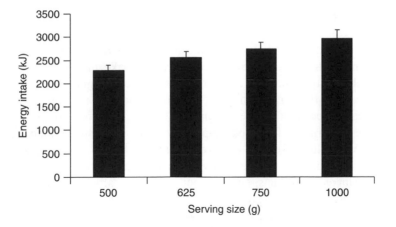

Figure 3.3 Increases in energy intake with increasing serving size of a macaroni cheese dish. Data from Rolls *et al.* [71]. Intakes in all conditions were significantly different from each other ($p < 0.05$) except 625 g and 750 g ($p = 0.097$)

Snacking

There is a clear secular decline in traditional three-meal-a-day eating patterns and a rise in more frequent, less formal eating occasions, commonly described as snacking [39,40]. Epidemiological associations between eating frequency and obesity yield mixed results and are heavily confounded by under-reporting of energy intake and hence potentially under-reporting of eating episodes too [41]. Indeed a study involving covert observation of food consumption in a metabolic facility while volunteers were allowed free access to food showed that volunteers specifically under-reported food consumed between formal meal eating episodes when asked to recall the food consumed [42].

Studies in the laboratory have shown that under isoenergetic conditions there is no effect of eating frequency on energy expenditure [43]. Eating frequency per se may not have any effect on energy intake either. In experimental conditions adding three mandatory snacks to the diet of eight lean men was not associated with an increase in overall energy intake. Total energy intake did not vary between the control and snack conditions suggesting that intake was reduced at other meal times to account for the extra snack energy between meals [44].

However, in free-living conditions, imposed consumption of high-fat or high-sugar snacks led to a modest increase in total energy intake over 1 day with a greater impact observed in those who did not habitually eat between meals [45]. A second, longer study lasting 2 weeks, introduced six mandatory commercially available snack-foods (including crisps, cakes, chocolate and confectionery) into the daily diet of 18 adults. Over 2 weeks total energy intake was increased when snacks were imposed compared to a control condition with no snacks [46]. These two studies suggest that it may not be a higher eating frequency that is the problem but rather composition of commercially available snack-foods (which are typically energy dense) that may lead to an increase in total energy intake and long-term weight gain.

Dietary patterns

Looking at the impact of the whole diet on obesity acknowledges the complexity of 'real life' food consumption. Combinations of nutrients make up foods and foods are consumed collectively to make up a dietary pattern. The amalgamation of many small effects from large portion sizes, a high dietary energy density, increased intake of soft drinks and snack foods could have an important impact on body weight.

Two major patterns of food consumption tend to encapsulate diets in Western populations. A so-called 'Western' diet is characterized by high consumption of cakes, pastries, biscuits, chocolate, confectionary, sugar sweetened drinks, refined grains, fast foods and high fat dairy products. The 'Prudent' diet is typically high in fruit, vegetables, whole grains and low-fat dairy products [47]. Consuming the 'Prudent' pattern of diet has been consistently related, in prospective analyses, to a lower risk of obesity in adults [48–53]. A prospective study of the diets of children has shown that those consuming the most energy dense, lowest fibre, highest fat foods – characterized by a low intake of fruits, vegetables and wholemeal bread but a high intake of white bread, crisps, sweets and chocolate – were four times more likely to have excess adiposity 2 years later than those children consuming the least energy dense, highest fibre, lowest fat foods [54]. Overall this supports the hypothesis that a conventionally 'healthy' diet, rich in fruit, vegetables, fibre and low-fat foods, protects against the development of obesity.

3.4   An integrated analysis

Secular increases in mean body weight show that at a population level there is a sustained small positive energy imbalance. Evidence cited previously suggests that this is driven by the two discretionary components of energy balance, namely food intake and physical activity. In the past too much emphasis has been placed on the study of each factor in isolation. For example, many people cite a paper that documented the decline in energy intake and rise in sedentary lifestyles between 1970 and 1990 [55] as support for the hypothesis that physical inactivity is the major determinant of obesity. However, inactivity per se does not cause obesity. Obesity only develops when energy intake is not precisely down-regulated to match the low energy needs of modern living. It is the coupling between intake and expenditure that is at the heart of the obesity epidemic [56].

The physiological coupling between intake and expenditure across the intermediary range of energy needs is clearly demonstrated in a study in laboratory animals, dating from the 1950s (Figure 3.4) [57]. Here, animals were required to exercise for progressively increasing periods of time, increasing energy needs. Spontaneous energy intake increased in parallel and body weight was maintained. However, at extremely high levels of exercise, insufficient food was consumed and weight was gradually lost, while at very low levels of activity the animals were unable to constrain their consumption to match their excessively low energy needs and weight increased.

A study of human energy balance conducted under controlled conditions in a whole-body calorimeter provides insight into the limits of the homeostatic mechanisms that

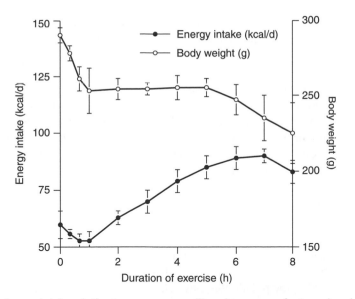

Figure 3.4 Energy intake relative to energy expenditure in a group of rats undergoing different levels of imposed exercise. Data from [56]

regulate body weight. Over 2 days a group of lean young men were exposed to a low or high fat diet, together with either sufficient exercise to maintain habitual activity levels or only sedentary activities in a 2×2 design [58]. Energy balance was close to zero on the low-fat diet with habitual activity condition. Whereas the imposition of sedentary behaviour or a high-fat diet each created net energy gains (of $+2.55$ and $+1.07\,$MJ/d respectively). When imposed together, the two effects appeared to interact, creating a positive imbalance of $+5.13\,$MJ/d, which is equal to nearly 50% of the subjects' daily energy requirements and would result in about 130 g fat gain per day.

The integrated effects of these two behaviours are critical since poor dietary habits and low levels of physical activity frequently co-exist. Television viewing is frequently observed to be strongly associated with an increased risk of obesity [59]. Many people assume that this effect is a result of an overall reduction in activity levels; however there is little evidence of this [60]. A more likely explanation is the interaction between TV watching and food intake. An obesogenic dietary pattern characterized by a higher consumption of savoury snack foods, high fat foods, fast foods and a lower consumption of fruits and vegetables has been associated with higher levels of TV watching in many studies [54,61–63]. Television viewing may be causally linked to such eating habits through increased exposure to food adverts [64] and the association with obesity may reflect the effects of distraction on the development of satiety [65].

Environmental impacts on lifestyle

The world we live in has changed and this transition has occurred at a rate far greater than man is able to evolve and adapt. Our genetic makeup has been moulded by an environment in which food was scarce and the physical demands for survival were high [66]. Today the decline in manual occupations and the rise in motorized transport, sedentary leisure pursuits such as television, computers and electronic toys have reduced our energy needs to a level below which innate appetite control systems are no longer able to precisely match energy intake to energy needs. A huge variety of highly palatable foods are more available to us than ever before, and we spend a smaller proportion of our disposable income on food than ever before. There has been a marked increase in the proportion of food consumed outside the home which contains a greater proportion of fat and is frequently more energy dense than household food. Consumption is encouraged through a variety of marketing strategies including advertisements and economic incentives to purchase larger or additional items. Portion sizes are standardized and not tailored to personal needs and individuals have limited understanding of the composition of food items which impairs any cognitive control over food intake. It has been argued that excess weight gain is a predictable response to this changed environment [67], yet some individuals, families and subgroups of the population are remaining lean. But how is this achieved?

Differences within the population may reflect variation in genetic susceptibility to obesity. Research into gene–environment interactions is in its infancy but evidence is emerging. For example, high fat diets may be a more potent risk factor for obesity among individuals with a specific mutation in the peroxisome proliferator activated γ receptor gene (PPARγ, a critical regulator of adipogenesis) [68]. It is important to acknowledge that differences in cognitive coping strategies or psychological ambivalence can also modify an individual's response to the obesogenic environment. Given that genetic pathways are not readily amenable to change a focus on effective behaviour change methods is perhaps the way forward in order to help people adopt a healthy lifestyle.

A comprehensive review in the Government's Foresight report identified a series of contributory factors through which the environment may modulate the risk of obesity [4]. These include food availability, which may be limited by the location of fast food restaurants or supermarkets; food costs, which are often higher when following a 'healthy' diet; neighbourhood density of sports facilities and the 'walkability' of the built environment, which may limit the opportunity to be physically active; media exposure and food marketing, can be a powerful tool to increase consumption. Broader environmental changes could facilitate the avoidance of weight gain, especially in low-income communities that maybe disproportionately exposed to these factors.

Prevention strategies to date that have focused largely on modifying lifestyles, for example by encouraging physical activity and the consumption of fruits and vegetables. Few interventions have been successful in reducing the incidence of obesity [69]. This does not mean that lifestyles are not the cause of obesity but rather that such interventions need to be designed and implemented in more effective ways. There is a need for large-scale, community-based initiatives supported by both the public and private sectors that take an integrated approach to behaviour change that enables consistent messages about healthy living to be delivered over a sustained period of time [4].

3.5 Conclusions

Obesity is a complex heterogeneous disease. It is well accepted that there is an underlying genetic susceptibility to disease, but this is modified by environmental circumstances and individual lifestyle choices. Figure 3.5 illustrates how individual diet, activity and psychology interact with the basic biological drive for energy balance. Ultimately the risk of obesity is determined by energy balance, but the critical exposures (diet, activity and behaviour) are difficult to measure reliably. In this scenario it is not surprising that direct, incontrovertible evidence of the specific lifestyle determinants of excess weight gain is lacking. However, this integrated analysis of data from diverse sources points towards a number of factors that are likely to be important. These include energy dense

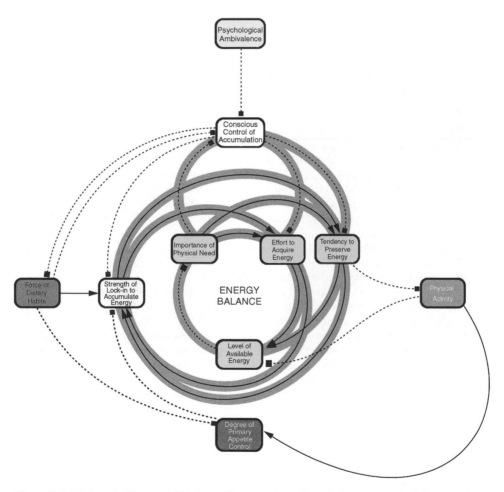

Figure 3.5 Integrated impact of biology, diet, activity and psychology on energy balance and the risk of obesity. Reproduced from Foresight. Tackling Obesities: Future Choices – Project Report. London, Government Office for Science, GOS, 2007 [4]

foods, large portions, a healthy dietary pattern and physical inactivity. Importantly a number of these factors may come together in an additive, or possibly even synergistic manner, to influence the risk of obesity. Together they provide a compelling case for lifestyle interventions to tackle the epidemic of obesity.

References

1. Department of Health & The Information Centre For Health and Social Care (2006) Health Survey for England – updating of trend tables to include 2005 data. London.
2. Jebb, S. (1997) Aetiology of obesity. *British Medical Bulletin*, **53**, 264–85.
3. Goldberg, G.R., Black, A.E., Jebb, S.A. *et al.* (1991) Critical evaluation of energy intake data using fundamental principles of energy physiology: 1. Derivation of cut-off limits to identify under-recording. *European Journal of Clinical Nutrition*, **45**, 569–81.
4. Foresight. Tackling Obesities: Future Choices – Project Report. London, Government Office for Science, GOS (2007).
5. Wareham, N. and Rennie, K.L. (1998) The assessment of PA in individuals and populations: why try to be more precise about how PA is assessed? *International Journal of Obesity*, **22**, S30–S38.
6. Ness, A.R., Leary, S.D., Mattocks, C. *et al.* (2007) Objectively measured physical activity and fat mass in a large cohort of children. *PLoS Medicine*, **4**, e97.
7. Ekelund, U., Sardinha, L.B., Anderssen, S.A. *et al.* (2004) Associations between objectively assessed physical activity and indicators of body fatness in 9- to 10-y-old European children: a population-based study from 4 distinct regions in Europe (the European Youth Heart Study). *American Journal of Clinical Nutrition*, **80**, 584–590.
8. Wareham, N. (2007) Physical activity and obesity prevention. *Obesity Reviews*, **8**, 109–14, 10.1111/j.1467-789X.2007.00328.x.
9. Ekelund, U., Brage, S., Franks, P.W. *et al.* (2005) Physical activity energy expenditure predicts changes in body composition in middle-aged healthy whites: effect modification by age. *American Journal of Clinical Nutrition*, **81**, 964–690.
10. Kinmonth, A.-L., Wareham, N.J., Hardeman, W. *et al.* (2008) Efficacy of a theory-based behavioural intervention to increase physical activity in an at-risk group in primary care (ProActive UK): a randomised trial. *Lancet*, **371**, 41–8.
11. King, N.A., Hopkins, M., Caudwell, P. *et al.* (2007) Individual variability following 12 weeks of supervised exercise: identification and characterization of compensation for exercise-induced weight loss. *International Journal of Obesity*, **32**, 177–84.
12. Hardeman, W., Griffin, S., Johnston, M. *et al.* (2000) Interventions to prevent weight gain: a systematic review of psychological models and behaviour change methods. *International Journal of Obesity and Related Metabolic Disorders*, **24**, 131–43.
13. Jebb, S.A. (2007) Dietary determinants of obesity. *Obesity Reviews*, **8** (Suppl 1), 93–7.
14. Goris, A.H., Westerterp-Plantenga, M.S. and Westerterp, K.R. (2000) Undereating and under-recording of habitual food intake in obese men: selective underreporting of fat intake. *American Journal of Clinical Nutrition*, **71**, 130–4.
15. Prentice, A.M., Black, A.E., Coward, W.A. *et al.* (1986) High levels of energy expenditure in obese women. *British Medical Journal (Clinical Research Ed.)*, **292**, 983–7.
16. Poppitt, S.D. and Prentice, A.M. (1996) Energy density and its role in the control of food intake: evidence from metabolic and community studies. *Appetite*, **26**, 153–74.
17. Stubbs, R.J., Harbron, C.G., Murgatroyd, P.R. and Prentice, A.M. (1995) Covert manipulation of dietary fat and energy density: effect on substrate flux and food intake in men eating ad libitum. *American Journal of Clinical Nutrition*, **62**, 316–29.

18. Stubbs, R.J., Harbron, C.G. and Prentice, A.M. (1996) Covert manipulation of the dietary fat to carbohydrate ratio of isoenergetically dense diets: effect on food intake in feeding men ad libitum. *International Journal of Obesity*, **20**, 651–60.
19. Ello-Martin, J.A., Roe, L.S., Ledikwe, J.H. *et al.* (2007) Dietary energy density in the treatment of obesity: a year-long trial comparing 2 weight-loss diets. *American Journal of Clinical Nutrition*, **85**, 1465–77.
20. Ledikwe, J.H., Blanck, H.M., Kettel Khan, L. *et al.* (2006) Dietary energy density is associated with energy intake and weight status in US adults. *American Journal of Clinical Nutrition*, **83**, 1362–8.
21. Kant, A.K. and Graubard, B.I. (2005) Energy density of diets reported by American adults: association with food group intake, nutrient intake, and body weight. *International Journal of Obesity*, **29**, 950–6.
22. Mendoza, J.A., Drewnowski, A. and Christakis, D.A. (2007) Dietary energy density is associated with obesity and the metabolic syndrome in US Adults 10.2337/dc06-2188. *Diabetes Care*, **30**, 974–979.
23. Kral, T.V.E., Berkowitz, R.I., Stunkard, A.J. *et al.* (2007) Dietary energy density increases during early childhood irrespective of familial predisposition to obesity: results from a prospective cohort study. *International Journal of Obesity*, **31**, 1061–7.
24. Johnson, L., Mander, A.P., Jones, L.R. *et al.* (2007) A prospective analysis of dietary energy density at age 5 and 7 years and fatness at 9 years among UK children. *International Journal of Obesity*, **32**, 586–93.
25. Mattes, R.D. and Rothacker, D. (2001) Beverage viscosity is inversely related to postprandial hunger in humans. *Physiology & Behavior*, **74**, 551–7.
26. Tordoff, M.G. and Alleva, A.M. (1990) Effect of drinking soda sweetened with aspartame or high-fructose corn syrup on food intake and body weight. *American Journal of Clinical Nutrition*, **51**, 963–9.
27. Raben, A., Vasilaras, T.H., Moller, A.C. and Astrup, A. (2002) Sucrose compared with artificial sweeteners: different effects on ad libitum food intake and body weight after 10 wk of supplementation in overweight subjects. *American Journal of Clinical Nutrition*, **76**, 721–9.
28. Prynne, C.J., Paul, A.A., Price, G.M. *et al.* (1999) Food and nutrient intake of a national sample of 4-year-old children in 1950: comparison with the 1990s. *Public Health Nutrition*, **2**, 537–47.
29. Gregory, J., Foster, K., Tyler, H. and Wiseman, M. (1990) *The Dietary and Nutritional Survey of British Adults*, HMSO, London.
30. Henderson, L. and Gregory, J. (2002) *National Diet and Nutritional Survey: adults aged 19 to 64 years*, HMSO, London.
31. Vartanian, L.R., Schwartz, M.B. and Brownell, K.D. (2007) Effects of soft drink consumption on nutrition and health: a systematic review and meta-analysis. *American Journal of Public Health*, **97**, 667–75.
32. Nielsen, S.J. and Popkin, B.M. (2003) Patterns and trends in food portion sizes, 1977–1998. *Journal of the American Medical Association*, **289**, 450–3.
33. Rolls, B.J. (2003) The supersizing of America: portion size and the obesity epidemic. *Nutrition Today*, **38**, 42–53.
34. Rolls, B.J., Roe, L.S. and Meengs, J.S. (2006) Larger portion sizes lead to a sustained increase in energy intake over 2 days. *Journal of the American Dietetic Association*, **106**, 543–9.
35. Rolls, B.J., Roe, L.S. and Meengs, J.S. (2007) The effect of large portion sizes on energy intake is sustained for 11 days. *Obesity (Silver Spring)*, **15**, 1535–43.
36. Kral, T.V., Roe, L.S. and Rolls, B.J. (2004) Combined effects of energy density and portion size on energy intake in women. *American Journal of Clinical Nutrition*, **79**, 962–8.

37. Fisher, J.O., Liu, Y., Birch, L.L. and Rolls, B.J. (2007) Effects of portion size and energy density on young children's intake at a meal. *American Journal of Clinical Nutrition*, **86**, 174–9.
38. Zizza, C., Siega-Riz, A.M. and Popkin, B.M. (2001) Significant increase in young adults' snacking between 1977–1978 and 1994–1996 represents a cause for concern! *Preventive Medicine*, **32**, 303–10.
39. Jahns, L., Siega-Riz, A.M. and Popkin, B.M. (2001) The increasing prevalence of snacking among US children from 1977 to 1996. *Journal of Pediatrics*, **138**, 493–8.
40. Bellisle, F., Mcdevitt, R. and Prentice, A.M. (1997) Meal frequency and energy balance. *British Journal of Nutrition*, **77** (Suppl 1), S57–S70.
41. Poppitt, S.D., Swann, D., Black, A.E. and Prentice, A.M. (1998) Assessment of selective under-reporting of food intake by both obese and non-obese women in a metabolic facility. *International Journal of Obesity*, **22**, 303–11.
42. Dallosso, H.M., Murgatroyd, P.R. and James, W.P. (1982) Feeding frequency and energy balance in adult males. *Human Nutrition – Clinical Nutrition*, **36**, 25–39.
43. Johnstone, A.M., Shannon, E., Whybrow, S. *et al.* (2000) Altering the temporal distribution of energy intake with isoenergetically dense foods given as snacks does not affect total daily energy intake in normal-weight men. *British Journal of Nutrition*, **83**, 7–14.
44. Green, S.M. and Blundell, J.E. (1996) Effect of fat- and sucrose-containing foods on the size of eating episodes and energy intake in lean dietary restrained and unrestrained females: potential for causing overconsumption. *European Journal of Clinical Nutrition*, **50**, 625–35.
45. Whybrow, S., Mayer, C., Kirk, T.R. *et al.* (2007) Effects of two weeks' mandatory snack consumption on energy intake and energy balance. *Obesity*, **15**, 673–85.
46. Kant, A.K. (2004) Dietary patterns and health outcomes. *Journal of the American Dietetic Association*, **104**, 615–35.
47. Schulze, M.B., Fung, T.T., Manson, J.E. *et al.* (2006) Dietary patterns and changes in body weight in women. *Obesity (Silver Spring)*, **14**, 1444–53.
48. Schulz, M., Nothlings, U., Hoffmann, K. *et al.* (2005) Identification of a food pattern character-ized by high-fiber and low-fat food choices associated with low prospective weight change in the EPIC-Potsdam cohort. *Journal of Nutrition*, **135**, 1183–9.
49. Quatromoni, P.A., Copenhafer, D.L., D'Agostino, R.B. and Millen, B.E. (2002) Dietary patterns predict the development of overweight in women: The Framingham Nutrition Studies. *Journal of the American Dietetic Association*, **102**, 1239–46.
50. Newby, P.K., Muller, D., Hallfrisch, J. *et al.* (2003) Dietary patterns and changes in body mass index and waist circumference in adults. *American Journal of Clinical Nutrition*, **77**, 1417–25.
51. Mcnaughton, S.A., Mishra, G.D., Stephen, A.M. and Wadsworth, M.E.J. (2007) Dietary patterns throughout adult life are associated with body mass index, waist circumference, blood pressure, and red cell folate. *Journal of Nutrition*, **137**, 99–105.
52. Park, S.Y., Murphy, S.P., Wilkens, L.R. *et al.* (2005) Dietary patterns using the Food Guide Pyramid groups are associated with sociodemographic and lifestyle factors: the multiethnic cohort study. *Journal of Nutrition*, **135**, 843–9.
53. Johnson, L., Mander, A.P., Jones, L.R. *et al.* (2008) An energy dense, low fibre, high fat dietary pattern is associated with increased fatness in childhood. *American Journal of Clinical Nutrition*, **84**, 846–54.
54. Prentice, A.M. and Jebb, S.A. (1995) Obesity in Britain: gluttony or sloth? *British Medical Journal*, **311**, 437–9.
55. Prentice, A. and Jebb, S. (2004) Energy intake/physical activity interactions in the homeostasis of body weight regulation. *Nutrition Reviews*, **62**, S98–S104.
56. Mayer, J. (1966) Some aspects of the problem of regulation of food intake and obesity. *New England Journal of Medicine*, **274**, 610–16, contd.

57. Murgatroyd, P.R., Goldberg, G.R., Leahy, F.E. *et al.* (1999) Effects of inactivity and diet composition on human energy balance. *International Journal of Obesity and Related Metabolic Disorders*, **23**, 1269–75.

58. Crespo, C.J., Smit, E., Troiano, R.P. *et al.* (2001) Television Watching, Energy Intake and Obesity in US Children. *Archives of Pediatrics & Adolescent Medicine*, **155**, 360–5.

59. Marshall, S.J., Biddle, S.J., Gorely, T. *et al.* (2004) Relationships between media use, body fatness and physical activity in children and youth: a meta-analysis. *International Journal of Obesity*, **28**, 1238–46.

60. Rennie, K.L., Johnson, L. and Jebb, S.A. (2005) Behavioural determinants of obesity. *Best Practice & Research. Clinical Endocrinology & Metabolism*, **19**, 343–58.

61. Vereecken, C.A., Todd, J., Roberts, C. *et al.* (2006) Television viewing behaviour and associations with food habits in different countries. *Public Health Nutrition*, **9**, 244–50.

62. Coon, K.A. and Tucker, K.L. (2002) Television and children's consumption patterns. A review of the literature. *Minerva Pediatrica*, **54**, 423–36.

63. Halford, J.C., Gillespie, J., Brown, V. *et al.* (2004) Effect of television advertisements for foods on food consumption in children. *Appetite*, **42**, 221–5.

64. Brunstrom, J.M. and Mitchell, G.L. (2006) Effects of distraction on the development of satiety. *British Journal of Nutrition*, **96**, 761–9.

65. Peters, J.C., Wyatt, H.R., Donahoo, W.T. and Hill, J.O. (2002) From instinct to intellect: the challenge of maintaining healthy weight in the modern world. *Obesity Reviews*, **3**, 69–74.

66. Prentice, A.M. (1997) Obesity–the inevitable penalty of civilisation? *British Medical Bulletin*, **53**, 229–37.

67. Loos, R.J.F. and Rankinen, T. (2005) Gene–diet interactions on body weight changes. *Journal of the American Dietetic Association*, **105**, 29–34.

68. Summerbell, C.D. (2007) The identification of effective programs to prevent and treat overweight preschool children. *Obesity*, **15**, 1341–2.

69. Rolls, B.J., Morris, E.L. and Roe, L.S. (2002) Portion size of food affects energy intake in normal-weight and overweight men and women. *The American Journal of Clinical Nutrition*, **76**, 1207–13.

4

Pathophysiology of obesity-induced T2DM

Konstantinos Lois, Phillip McTernan and Sudhesh Kumar

WISDEM, University Hospital, Coventry and CSRI, Warwick Medical School, Coventry, UK

4.1   Introduction

The obesity and diabetes epidemics continue to escalate. There is a wealth of data that reveal their close relationship to each other, expressed recently by the term 'diabesity'. Although intensively researched, a unifying hypothesis linking different pathogenic mechanisms that make obese individuals resistant to insulin and their pancreatic β-cells to fail leading eventually to frank diabetes, remains elusive. The distribution of body fat seems to be more important than the body weight itself [1] and central adiposity, estimated in clinical practice with the evaluation of waist circumference, is considered an independent risk factor for the development of insulin resistance and type 2 diabetes (T2DM) later in life (Figure 4.1).

4.2   Potential mechanisms linking central obesity to T2DM

Obesity is a heterogeneous condition with respect to regional distribution and biological properties of fat tissue [2]. Visceral adipose tissue refers to fat accumulation within omental and mesenteric fat depots, and constitutes about 6–20% of total body fat tissue. It is less receptive to the anabolic effects of insulin and metabolically–lipolytically more active than the peripheral fat tissue, which refers to subcutaneous fat accumulation and comprises 80% of total adipose tissue.

The traditional views on metabolic derangements of diabetes have been largely 'glucocentric', considering hyperglycaemia the main underlying cause. However, the recognition that obese individuals who usually suffer from hyper- or dyslipidaemia

Obesity and Diabetes, Second Edition   Edited by Anthony H. Barnett and Sudhesh Kumar
© 2009 John Wiley & Sons, Ltd

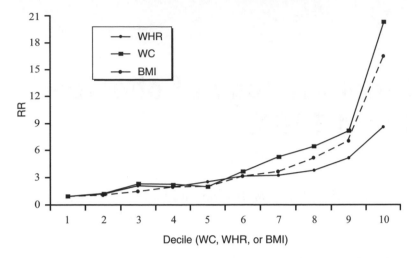

Figure 4.1 Age-adjusted relative risk (RR) of type 2 diabetes by baseline waist circumference (WC), waist-to-hip ratio (WHR), and BMI deciles. Source: Youfa Wang *et al. American Journal of Clinical Nutrition*, Vol. 81, No. 3, 555–63, March 2005

develop insulin resistance and diabetes much more frequently than lean people and also that people with T2DM almost invariably manifest serious breakdown in lipid dynamics, reflected by elevated levels of circulating non-esterified fatty acids (NEFAs) and triglycerides (TG), led researchers to investigate the potential role of altered lipid metabolism in the pathogenesis of T2DM. Two theories mainly explain the close relationship between fat excess and impaired glucose metabolism; the 'Randle's cycle' that provides the reciprocal relationship between fatty acid oxidation and glucose oxidation and the 'ectopic fat storage hypothesis' according to which the impaired insulin effect is due to deposition of lipids within insulin-target tissues. They both suggest the so called 'lipotoxicity theory' that proposes a probable metabolic model by which prolonged fat excess is positively correlated with both insulin resistance and decreased insulin secretory capacity of beta cells, in the context of concomitant hyperglycaemia.

Recently, two more hypotheses were added to the suggested theories by which obesity may lead to T2DM; first, the identification of adipose tissue as an endocrine organ that produces and metabolizes multiple bioactive factors, which may potentially impair glucose metabolism and second, change of adipose tissue phenotype due to a low-grade inflammatory state that impairs insulin effectiveness. Although these theories provide metabolic mechanisms that seem to be different in origin and nature, the underlying trigger factor may be related to effect of substrate excess relative to what adipose tissue has the genetically determined capacity to store. As a result, obese individuals develop insulin resistance, which is initially compensated for by hyper-insulinaemia, through which normal glucose tolerance is preserved. However, over time further deterioration of glucose metabolism, either by increased insulin resistance or by decreased compensatory insulin secretory responses or by both, accelerates the progression to impaired glucose tolerance and eventually to overt T2DM.

4.3   Sources of increased plasma NEFA in obesity

Obese individuals have two main sources of plasma NEFA excess: meal-derived fatty acids and adipose tissue lipolysis. High-calorie diets increase plasma concentration of TG-rich lipoproteins (very low density lipoproteins and chylomicrons), which are in turn hydrolysed by the lipoprotein lipase in endothelial cells lining the capillaries, releasing large amounts of fatty acids to the bloodstream.

The role of visceral fat in NEFA flux to the liver is also of considerable significance; the adipose tissue stores energy in postabsorptive states as triglycerides, which can be quickly released in the form of fatty acids when energy is needed elsewhere in the body. However, it has been demonstrated that although in lean individuals the adipose tissue can switch from a negative to a positive NEFA balance during the transition from fasting to the postprandial state, in obese individuals, adipocyte NEFA balance remains negative even postprandially [3]. Furthermore, in comparison to the peripheral–gluteal adipose tissue, central abdominal fat is metabolically and lipolytically more active, producing more NEFAs, while obese individuals' visceral adipocytes have markedly higher NEFA release than lean controls [4]. Regional differences in the number and sensitivity of adrenoreceptors [5], the activity of 11β-hydroxysteroid dehydrogenase type 1 (11β-HSD1) [6] and the adipocytes' response to lipogenic/antilipolytic effects of insulin, are considered the main underlying causes for the variation in biological properties of fat tissue from different depots.

Despite substantial increase in adipose tissue mass in obesity, plasma NEFAs are initially kept close to physiological ranges, via hyperisulinaemia that accompanies obesity. However, over time, as obesity becomes a chronic state, there is deregulation of this process and day-long elevation of plasma NEFA concentration in obese individuals ensues [7]. The latter is considered a crucial link between central obesity and T2DM, as it impairs liver and pancreatic beta cell function and reduces peripheral tissues sensitivity to insulin (Randle's cycle).

4.4   'Randle's glucose-fatty acid' hypothesis

Glucose and fatty acids are the major fuels for mammalian metabolism, accounting for about 80% of oxidative metabolism. Therefore, powerful regulatory mechanisms are in place to co-ordinate their appropriate utilization in the body, perhaps as a means of protecting cells against excess fuel utilization.

In 1963 Philip Randle first proposed one set of metabolic pathways by which carbohydrate and fat metabolism interact. He called it 'cycle' because it describes a series of events that interlink glucose and fat utilization within the cells. Its basic outline is simple; carbohydrates, when available (postprandially), are preferred as fuels than lipids, which are stored in adipose tissue for future use. Insulin plays a primary role in this regulation, facilitating glucose peripheral uptake and utilization, while at the same time it inhibits NEFA mobilization from the adipose tissue, inactivating hormone-sensitive lipase and thus it removes the competition for substrate utilization in peripheral tissues. On the other hand, when carbohydrates are decreased (fasting), serum insulin levels fall, permitting lipolysis and NEFA mobilization, which then become the major fuel for peripheral tissues. Randle *et al.* went a step further, demonstrating the inhibitory effect of enhanced NEFA oxidation on glucose metabolism. This particular metabolic effect takes place in body situations with lipid excess, as in obesity and is considered pathogenic in the development of insulin resistance and eventually T2DM in obese individuals. It is suggested that by mass action, the increased plasma NEFAs augment their cellular uptake and induce their mitochondrial β-oxidation. As a result, the cellular metabolism may be altered at the level of substrate competition, intermediates accumulation, enzyme regulation, intracellular signalling and/or gene transcription, affecting among others glucose metabolism. Clinical studies in healthy volunteers, in which acute elevation of plasma NEFAs resulted in whole body insulin resistance, confirmed the proposed metabolic model [7].

The liver is considered of great importance in the regulation of glucose metabolism as in fasted states when blood concentrations of glucose and insulin begin to decline, it depolymerizes glycogen (glycogenolysis) or even synthesizes glucose out of non-sugar carbon substrates (gluconeogenesis) and exports glucose back into the blood, so that hypoglycaemia is prevented (hepatic glucose production, HGP). On the other hand, when plasma glucose is adequate, as in postprandial states, under the effect of insulin, HGP is decreased and liver rapidly takes up the excess glucose entering the blood and stores it as the large polymer glycogen (glycogenesis), hence restricting excessive postprandial increases in plasma glucose concentrations. Insulin is considered a potent inhibitor of HGP and stimulator of glycogenesis. Thus, in patients with T2DM in whom early phase insulin secretion is impaired, defective liver disposal of glucose and postprandial HGP significantly worsen hyperglycaemia. Ferrannini [7] first demonstrated that NEFAs excess impair insulin effect on the liver. It has been suggested that by mass action, NEFAs augment their hepatic uptake and utilization, leading to intracellular accumulation of acetyl-coenzyme A. The later stimulates even in post-absorptive states gluconeogenesis and glycogenolysis (via pyruvate carboxylase and glucose-6-phosphatase, respectively) worsening hyperglycaemia, while NEFA oxidation provides hepatocytes the necessary energy for these metabolic events. In support of this is the finding that a significant portion of the suppressive effect of insulin on HGP is mediated by inhibition of lipolysis and reduction of circulating NEFAs, confirming the primary role of NEFAs in liver-dependent glucose metabolism.

The pancreatic beta cells are also targets of a biphasic NEFA effect. β-cells are responsible for sensing and secreting the appropriate amount of insulin in response to a glucose stimulus. Although this process is complex and dependent on many factors, the critical importance of mitochondrial glucose metabolism in linking stimulus to secretion is well established. While short-term exposure to NEFAs increases glucose-induced insulin secretion (GIIS), prolonged exposure suppresses it. The accumulation of NEFAs oxidation metabolites (acetyl coenzyme A) within the beta cells [8] is considered the underlying cause for this effect. It is suggested that the accumulated acetyl coenzyme A blocks via phosphate dehydrogenase inhibition and citrate formation, glycolysis. Since glycolysis is an essential source of ATP requisite for GIIS, chronic beta cell exposure to NEFA excess eventually impairs insulin secretion. Furthermore, it is supported that it also stimulates ceramide synthesis, which in turn affects beta cell function and promotes apoptosis.

In obesity, a vicious cycle between increased circulating NEFAs, insulin resistance and NEFA mobilization from the adipose tissue ensues, which eventually exaggerates any impairment in the whole body's glucose metabolism. The high correlation between disturbances in normal metabolism of adipose tissue (obesity, lipodystrophy) and the manifestation of insulin resistance indicates the important role of adipose tissue in its aetiology. Recent findings show that insulin resistance and impaired insulin action occur early in adipose tissue, long before glucose intolerance develops and adipose tissue is now recognized by many as the primary site of insulin resistance. It is proposed that plasma NEFA excess ameliorate, via intracellular long-chain saturated fatty acid formation, the insulin effect in fat tissue [9]. As a result, the hormone sensitive lipase remains active, mobilizing more NEFAs from the adipocytes to the bloodstream, with subsequent detrimental effects on insulin production and peripheral tissues response to it.

Skeletal muscle is considered a crucial metabolic target of NEFAs, as it is thought to be the most important tissue in determining whole-body insulin resistance, accounting for approximately 70–80% of the whole-body glucose disposal rate in normal humans [10]. Although the excessive NEFA β-oxidation as proposed by Randle could provide several abnormal metabolic pathways by which it eventually impairs glucose metabolism and insulin action in myocytes leading to hyperglycaemia (e.g. inhibition of hexokinase, glucose utilization and glucose transporter 4 (GLUT4) synthesis and translocation, by acetyl coenzyme A and citrate accumulation), recent data do not entirely support this hypothesis. It seems that the 'metabolic inflexibility' proposed by Kelley and colleagues [11] is the key underlying metabolic condition that explains the development of myocellular insulin resistance in obese individuals. According to this theory lean healthy individuals myocytes display substantial metabolic flexibility, with the capacity to switch from predominantly lipid oxidation and high rates of fatty acid uptake during fasting conditions [12] to the suppression of lipid oxidation and increased glucose uptake, oxidation and storage under insulin stimulated conditions [13]. In obese patients however skeletal muscles present fixed lipid oxidation in comparing fasting and insulin-stimulated conditions. It is suggested that the inhibition of CTP1 (the enzyme that enables NEFA entry into mitochondria and thus their oxidation) by the hyperglycaemia/hyperinsulinaemia-induced increased malonyl coenzyme A intracellular concentration, is the underlying cause. As a result, skeletal muscles fail to augment lipid oxidation during fasting conditions resulting in intracellular lipid accumulation and insulin resistance (ectopic fat storage theory).

Finally, a vascular-endothelium related explanation for NEFA-induced insulin resistance has been suggested by several researchers. It is well known that insulin acts on endothelial cells enhancing nitric oxide (NO) synthase activity and NO production, which is a very potent vasodilator. Further to its vasodilatory effect, insulin also possesses microvascular-recruitment properties, by which it facilitates its access (as well as glucose access and uptake) to the peripheral tissues. Baron *et al.* [14] showed that NEFAs reduce the endothelial cells sensitivity to insulin, impairing NO production and thus the access and effect of insulin on peripheral tissues.

By the above metabolic pathways, obesity-associated prolonged or even chronic NEFA excess causes beta cell dysfunction and impairs peripheral tissues glucose uptake and utilization, leading to hyperglycaemia and eventually T2DM once the pancreatic beta cells fail to compensate for the increased needs on insulin.

4.5   Ectopic fat storage hypothesis

Until recently, adipose tissue was considered the only tissue in the human body that stores fat. Normally, the adipocytes take up lipids from fat-rich plasma lipoproteins, through the effect of fat cell-derived lipoprotein lipase and store almost pure triglycerides in quantities of up to 95% of their volume. This process called lipogenesis is enhanced by insulin [15]. On the other hand, when energy is needed elsewhere in the body, the stored fat is mobilized (lipolysis) in the form of NEFAs by the hormone sensitive lipoprotein lipase, against the effect of insulin. It is estimated that the rate of this exchange is so high, that the entire content of each fat cell is renewed approximately every 2–3 weeks. However, when the diet-derived fat intake is increased, as in obesity, fat storage within and around other tissues and organs, including liver, skeletal muscle and pancreatic beta cells, which under normal conditions do not store lipids, has been demonstrated [16]. The increased fat intake, the impaired fat oxidation and the inadequate fat cell proliferation are considered the main underlying causes of the obesity-associated diversion of fat to non-adipose organs, which in turn deregulates glucose metabolism (ectopic fat storage hypothesis).

In obese individuals, adipose tissue grows to store the fat excess. Its growth consists of hyperplasia and lipid-filling differentiation of preadipocytes, coupled with hypertrophic changes of the mature adipocytes. However, adipocytes do not have limitless capacity to store TG. There is probably a critical visceral adipose tissue threshold (CVATT), after which fat deposition is diverted to extra-adipose tissues. In addition, it is supported that the metabolic properties of the engorged adipocytes are changed. They are reprogrammed and secrete an array of bioactive factors such as cytokines, growth factors and adipocytokines, while they also become fragile, releasing factors such as macrophage colony-stimulating factor (M-CSF) and monocyte chemoattractant protein-1 (MCP-1) that attract locally macrophages. The resultant changes in the adipose tissue microenvironment (inflammation and insulin resistance), inhibit proliferation and differentiation of pre-adipocytes, restrict further TG storage within the already over-filled adipocytes and divert fat excess to non-adipose tissues. It has been demonstrated that although initially the peripheral organs facilitate the storage-esterification of the surplus in the form of TG, their limited TG buffer capacity soon becomes saturated and the excess of lipids enter alternative non-oxidative pathways. As a result, excessive mitochondrial production of toxic reactive lipid species ensues, which mediate organ-specific oxidative damage and cellular dysfunction, leading progressively to the development of insulin resistance, impaired glucose metabolism and finally T2DM [17]. What determines the CVATT level, as well as which is the underlying mechanism that leads to ectopic fat storage, remains unclear.

The ectopic fat storage theory has gained a significant body of supporting experimental data in the last few years. The inherited or human immunodeficiency virus-related forms of lipodystrophy, where the selective loss of subcutaneous and visceral fat is associated with ectopic fat storage and subsequent severe insulin resistance and T2DM, indicates the detrimental effect of ectopic fat deposition in glucose metabolism. [18, 19]. On the other hand adipogenic promoters, such as peroxisome proliferator activator receptor-γ (PPAR-γ) agonists, improve insulin sensitivity, underlying the importance of adipose tissue-restricted fat storage in whole body metabolism.

Non-alcoholic fatty liver disease (NAFLD) remains the most common model of the ectopic fat storage adverse effects on glucose metabolism. It is estimated that patients with fatty liver have insulin resistance comparable to that of those with T2DM [20], while on the other hand only a minority of patients who are insulin resistant have NAFLD. Several pathogenic pathways have been implicated in the pathogenesis of NAFLD-related defective insulin action, including the cytotoxic effect of TG oxidation-generated free radicals, the mitochondrial malfunction and the failure of receptors in the cell nucleus that are involved in triggering the effects of insulin (PPARs). NAFLD clearly demonstrates the key role of visceral fat in the pathogenesis on insulin resistance, as liver is directly affected by NEFAs mobilized mainly from the central adipose tissue.

Diacylglycerol and long chain fatty acyl-CoA (LC-AcCoA) seem to mediate the ectopic fat-induced insulin resistance in skeletal muscles. They both activate the protein kinase C-theta, which in turn inactivates, via serine phosphorylation, the insulin receptor substrate 1 (IRS-1) protein and uncouples the insulin signalling pathway. In addition LC-AcCoA inhibits hexokinase and thus glucose oxidation, leading to intracellular accumulation of free glucose and subsequent inhibition of GLUT4 translocation and glucose uptake by muscles [21].

Several studies also cast light on the metabolic pathways by which excessive TG stores within beta cells may lead to secretory defects that characterize T2DM. The identification of hormone sensitive lipase (HSL) in β-cells [22] showed the potential key enzyme that regulates the NEFA mobilization from the ectopic fat and mediates lipotoxic effect in pancreas. It is suggested that via the uncoupling protein 2 gene (*UCP2*), ceramide and nitric oxide synthesis, HSL not only deprives beta cells from the required energy for GIIS but also leads to intracellular accumulation of toxic metabolites (oxidative stress) that eventually induce beta cell apoptosis.

Obviously, the metabolic pathways by which elevated plasma NEFAs and ectopic fat stores worsen both insulin action and secretion, thereby accelerating the progression to overt T2DM, largely interact. The 'lipotoxic theory' describes the detrimental effect of excess fat as a unit on glucose metabolism.

4.6 'Oxidative stress'

During the last few years, there has been considerable debate regarding the importance of oxidative stress in the pathogenesis of insulin resistance and β-cell dysfunction in obese individuals. It refers to a condition in which imbalance between oxidant generation and antioxidant protection or repair of oxidative damage exists. Normally, during the aerobic cellular metabolic processes, several reactive oxygen species (ROS) are produced. Although in normal concentrations, these elements act as necessary messengers in biological systems (redox signalling), when abnormally high, they become cytotoxic, damaging cellular structures and organelles, impairing cellular metabolism and inducing cellular apoptosis.

A currently favoured hypothesis is that oxidative stress, through a single unifying mechanism of superoxide production, is the common pathogenic factor leading to insulin resistance, beta cell dysfunction, impaired glucose tolerance and ultimately to T2DM. It is suggested that excessive intracellular ROS activate multiple stress-sensitive serine/threonine kinase signalling cascades, including kinase-β (IKKβ) and c-Jun NH2-terminal kinase (JNK)/stress-activated protein kinase, which in turn phosphorylate on discrete serine or threonine sites and thus inactivate insulin receptor and IRS proteins, inhibiting insulin action [23]. As the peroxisomal β-oxidation of NEFAs generates oxidants in states with NEFA excess, as in obesity, their enhanced oxidation results in excessive production of cytotoxic agents that eventually ameliorate insulin effect. B-cells are considered very sensitive to oxidative stress as they are low in antioxidant enzymes. The critical importance of mitochondrial glucose metabolism in GIIS is well established and as oxidative stress damages mitochondria, the markedly blunt insulin secretion in these cases is not surprising [24]. Beta cell apoptosis is also markedly enhanced by the effect of accumulating free radicals, developing a vicious cycle between fat excess, oxidative stress and hyperglycaemia that may eventually lead to T2DM.

4.7 The role of adipose tissue as an 'endocrine organ' in the pathogenesis of T2DM

Adipose tissue was previously regarded as inert storage depot. However, the recognition of various receptors that are expressed in fat tissue and of a vast array of bioactive factors (Table 4.1) with local (autocrine/paracrine) and systemic (endocrine) effects that are produced by the fat cells, revealed humoral and neuronal cross-talk between adipocytes, as well as between adipose tissue and distant organs; this seems to play an essential role in the regulation of whole body metabolism and energy homeostasis [25]. Current research has identified over 50 adipocyte-secreted factors, and more are yet to be discovered. Various adipocyte-released compounds profoundly affect insulin sensitivity and might potentially link obesity with T2DM.

In obesity the adipocytes become enlarged, due to storage of excessive fat. Some researchers consider the extreme enlargement of adipocytes in which the fatty lipids that crowd in squash their cytoplasm against the stretched membrane, is a 'distressing' metabolic state. It is believed that the bloated adipocytes express their distress by turning down insulin signalling that tends to increase the intracellular fat storage and by

Table 4.1   Differences between adipocytes from subcutaneous (Sc) and visceral depots

Factor	Regional difference	Reference
Leptin mRNA and protein	Visceral < Sc	[50, 51]
TNF-α	Visceral < Sc	[52]
IL-6	Visceral > Sc	[53]
PAI-1	Visceral > Sc	[54]
Angiotensinogen mRNA	Visceral > Sc	[55]
Resistin	Visceral = Sc	[56]
Adiponectin	Visceral < Sc	[57]
Androgen receptor mRNA	Visceral > Sc	[58]
PPARγ	visceral = Sc	[59]
TZD stimulated pre-adipocyte differentiation	Visceral < Sc	[60]
Lipolytic response to catecholamines	Visceral > Sc	[61]
Antilipolytic effect of insulin	Visceral < Sc	[62, 63]
β1 and β2-adrenergic receptor binding and mRNA	Visceral > Sc	[64, 65]
Dexamethasone-induced increase in LPL	Visceral > Sc	[66]
α2-Adrenergic receptor agonist inhibition of cAMP	Visceral < Sc	[67]
Insulin receptor affinity	Visceral < Sc	[68]
IRS-1 protein expression	Visceral < Sc	[62]
Insulin receptor (exon 11 deleted)	Visceral > Sc	[68]
Glucocorticoid receptor mRNA	Visceral > Sc	[69]

Source: Montague and O'Rahilly (1998) [59].
PAI-1, plasminogen activator inhibitor-1.

releasing agents, including fatty acids, inflammatory mediators and proteins termed adipocytokines that alter insulin sensitivity in insulin-targeted organs and participate in the development of obesity-associated T2DM [26]. Here, we focus on certain adipocytokines and how they influence insulin sensitivity.

Leptin is an adipokine whose levels increase with increasing fat mass. For many years it was considered part of a negative feedback loop that restricts food intake and enhances energy expenditure. However, the identification of leptin receptors in peripheral tissues with important role in nutrient metabolism, for example myocytes, liver and pancreas, implies a more complex role of this adipocytokine on metabolism and energy homeostasis. It has been demonstrated that in skeletal muscles, leptin has a beneficial effect on glucose metabolism, as it stimulates the 5'AMP-activated protein kinase (AMPK)-mediated reduction of the ectopic lipid content [27]. Furthermore, in hepatocytes leptin seems to have additive effects with insulin in glycogen storage enhancement and glycogenolysis inhibition, by which it eventually reduces HGP and keeps off hyperglycaemia [28]. In addition, via the so-called 'adipo-insular axis', the insulin-stimulated leptin production inhibits the excessive beta cell insulin biosynthesis and secretion, and confers protection from the development of hyperinsulinaemia, which could subsequently downregulate insulin receptors, promoting insulin resistance [29].

In obesity however, leptin's action seems to be selectively disturbed, leading to hyperleptinaemia. The saturation of its central transport system and the inhibition of its intracellular pathway of action (Janus kinase/signal transducers and activators of transcription, JAK/STAT) pathway) are considered the two most probable underlying mechanisms for that. However, although leptin's central appetite-suppressant effect is impaired, its stimulatory effect on the sympathetic nervous system is maintained, leading to enhanced catecholamine NEFA mobilization from the adipose tissue and subsequent insulin resistance (Randle's cycle). Some studies also support a direct lipolytic effect of hyperleptinaemia upon adipocytes [30], while experimental data demonstrate hyperleptinaemia-induced over-phosphorylation of IRS-1/IRS-2 and depletion of phosphatidylinositol-3 kinase, by which it eventually ameliorates insulin action. In addition, confluent data support prolonged hyperleptinaemia-induced pancreatic beta cells interleukin (IL)-1β production, which in turn decreases their insulin secretory capacity and enhances their apoptosis. Thus, although the adipocytes seem to produce leptin in an attempt to adapt quickly to metabolic challenges in a way that is beneficial for body's metabolism, very prolonged excess in energy intake, results in fine derangement of its central or peripheral effects, so that it eventually aggravates glucose metabolism and contributes to insulin resistance and type 2 diabetes development (Figure 4.2).

Recently, the identification of adiponectin has dramatically changed our view of adipocytes. Potent insulin-mimetic, insulin-sensitizing and anti-inflammatory properties have been attributed to this adipocytokine, making adiponectin seem the most interesting and promising molecule released from fat cells (Figure 4.3). In case–control studies, low plasma adiponectin was an independent risk factor for future development of T2DM [31], while administration of adiponectin reverses insulin resistance in rodent models of obesity and T2DM [32], suggesting an important link between adiponectin

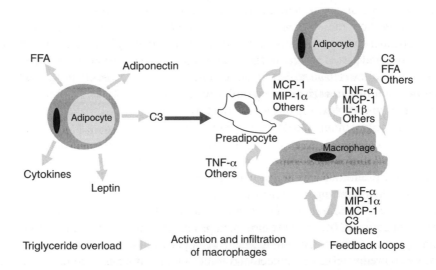

Figure 4.2 Hypothetical model of chronic inflammation and adipocyte insulin resistance. Source: Xu *et al. Journal of Clinical Investigation*, 2003. Reproduced with permission

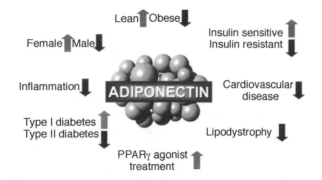

Figure 4.3 Summary of established effects influencing circulating adiponectin levels. Copyright © 2006 American Diabetes Association. From *Diabetes*, Vol. 55, 2006; 1537–1545. Reprinted with permission from The American Diabetes Association

and insulin resistance. The mechanism by which adiponectin ameliorates insulin resistance has not been fully elucidated. However it seems to be AMPK-mediated, by which adiponectin regulates lipid metabolism (increases fuel oxidation and reduces NEFA influx/ectopic fat storage) and carbohydrate metabolism (improves hepatic insulin sensitivity and peripheral glucose uptake) [33]. Unfortunately, its plasma concentration is markedly reduced with increasing body weight [34] and visceral fat mass, while its receptors are markedly downregulated in hyperinsulinaemic states, depriving obese individuals of its beneficial metabolic effects. The underlying mechanisms seem to be the obesity-associated insulin resistance due to which the stimulatory effect of insulin upon adiponectin gene transcription is ameliorated, as well as the enhanced effect of tumour necrosis factor-α (TNF-α) and IL-6 that repress adiponectin production [35].

Resistin, is another hormone secreted by the adipose tissue, specifically the central fat tissue [36], whose serum levels increase with increasing body weight (Figure 4.4). Although about 7 years have past since its identification, the physiological role of this hormone is still the subject of much controversy. It is reputed to be key link between obesity and insulin resistance, as it increases the production of several adipocyte-derived chemotactive agents (intracellular adhesion molecule-1, vascular cell adhesion molecule-1 and CCL2) and pro-inflammatory cytokines (IL-1, IL-6, IL-12, TNF-α, etc.), which by direct effect or via exacerbation of the obesity-related whole body's proinflammatory state, impair insulin action [37]. Furthermore, it is also suggested that in hepatocytes, resistin represses IRS-2, and stimulates the suppressor of cytokine signalling-3 (SOCS-3) expression, thus uncouples the insulin signalling pathway [38], while in skeletal muscles, it impairs glucose uptake and blocks insulin transduction pathway, by inhibiting GLUT4 translocation and IRS-1 tyrosine phosphorylation, respectively [39]. It is postulated that the insulin-sensitizing effect of thiazolidinediones (TZDs) is mediated at least in part by its suppressive effect on resistin expression, while a direct correlation between resistin levels and subjects with T2DM has been documented, confirming the detrimental effect of resistin on glucose metabolism [40].

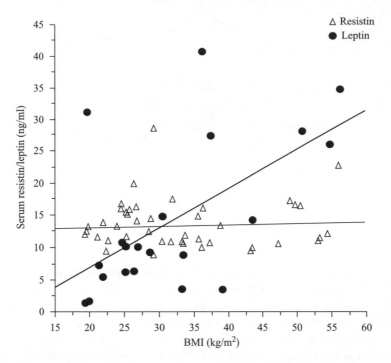

Figure 4.4 Serum resistin and leptin levels in nondiabetic and diabetic subjects were correlated with their corresponding BMIs. Source: McTernan *et al.* [40]

Recently, two more adipocytokines, omentin and visfatin, have been described. They both seem to exert hypoglycaemic effects by reducing glucose release from hepatocytes and stimulating glucose utilization in peripheral tissues. However, the physiological relevance of these adipocytokines with the obesity-associated metabolic defects is still in question.

Further to its role as tissue that produces bioactive agents that affect whole body metabolism, studies have also proven that adipose tissue modifies the metabolism of circulating hormones. The strong morphological and metabolic similarities between Cushing's syndrome and visceral adiposity/metabolic syndrome have been well recognized for many years. The cortisol excess in patients with Cushing's syndrome results in secondary development of central fat deposition and insulin resistance, while people who are primarily centrally obese develop over time Cushing-associated metabolic disorders including insulin resistance. Thus, a potential role of hyper-cortisolaemia in the pathogenesis of metabolic defects that follow central obesity has been proposed.

Glucocorticoids antagonize insulin effects by reducing the translocation of GLUT4 to the cell membrane and thus the glucose uptake by the peripheral tissues, while they also induce lipolysis and NEFA flux to the bloodstream, uncoupling, via Randle's cycle the insulin's transduction signalling pathway. Several studies also suggest that glucocorticoids suppress insulin-induced endothelium-mediated peripheral vasodilatation and subsequently insulin access and effect on peripheral tissues. As far as the effect of glucocorticoids on adipose tissue, they increase central adiposity by stimulating the preadipocyte differentiation and the substrate flux in favour of gluconeogenesis and TG synthesis in visceral fat tissue and reduce peripheral adiposity by increasing lipolysis and downregulating lipoprotein lipase – thereby liberating NEFAs from peripheral fat.

Although the presence of hypercortisolaemia could explain the pathogenesis of central obesity-related metabolic defects, it has been found that the plasma concentration of glucocorticoids in obese individuals is normal. Suspicion has therefore fallen on impaired metabolism and function of glucocorticoids within tissues with important role in the whole body's metabolism. Stewart *et al.* [6] identified increased concentration of glucocorticoids in the visceral fat tissue of obese individuals – at the same time that their plasma levels were within the normal range. They related the increased local concentration of glucocorticoids to the expression of 11β-HSD1 which was similarly enhanced within the tissue. The latter is the microsomal enzyme that converts inactive steroid cortisone to the active steroid cortisol and is expressed in both hepatocytes and adipocytes. It has been demonstrated that with increasing adiposity, the expression of 11β-HSD1 is reduced in the liver (maybe as a protective mechanism in obesity, reducing insulin resistance and ongoing adipogenesis, [41]), but it is markedly increased in fat tissue (especially in omental tissue) a finding that is compatible with the detrimental effects of central obesity on glucose metabolism. In support are data from animal experiments where transgenic mice that overexpress 11β-HSD1 specifically in adipocytes develop visceral adiposity, high plasma NEFA levels, insulin resistance and hypertension, while others that over-express 11β-HSD1 in the liver alone develop an attenuated phenotype without glucose intolerance, suggesting that the complete metabolic syndrome requires excessive glucocorticoid production in adipocytes. It is postulated that the enhanced 11β-HSD1 activity in the visceral fat tissue, is due to the high regional production of cytokines (e.g. TNF-α) that exert stimulatory effect on it.

Recently, an alternative metabolic pathway that may enhance adipose tissue glucocorticoid activity in obesity has been proposed. The adipocytes express 5-alpha reductase type 1 that generates glucocorticoid metabolites, which retain glucocorticoid activity. It has been estimated that the expression of this enzyme increases with increasing obesity, representing an additional abnormal pathway that leads to persistent glucocorticoid effects in obese individuals. [42].

4.8 Obesity as a low-grade inflammatory state

In the last decade, scientists have come to view obesity as a low-grade inflammatory state. The increased plasma circulating mononuclear cells and lymphocytes, as well as the increased concentration of C-reactive protein, TNF-α, IL-1 and IL-6 in obese individuals' blood, are compatible with this suggestion. It has been proposed that source of the pro-inflammatory molecules is the adipose tissue and more specifically the enlarged adipocytes which appear to produce increased concentration of molecules that induce low-grade inflammation locally in the adipose tissue, but also in the whole body [43]. Furthermore, an overlap between metabolic and inflammatory signalling pathways that impair insulin effect in peripheral tissues has been demonstrated, associating the obesity-related pro-inflammatory state with insulin resistance and T2DM. Visceral fat appears to produce pro-inflammatory markers more actively than subcutaneous adipose tissue, confirming the crucial role of central obesity in the pathogenesis of the obesity-associated morbidities (Figure 4.2).

Initially, the adipocytes have been exclusively blamed for the fat tissue-derived pro-inflammatory molecules. Recent studies [44], however, suggest that obesity is associated with increased macrophage infiltration into adipose tissue (Figure 4.5), which in some cases may account for about 40% of all fat tissue cells, as in severely obese individuals with body mass index (BMI) around 50; the latter also secrete in high concentrations bioactive agents with inflammatory properties, which in turn fuel systemic inflammation. Several hypotheses have been suggested to explain the accumulation of macrophages in fat tissue. The most widely accepted suggests that the enlarged adipocytes become 'fragile', leaking chemotactive agents such as M-CSF and MCP-1 that activate and recruit macrophages in adipose tissue, even from the early stages of obesity [45]. Scherer's group has also demonstrated that adipocytes exert a strong inflammatory stimulus on macrophages, suggesting a 'cross talk' between adipocytes and interstitial macrophages in adipose tissue *in vivo*. The resultant whole body's inflammatory state deregulates nutrient homeostasis and leads to diabetes. Meanwhile the local, within the fat tissue, inflammation affects the adipocytes which become less insulin sensitive and increase the NEFA efflux to the bloodstream (Randle's cycle) and suppresses the differentiation of pre-adipocytes, leading to excessive ectopic fat storage and subsequently to impairment of glucose metabolism in the whole body.

In recent years, the role of the enlarged adipocytes- and adipose tissue macrophages (ATMs) produced pro-inflammatory molecules (e.g. IL-1, IL-6, TNF-α), has been

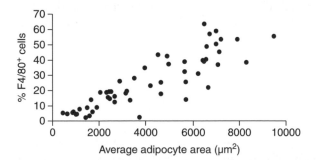

Figure 4.5   The relationship between adipocyte size and the percentage of macrophages (F4/80[+]) in adipose tissue (in mice). Source: Weisberg *et al.* [44]

extensively investigated. The close relationship between metabolic and inflammatory signalling pathways has been more or less revealed, demonstrating their crucial role in the pathogenesis of T2DM. It has been shown that IL-1 down-regulates IRS-1 mRNA and GLUT4 translocation and thus reduces peripheral tissues response to insulin, while it also activates IKK and JNK which in turn phosphorylate IRS-1 in serine-position and thus uncouple the insulin transduction pathway and block insulin action [46]. Additionally, IL-1 decreases the pancreatic beta cells' insulin secretory capacity and enhances (via caspase-3 activation) their apoptosis, accelerating the progression to overt type 2 diabetes.

IL-6 is another cytokine that increases with increasing obesity and which is considered to inhibit insulin receptor signal transduction and insulin action, mainly by enhancing SOCS-3 expression. The later promotes specifically degradation of IRS1 and IRS2, two critical signalling molecules for insulin action, and blocks insulin effect. It was also demonstrated that IL-6 inhibits in a large portion, the insulin-induced glycogen synthesis in human hepatocytes, depriving obese individuals from a quick and effective way to dispose glucose from the bloodstream [47].

TNF-α, whose circulating levels are elevated in obese subjects, is considered important mediator in the central obesity-induced impaired glucose metabolism. Studies have shown that TNF-α, increases the serine phosphorylation of IRS-1 and IRS-2 ameliorating insulin's action, while at the same time it downregulates the GLUT-4 molecules, reducing more the transportation of glucose into the cells. Several studies in insulin resistant animals, demonstrated marked improvement in insulin action after TNF-α neutralization, confirming its detrimental effect on glucose metabolism, while TZDs suppress TNF-α, which may partially account for their insulin-sensitizing effect.

A role for JNK-1, in the pathogenesis of T2DM has been also proposed. JNK-1 belongs to the family of mitogen-activated protein kinases, better known in apoptosis, regeneration and inflammation processes. It has been demonstrated that NEFAs and inflammatory cytokines, directly activate JNK-1 in tissues, such as fat, muscle and liver, which in turn phosphorylates serine residues on IRS-1 and blocks insulin effect. In support of this theory, animal studies confirmed that activated JNK-1 is elevated in obesity, especially in the central obesity, whilst its absence improves insulin sensitivity and enhances insulin receptor signalling capacity, thus proposing JNK-1 as another potential link in the pathogenesis and maintenance of the vicious cycle between central obesity, inflammation and insulin resistance [48].

Recently, another inflammatory pathway between obesity and insulin resistance was identified. IKK-β is a kinase that acts as central coordinator of inflammatory responses through activation of nuclear factor-κB, a family of cellular transcription factors involved in the inducible expression of a variety of cellular genes with crucial role in the pathogenesis of the inflammatory response including IL-1, IL-6 and adhesion molecules. It has been determined that TNF-α and NEFAs stimulate IKK-β activity and thus exacerbate the obesity-associated inflammatory state and its detrimental effect on insulin effect. Now it turns out that IKK-β also diverts IRS phosphorylation and subsequently the insulin signal transduction deep into the cell. Since the late 1800s, clinical observations have indicated that high-dose aspirin lowers blood glucose in

T2DM, but the mechanism was not understood. This effect is now considered to be mediated by the inhibitory effect of high doses of salicylates on IKK-β [49].

Finally, it should be noted that further to their direct adverse effect on insulin action, the proinflammatory cytokines affect glucose metabolism by additional pathways. They suppress adipogenesis, diverting fat excess to ectopic storage, while they also increase the central adipose tissue activity of 11β-HSD1, which in turn increases regional production of cortisol and thus insulin resistance.

4.9 Summary

The prevalence of obesity is dramatically increasing across the world. The recent increase in the prevalence of metabolic syndrome, insulin resistance and diabetes has paralleled this increase; therefore, it would seem intuitive to blame excess body weight and excess adipose tissue mass for the increased prevalence of T2DM. The term 'diabesity' has been suggested as providing the point that T2DM and obesity often go hand in hand. The results of large epidemiological studies are compatible with this hypothesis and it is estimated that in the UK, there are currently over 2 million people with diabetes, while over 80% of them are overweight. Yet, not all obese individuals develop insulin resistance. In the 1950s, Vague [2] first proposed that excess fat stored on the trunk could be metabolically more damaging than fat stored on the limbs. This proposal has been confirmed by a large number of cross-sectional and prospective studies (e.g. Nurses Health Study cohort, Third National Health and Nutrition Survey) and it is now recognized that central obesity is a cardinal feature of the metabolic syndrome, with insulin resistance as a key link between abdominal fat and risks for chronic diseases. Most studies suggest that increased visceral adiposity leads to overexpression of specific adipokines, free fatty acids and proinflammatory peptides that adversely affect peripheral tissues sensitivity to insulin and pancreatic beta cell insulin production. In addition, emerging evidence has also drawn attention towards the novel concept of ectopic fat accumulation, according to which with progressive obesity, lipid is deposited into other non-adipose organs including liver, pancreas and skeletal muscle, leading to cell dysfunction (lipotoxicity) and lipid-induced cell death (lipoapoptosis). It is proposed that by these metabolic pathways, central obesity impairs glucose metabolism and leads to hyperglycaemia and eventually T2DM once the pancreatic beta cells fail to compensate for the increased needs of insulin.

References

1. Kissebah, A.H. and Krakower, G.R. (1994) Regional adiposity and morbidity. *Physiological Reviews*, **74**, 761–809.
2. Vague, J. (1956) The degree of masculine differentiation of obesities: a factor determining predisposition to diabetes, atherosclerosis, gout and uric calculous disease. *American Journal of Clinical Nutrition*, **4**, 20–34.

3. Frayn, K., Humphreys, S. and Coppack, S. (1996) Net carbon flux across subcutaneous adipose tissue after a standard meal in normal weight and insulin resistant obese subjects. *International Journal of Obesity and Related Metabolic Disorders*, **20**, 795–800.

4. Lönnqvist, F., Thörne, A., Nilsell, K. *et al.* (1995) A pathogenic role of visceral ß3-adrenoceptors in obesity. *Journal of Clinical Investigation*, **95**, 1109–16.

5. Van Harmelen, V., Lonnqvist, F., Thorne, A. *et al.* (1997) Noradrenaline-induced lipolysis in isolated mesenteric, omental and subcutaneous adipocytes from obese subjects. *International Journal of Obesity and Related Metabolic Disorders*, **21**, 972–9.

6. Stewart, P.M., Boulton, A., Kumar, S. *et al.* (1999) Cortisol metabolism in human obesity: impaired cortisone–cortisol conversion in subjects with central adiposity. *Journal of Clinical Endocrinology and Metabolism*, **84**, 1022–7.

7. Ferrannini, E., Barrett, E.J., Bevilacqua, S. and DeFronzo, R.A. (1983) Effect of fatty acids on glucose production and utilization in man. *Journal of Clinical Investigation*, **72** (5), 1737–47.

8. Unger, R.H. (1994) Lipotoxicity in the pathogenesis of obesity-dependent NIDDM. Genetic and clinical implications. *Diabetes*, **44**, 863–70.

9. Van Epps-Fung, M., Williford, Jodie, Hardy, Robert, W. *et al.* (1997) Fatty acid-induced insulin resistance in adipocytes. *Endocrinology*, **138** (10), 4338–45.

10. Defronzo, R.A., Bonadonna, R.C. and Ferrannini, E. (1992) Pathogenesis of NIDDM. A balanced overview. *Diabetes Care*, **15**, 318–68.

11. Kelley, D. and Mandarino, L. (2000) Fuel selection in human skeletal muscle in insulin resistance. *Diabetes*, **49**, 677–83.

12. Andres, R., Cader, G. and Zierler, K. (1956) The quantitatively minor role of carbohydrate in oxidative metabolism by skeletal muscle in intact man in the basal state. Measurement of oxygen and glucose uptake and carbon dioxide production in the forearm. *Journal of Clinical Investigation*, **35**, 671–682.

13. Kelley, D.E., Reilly, J., Veneman, T. and Mandarino, L.J. (1990) Effect of insulin on skeletal muscle glucose storage, oxidation and glycolysis in humans. *American Journal of Physiology*, **258**, E923–E929.

14. Baron, A.D. (1994) Hemodynamic actions of insulin. *American Journal of Physiology*, **267**, E187–E192.

15. Frayn, K., Shadid, S., Hamlani, R. *et al.* (1994) Regulation of fatty acid movement in human adipose tissue in the postabsorptive-to-postprandial transition. *Te American Journal of Physiology*, **266**, E308–E317.

16. Ravussin, E. and Smith, S.R. (2002) Increased fat intake, impaired fat oxidation, and failure of fat cell proliferation result in ectopic fat storage, insulin resistance, and type 2 diabetes mellitus. *Annals of the New York Academy of Sciences*, **967**, 363–78.

17. Lewis, G.F., Carpentier, A., Adeli, K. and Giacca, A. (2002) Disordered fat storage and mobilization in the pathogenesis of insulin resistance and type 2 diabetes. *Endocrine Reviews*, **23**, 201–229.

18. Hegele, R.A., Cao, H., Frankowski, C. *et al.* (2002) PPARG F388L, a transactivation-deficient mutant, in familial partial lipodystrophy. *Diabetes*, **51**, 3586–90.

19. Sutinen, J., Hakkinen, A.M., Westerbacka, J. *et al.* (2002) Increased fat accumulation in the liver in HIV-infected patients with antiretroviral therapy-associated lipodystrophy. *AIDS (London, England)*, **16**, 2183–93.

20. Marchesini, G., Brizi, M., Bianchi, G. *et al.* (2001) Nonalcoholic fatty liver disease. A feature of the metabolic syndrome. *Diabetes*, **50**, 1844–50.

21. Defronzo, R.A. and Mandarino, L.J. (2003) Pathogenesis of type 2 diabetes mellitus. Chapter 9. www.endotext.org. (accessed January 20, 2008).

22. Mulder, H., Holst, L.S., Holm, C. *et al.* (1999) Hormone-sensitive lipase, the rate-limiting enzyme in triglyceride hydrolysis, is expressed and active in β- cells. *Diabetes*, **48**, 228–32.

23. Ceriello, A. and Motz, E. (2004) Is oxidative stress the pathogenic mechanism underlying insulin resistance, diabetes, and cardiovascular disease? The common soil hypothesis revisited. *Arteriosclerosis, Thrombosis, and Vascular Biology*, **24**, 816–23.

24. Lameloise, N., Boss, O., Pralong, W.-F. *et al.* (1998) Fatty acid-regulation of the expression of uncoupling protein-2 in insulin-producing cells. *Diabetologia*, **41** (Suppl 1), 570.

25. Ahima, R.S. and Flier, J.S. (2000) Adipose tissue as an endocrine organ. *Trends in Endocrinology and Metabolism*, **11**, 327–32.

26. Mohammed-Ali, V., Pinkney, J.H. and Coppack, S.W. (1998) Adipose tissue as an endocrine and paracrine organ. *International Journal of Obesity and Related Metabolic Disorders*, **22** (12), 1145–58.

27. Winder, W.W. (2001) Energy-sensing and signaling by AMP-activated protein kinase in skeletal muscle. *Journal of Applied Physiology (Bethesda, Md: 1985)*, **91** (3), 1017–28.

28. Aiston, S. and Agius, L. (1999) Leptin enhances glycogen storage in hepatocytes by inhibition of phosphorylase and exerts an additive effect with insulin. *Diabetes*, **48** (1), 15–20.

29. Kieffer, T.J., Heller, R.S., Leech, C.A. *et al.* (1997) Leptin suppression of insulin secretion by the activation of ATP-sensitive K+ channels in pancreatic-cells. *Diabetes*, **46**, 1087–93.

30. Martínez, J.A., Aguado, M. and Frühbeck, G. (2000) Interactions between leptin and NPY affecting lipid mobilization in adipose tissue. *Journal of Physiology and Biochemistry*, **56** (1), 1–8.

31. Lindsay, R.S., Funahashi, T., Hanson, R.L. *et al.* (2002) Adiponectin and development of type 2 diabetes in the Pima Indian population. *Lancet*, **360**, 57–8.

32. Yamauchi, T., Kamon, J., Waki, H. *et al.* (2001) The fat-derived hormone adiponectin reverses insulin resistance associated with both lipoatrophy and obesity. *Nature Medicine*, **7**, 941–6.

33. Yamauchi, T., Kamon, J., Minokoshi, Y. *et al.* (2002) Adiponectin stimulates glucose utilization and fatty-acid oxidation by activating AMP-activated protein kinase. *Nature Medicine*, **8**, 1288–95.

34. Arita, Y., Kihara, S., Ouchi, N. *et al.* (1999) Paradoxical decrease of an adipose-specific protein, adiponectin, in obesity. *Biochemical and Biophysical Research Communications*, **257**, 79–83.

35. Bruun, J.M., Lihn, A.S., Verdich, C. *et al.* (2003) Regulation of adiponectin by adipose tissue-derived cytokines: in vivo and in vitro investigations in humans. *American Journal of Physiology. Endocrinology and Metabolism*, **285**, E527–E533.

36. McTernan, C.L., McTernan, P.G., Kumar, S. *et al.* (2002) Resistin, central obesity, and type 2 diabetes. *Lancet*, **359**, 46–7.

37. Flier, J.S. (2001) Diabetes. The missing link with obesity? *Nature*, **409**, 292–3.

38. Muse, E.D., Obici, S., Bhanot, S. *et al.* (2004) Role of resistin in diet-induced hepatic insulin resistance. *Journal of Clinical Investigation*, **114**, 232–9.

39. Bajaj, M., Suraamornkul, S., Hardies, L.J. *et al.* (2004) Plasma resistin concentration, hepatic fat content, and hepatic and peripheral insulin resistance in pioglitazone- treated type II diabetic patients. *International Journal of Obesity and Related Metabolic Disorders*, **28**, 783–9.

40. McTernan, P.G., Fisher, F.M., Kumar, S. *et al.* (2003) Resistin and type 2 diabetes: regulation of resistin expression by insulin and rosiglitazone and the effects of recombinant resistin on lipid and glucose metabolism in human differentiated adipocytes. *Journal of Clinical Endocrinology and Metabolism*, **88**, 6098–106.

41. Valsamakis, G., Anwar, A., Kumar, S. *et al.* (2004) 11ß-Hydroxysteroid dehydrogenase type 1 activity in lean and obese males with type 2 diabetes mellitus. *Journal of Clinical Endocrinology & Metabolism*, **89** (9), 4755–61.

42. Westerbacka, J., Yki-Järvinen, H., Vehkavaara, S. *et al.* (2003) Body fat distribution and cortisol metabolism in healthy men: enhanced 5beta-reductase and lower cortisol/cortisone metabolite ratios in men with fatty liver. *Journal of Clinical Endocrinology and Metabolism*, **88** (10), 4924–31.

43. Xu, H., Barnes, G.T., Yang, Q. *et al.* (2003) Chronic inflammation in fat plays a crucial role in the development of obesity-related insulin resistance. *Journal of Clinical Investigation*, **112**, 1821–30.

44. Ferrante, W., Weisberg, S.P. and McCann, D. *et al.* (2003) Obesity is associated with macrophage accumulation in adipose tissue. *Journal of Clinical Investigation*, **112** (), 1796–808.

45. Sbarbati, A., Osculati, Francesco, Maffeis, Claudio *et al.* (2006) Obesity and inflammation: evidence for an elementary lesion. *Pediatrics*, **117** (1), 220–23.

46. Jager, J., Grémeaux, Thierry, Tanti, Jean-Franois *et al.* (2006) Interleukin-1β-induced insulin resistance in adipocytes through down-regulation of insulin receptor substrate-1 expression. *Endocrinology*, **148** (1), 241–51.

47. Senn, J.J., Klover, P.J., Nowak, I.A. and Mooney, R.A. (2002) Interleukin-6 induces cellular insulin resistance in hepatocytes. *Diabetes*, **51** (12), 3391–9.

48. Hirosumi, J., Tuncman, G., Chang, L. *et al.* (2002) A central role for JNK in obesity and insulin resistance. *Nature*, **420**, 333–6.

49. Kopp, E. and Ghosh, S. (1994) Inhibition of NF-kappa B by sodium salicylate and aspirin. *Science*, **265** (5174), 956–59.

50. Montague, C.T., Prins, J.B., Sanders, L., Digby, J.E. and O'Rahilly, S. (1997) Depot and sex specific differences in human leptin mRNA expression. *Diabetes*, **46**, 342–7.

51. Van Harmelen, V., Reynisdottir, S., Eriksson, P. *et al.* (1998) Leptin secretion from subcutaneous and visceral adipose tissue in women. *Diabetes*, **47** (6), 913–17.

52. Hube, F., Birgel, M., Lee, Ym. and Hauner H. (1999) Expression pattern of tumour necrosis factor receptors in subcutaneous and omental human adipose tissue: role of obesity and non-insulin dependent diabetes mellitus. *European Journal of Clinical Investigation*, **29**, 672–8.

53. Fried, S.K., Bunkin, D.A., and Greenberg, A.S. (1998) Omental and subcutnaeous adipose tissues of obese subjects release interleukin-6: depot difference and regulation by glucocorticoid. *Journal of Clinical and Endocrinological Metabolism*, **83**, 847–50.

54. Shimomura, I., Funahashi, T., Takahashi, M. *et al.* (1996) Enhanced expression of PAI-1 in visceral fat: possible contributor to vascular disease in obesity. *Nature Medicine*, **2**, 800–3.

55. Van Harmalen, V., Elizalde, M., Ariapart, P., *et al.* (2000) The association of human adipose angiotensinogen gene expression with abdominal fat distribution in obesity. *International Journal of Obesity*, **24**, 673–8.

56. McTernan, P.G., McTernan, C.L., Kumar, S. *et al.* (2002) Increased resistin gene and protein expression in human abdominal adipose tissue. *Journal of Clinical Endocrinology and Metabolism*, **87**, 2407.

57. Fisher, F.M., McTernan, P.G., Valsamakis, G. *et al.* (2002) Differences in adiponectin protein expression: effect of fat depots and type 2 diabetic status. *Hormone and Metabolism Research*, **34** (11–12), 650–4.

58. Dieudonné, N., Pecquery, R., Boumediene, A. *et al.* (1998) Androgen receptors in human preadipocytes and adipocytes: regional specificities and regulation by sex steroids. *American Journal of Physiology: Cell Physiology*, **274**, C1645–C1652.

59. Montague, C., Prins, J., O'Rahilly, S. *et al.* (1998) Depot-related gene expression in human subcutaneous and omental adipocytes. *Diabetes*, **47**, 1384–91.

60. Adams, M., Montague, C.T., Prins, J.B., *et al.* (1997) Activators of peroxisome proliferator-activated receptor gamma have depot-specific effects on human preadipocyte differentiation. *Journal of Clinical Investigation*, **100**, 3149–53.

61. Rebuffe-Scrive, M., Andersson, B., Olbe, L. and Bjorntorp, P. (1989) Metabolism of adipose tissue in intraabdominal depots of nonobese men and women. *Metabolism*, **38**, 453–8.

62. Zierath, J., Livingston, J., Thorne, A., *et al.* (1998) Regional difference in insulin inhibition of non-esterified fatty acid release from human adipocytes: relation to insulin receptor

phosphorylation and intracellular signalling through the insulin recpetor substrate-1 pathway. *Diabeologia*, **41**, 1343–1354.

63. Lefebvre, A., Peinado-Onsurbe, M., Leitersdorf, J. *et al.* (1997) Regulation of lipoprotein metabolism by thiazolidinediones occurs through a distinct but complementary mechanism relative to fibrates. *Arteriosclerosis Thrombosis and Vascular Biology*, **17**, 1756–64.

64. Hellmer, J., Marcus, C., Sonnenfeld, T. and Arner, P. (1992) Mechanisms for differences in lipolysis between human subcutaneous and omental fat cells. *Journal of Clinical and Endocrinological Metabolism*, **75**, 15–20.

65. Arner, P. (1992) Adrenergic receptor function in fat cells. *American Journal of Clinical Nutrition*, **55**, 228S–236S.

66. Fried, S.K., Russell, C.D., Grauso, N.L. and Brolin, R.E. (1993) Lipoprotein lipase regulation by insulin and glucocorticoid in subcutaneous and omental adipose tissues of obese women and men. *Journal of Clinical Investigation*, **92** (5), 2191–8.

67. Vikman, H.-L., Savola, J.-M., Raasmaja, A. and Ohisalo, J.J. (1996) 2A-Adrenergic regulation of cyclic AMP accumulation and lipolysis in human omental and subcutaneous adipocytes. *International Journal of Obesity*, **20**, 185–9.

68. Lefebvre, A.M., Laville, M., Vega, N., *et al.* (1998) Depot-specific differences in adipose tissue gene expression in lean and obese subjects. *Diabetes*, **47**, 98–103.

69. Rebuffe-Scrive, M., Bronnegard, M., Nilsson, A., Eldh, J., Gustafsson, J.-A. and Bjorntorp, P. (1990) Steroid hormone receptors in human adipose tissues. *Journal of Clinical Endocrinological Metabolism*, **71**, 1215–19.

5
Obesity and prevention of type 2 diabetes

Jaakko Tuomilehto, Jaana Lindström and Karri Silventoinen

5.1 Obesity and the risk of type 2 diabetes

Several prospective studies have documented that obesity is probably the most powerful predictor of the development of type 2 diabetes ([1–3]). However, not every obese subject develops diabetes, that is obesity alone is not sufficient to cause type 2 diabetes; there are other factors that considerably modify the effect of obesity on diabetes risk. It is probable that the genetic susceptibility to diabetes is a necessary prerequisite for diabetes. This was demonstrated in the Pima Indians in whom the incidence increases more steeply with body mass index (BMI, kg/m^2) in those whose parents have diabetes than in these who do not [2]. Vice versa, in non-obese people the incidence of type 2 diabetes is low in the middle-aged even in populations such as the Pima Indians where the overall risk of the disease is very high. Today, a plethora of studies have demonstrated that family history of type 2 diabetes is increasing the risk of the disease. However, it is likely that a large proportion of the human populations possesses genes that permit type 2 diabetes to develop, well documented by a high prevalence of diabetes and impaired glucose regulation among the elderly [4,5]. Age-specific incidence rates of diabetes were also shown to vary according to BMI in the Pima Indians [2]: in younger age groups subjects with a high BMI have higher incidence rates than those with lower BMI. It is however possible that many genetically predisposed subjects will develop type 2 diabetes or milder forms of impaired glucose regulation in the elderly in absence of gross obesity, particularly with decreasing physical activity and other conditions that increase with ageing. There seems to be many genes predisposing to type 2 diabetes, of them about 20 have thus far confirmed [6], and many additional ones are under investigation.

Several studies indicate that other anthropometric indicators such as waist circumference or waist-to-hip ratio are strong risk factors for type 2 diabetes, independent of BMI, and may be better risk indicators than BMI alone [7–9]. Such

Obesity and Diabetes, Second Edition   Edited by Anthony H. Barnett and Sudhesh Kumar
© 2009 John Wiley & Sons, Ltd

data suggest that the distribution of body fat is an important determinant of risk as these measures reflect abdominal or visceral obesity. In Japanese American men, for example, the intra-abdominal fat, as measured from computed tomography scans, was the best anthropometric predictor of diabetes incidence [7]. More recent data indicate that intra-abdominal fat is more active than subcutaneous fat in secreting inflammatory cytokines that are associated with the development of type 2 diabetes [10]. However at population level, BMI is very highly correlated with waist circumference, and thus in epidemiological settings these obesity indicators can give largely similar risk estimates for type 2 diabetes [11].

Obesity has increased rapidly in most populations in recent years [12]. As expected, this increase has been accompanied by increasing prevalence of type 2 diabetes [13]. Since obesity is such a strong predictor of diabetes incidence, it appears that the rapid increases in the prevalence of type 2 diabetes seen in many populations in recent decades are almost certainly related to increasing obesity. Furthermore, interventions directed to reducing obesity have resulted in a decrease in the incidence of type 2 diabetes in obese individuals with impaired glucose tolerance [14].

Obesity is the outcome of a positive energy balance in which energy intake has exceeded energy expenditure over time. Although this implies that obese individuals are or have at some point consumed more energy than they need, there is increasing evidence to support the idea that there are genetically determined metabolic difference between individuals who gain excessive weight and those that do not [15]. Previous twin studies have revealed that heritability to body weight is very high [16] and a meta analyses of heritability of BMI in eight countries revealed that genetic differences explained 45–85% of the variation in BMI [17]. Recently, candidate genes for obesity have also been identified; however, even the most promising candidate gene, *FTO*, explained just 1% of the population level variation in BMI [18].

Nevertheless, endogenous factors alone do not explain the massive increase in the prevalence of obesity even though the recent weight gain in many populations probably results from interaction between genetically determined individual response to food and eating and environmental factors, food supply, palatability, for example [19]. The fundamental cause of this increasing prevalence can be ascribed largely to the increasing worlwide urbanization and its consequences. Some of the consequences have been the availability of 'affluent foods' (energy-dense foods which are high in fats and simple sugars and also low in dietary fibre) and an overall decrease in peoples' physical activity [20]. Decreased physical activity without simultaneous decrease in energy intake over a long period results in an imbalance of energy with excess energy being stored as fat in adipose tissue [21, 22]. In the presence of excess energy intake, the adaptive range is extremely small (<5%) and the body energy reserve as adipose tissue increases rapidly [23].

Yet, dietary studies in general have not revealed a direct relation between reported energy intakes and body weight. This could be due to several reasons: first, physically highly active individuals generally need and consume more energy than sedentary ones but do not become overweight. Second, obese people tend to under-report their energy intakes [24]. Third, increased obesity prevalence could be the result of a gradual reduction in physical activity over many years [23], and fourth, it could also be the result of metabolic differences between lean and obese individuals [21]. However, a previous study based on the World Health Organization (WHO) Multinational MONitoring of trends and determinants in CArdiovascular disease (MONICA) data revealed that trends in aggregate level energy consumption based on country level statistics on food production, import and export explained a major part of differences between the countries in trends of mean BMI and obesity [24]. This strongly suggests a causal link between increased energy consumption and increasing prevalence of obesity.

There is a tendency for weight gain with age [25,26]. Most of this increment in weight occurs in adipose tissue. Grundy [20] has estimated that that a relatively small energy imbalance underlies most relative obesity in the general population. About 1255 kJ (300 kcal) maintains about 10 kg (22 lb) of excess weight.

There has been a great deal of controversy regarding which macronutrients are responsible for causing a high prevalence of obesity in populations. Many investigators have favoured the causative effects of a high fat diet in this regard [27–29] and advocating low-fat diets has for past decades been the conventional approach to weight control. However, several studies have indicated that despite decreasing fat intakes, average body weight is increasing in the United States [30,31]. In contrast many countries in Europe, which have higher per capita consumption of fat than the United States, have lower prevalences of obesity [20]. Data from the National Health and Nutrition Examination Survey (NHANES) have shown a significant decrease in the mean percentage of total fat intake from fat since the 1970s [32], but still the prevalence of obesity has continued to rise [33]. The same NHANES report also revealed that as mean proportion of energy from fat has decreased, simultaneously total energy intake has increased [32]. Also other studies have shown increasing trends in energy consumption in the United States [34,35]. A meta-analysis in this regard by Swinburn *et al.* [36] showed that relatively simple messages regarding fat restriction could lead to weight loss. Another meta-analysis based on 19 controlled, low-fat 2–12 month intervention studies, showed that ad libitum, low-fat diets cause weight loss. The effect is more pronounced in subjects with a higher initial body weight [37]. Ultimately, however, the overall energy intake will determine whether weight is lost, regardless of the source [20].

Nutritional goals and guidelines are useful in community activities to prevent the pathological consequences of an excessive energy intake. WHO has identified energy density and fibre as important dietary factors for determining obesity risk [38]. Energy-density of diet can be reduced by restricting especially foods high in fats and simple sugars. With respect to ideal adult weight a BMI of less than 25 has been proposed [39]. However, more recently a population mean BMI of 21 has been promoted for some populations based on the fact that East Asian populations have a much lower BMI normal range [40].

Even though primary prevention of type 2 diabetes was first proposed 80 years ago [41] and more recently stressed by WHO [42], only a limited number of studies have attempted to assess the value of measures aimed at controlling its modifiable risk factors. To be able to prevent a chronic disease such as type 2 diabetes, certain requirements have to be met. Knowledge about its natural history with a pre-clinical phase, modifiable risk factors, effective and simple screening tool to identify high-risk subjects and effective intervention that is affordable and acceptable are necessary. In addition, the efficacy of the intervention has to be proven under a clinical trial setting. It is well known that obesity and physical inactivity are the major risk factors and in people genetically predisposed to the disease the probability to develop type 2 diabetes is very high once exposed to 'unhealthy' lifestyles. Type 2 diabetes results from as a dual process: a deficit in early insulin secretion and insulin resistance of liver, muscle and adipose tissue. During this process early prandial insulin secretion is blunted already in people with impaired glucose tolerance (IGT) [43–45], and it worsens with a longer duration of diabetes. Postprandial hyperglycemia per se may contribute to the progressive deterioration of beta-cells with early insulin secretion deficiency in type 2 diabetes as a vicious cycle. Thus, a detectable preclinical stage suitable for an intervention exists prior to the development of type 2 diabetes.

In testing the potential for prevention of type 2 diabetes, important questions must be answered:

1. Is lifestyle intervention efficacious to prevent type 2 diabetes?

2. What is the magnitude of the preventive intervention?

3. Does lifestyle intervention work in different ethnic groups and cultural settings?

Observational cross-sectional and prospective studies have provided a large body of data that leanness and physically active lifestyles are associated with a low prevalence of type 2 diabetes and vice versa communities where obesity and sedentary lifestyle are common have a high risk of diabetes [43–45]. A very high prevalence of type 2 diabetes in some communities was previously attributed to special genetic constellation in these populations, and also the 'thrifty genotype' hypothesis was formed [46,47]. Currently, however, type 2 diabetes has become common all over the world and is increasing in most countries [48]; the obvious inference is that there is no ethnic group with a particular genetic protection against the disease. While 'a thrifty genotype' may well exist, it is necessary to point out that such a genotype must have existed early on during the development of species since many animals also can develop hyperglycaemia and diabetes if obese and sedentary.

While observational data are important to identify risk factors for a disease and their possible independent role in the natural history of a disease, trials where risk factor exposures are modified are needed to determine their value in the prevention of the disease. Also, pharmacologic agents may be used to prevent hyperglycaemia or to halt the progressive increase in glucose levels in people with impaired glucose regulation. In the modern 'evidence-based medicine' era, the strongest evidence is considered to be coming from controlled clinical trials. Some of the earlier studies aiming intervening upon people with various types and degrees of impaired glucose regulation are summarized by Hamman [49]. Today, there is convincing evidence to suggest that the vicious circle in the natural history of type 2 diabetes can be stopped and the worsening from impaired glucose regulation to frank diabetes can be halted or delayed by influencing the causal environmental risk factors. Next we review the results from the major intervention studies for the prevention of diabetes and discuss their implications for public health applications and for the further research needs.

5.2 Lifestyle intervention studies

The main lifestyle issues that have been intervention targets in the prevention of type 2 diabetes are body weight, diet and physical activity. The intervention methods used to modify lifestyle have varied between the studies, since it is obvious that socio-cultural issues and the available facilities and personnel have dictated the application of the intervention. Also study designs have varied: both randomized and non-randomized studies have been conducted. The type of intervention, its duration and intensity has been very different in earlier preventive studies of type 2 diabetes [49]. One of the largest early intervention studies was the Malmöhus study in Sweden [45] comprised 267 men. A significant difference in the rates of development of type 2 diabetes was found between IGT subjects randomized to treatment and those randomized to no therapy. In an early intervention study in 10 years, the incidence of overt diabetes was 13% in treated subjects (diet alone, tolbutamide or combined) compared with 29% in the untreated subjects; the difference was statistically significant. The adherence with the treatment regimens was poor; for instance less than half of the people randomized to tolbutamide continued to take the drug throughout the study. Unclear also is what kind of dietary advice was actually given and how well the men randomized to diet group actually followed these. Nevertheless, this trial suggested that the worsening from IGT to diabetes could be prevented or delayed.

The malmö feasibility study [44]

The feasibility of diet and exercise intervention in 217 men with IGT was assessed in the Malmö feasibility study. The effect of exercise and diet was compared to a reference group with no intervention. The reference group consisted of men who themselves decided not to join the intervention programme. Thus, the groups were not assigned at random. By the end of the 5-year study period 10.6% of the intervention group and 28.6% of the reference group had developed diabetes. Thus the relative risk reduction in the incidence in the intervention group was 59% and the absolute risk reduction was 17%. This study was important in demonstrating the feasibility of carrying out a diet-exercise programme for 5-years among the volunteers, and furthermore it suggested that the incidence of type 2 diabetes might be halved with diet and exercise intervention. Overall, the progression to diabetes in these Swedish men was relatively low even in the reference group compared with the data from the observational studies. Even though the men who did not want to join the intervention programme, some of them may have changed their lifestyle as a result of the screening programme. Thus, these results based on intention-to-treat analysis may underestimate the true effect of lifestyle changes.

In this study, no difference was found between groups assigned to either diet alone, exercise alone or combined diet-exercise programmes. The intervention actually resulted in significant changes in lifestyle and physiological parameters. The estimated maximal oxygen uptake increased by 10% while it decreased by 5% in control men. BMI decreased by 2.5% in the intervention group but increased by 0.5% in the control group. While the results on diabetes risk in the Malmö feasibility study are likely to be due to the effects on diet and exercise, it is not possible to generalize these results since the men in the study were not assigned to the treatment groups randomly.

The 12-year follow-up of the Malmö study [50] revealed that the mortality rate among men in the former IGT intervention group was lower than among the men in the non-randomized IGT group who received 'routine care' only (6.5 vs. 14.0 per 1000 person years, $p = 0.009$). The findings suggest that a long-term intervention programme including dietary counselling and physical exercise, will reduce mortality in subjects with IGT who are at an increased risk of premature death due to IHD and other causes.

The da-qing study [51]

Another important study was carried out in Da-Qing, China based on a large population-based screening programme to identify people with IGT. The randomization of study subjects was not done by random, but the 33 participating clinics were randomized to carry out the intervention according to one of the four specified intervention protocols (diet alone, exercise alone, diet-exercise combined or none). Data on the preventive effect of a diet and exercise intervention have been reported from this cluster-randomized clinical trial on 577 subjects with IGT in 1986. The cumulative 6-year incidence of type 2 diabetes was lower in the three (diet alone, exercise alone, diet-exercise combined) intervention groups (41–46%) compared with the control group (68%). Because no individual allocation of study subjects to the intervention and control groups was done, but the participating clinics were allocated, the results based on individual data analysis must be interpreted with caution. Furthermore, the study subjects were relatively lean, the mean BMI 25.8 kg/m^2, making inferences for other ethnic groups, where IGT subjects are usually obese, difficult. Also, the progression from IGT to diabetes was high, more than 10% per year in the control group, which is more than usually reported by observational studies. In this study the relative risk reduction was approximately 40% while the absolute risk reduction was 22–26% during the 6-year period.

In clinics assigned to dietary intervention, the participants were encouraged to reduce weight if BMI was >25 kg/m^2 aiming at <24 kg/m^2, otherwise high-carbohydrate and low-fat diet was recommended. Counselling was done by physicians and also group sessions were organized weekly for the first month, monthly for 3 months and every 3 months thereafter. In clinics assigned to physical exercise, counselling sessions were arranged at a similar frequency. In addition, the participants were encouraged to increase their level of leisure-time physical activity by at least 1–2 'Units' per day. One unit would correspond for instance 30 minutes slow walking, 10 minutes slow running or 5 minutes swimming.

The overall changes in risk factor patterns were relatively small. Body weight did not change in lean subjects, and there was a modest, less than 1 kg reduction in subjects with baseline BMI >25 kg/m^2. Also the estimated changes in habitual dietary nutrient intakes were small and non-significant between groups. Exercise intervention seemed to produce best effects. Thus, it is not easy to determine the factors responsible for the beneficial effects on the risk of type 2 diabetes. It is nevertheless obvious that weight control was not the key issue. Thus, physical activity and qualitative changes in diet that are difficult to measure on individual level probably played a key role.

The 20-year follow-up of the original study cohort showed that the reduction in diabetes incidence persists in the combined intervention group compared with control participants with no intervention, and furthermore, the risk reduction remains essentially the same also during the post-intervention period [52].

Thus far no trial evidence exists regarding the effects of lifestyle changes on cardiovascular disease (CVD) morbidity or mortality in persons with IGT. Li et al. [52] observed no statistically significant differences in CVD events, CVD mortality, or total mortality either between the control group and the combined intervention groups. They found 17% (nonsignificant) reduction in CVD death, which can be seen at least suggestive for favouring of lifestyle intervention.

The finnish diabetes prevention study [53–57]

The Finnish Diabetes Prevention Study (DPS) is the first proper controlled trial on prevention of type 2 diabetes where the study subjects were individually randomly allocated into the intervention and control groups. The intervention of the DPS was carried out during 1993–2001 in five clinics in Finland, aiming at preventing type 2 diabetes with lifestyle modification alone. A total of 522 individuals at high risk to develop diabetes were recruited into the study, mainly by screening for IGT in middle-aged (age 40–64 years), overweight (BMI >25 kg/m^2) subjects. The presence of IGT before randomization was confirmed in two successive 75-g oral glucose tolerance tests; the mean of the two values had to be within the IGT range. From previous studies it was estimated that the cumulative diabetes incidence in such a high-risk group would be 35% in 6 years. The study subjects were randomly allocated either into the control group or the intensive intervention group. The subjects in the intervention group had frequent consultation visits with a nutritionist (seven times during the first year and every 3 months thereafter). They received individual advice about how to achieve the intervention goals: reduction in weight of 5% or more, total fat intake less than 30% of energy consumed, saturated fat intake less than 10% of energy consumed, fibre intake of at least 15 g/1000 kcal, and moderate exercise for 30 minutes per day or more. Frequent ingestion of wholemeal products, vegetables, berries and fruit, low-fat milk and meat products, soft margarines, and vegetable oils rich in monounsaturated fatty acids were recommended. The dietary advice was based on 3-day food records completed four times per year. The participants were also individually guided to increase their level of physical activity. Endurance exercise (walking, jogging, swimming, aerobic ball games, skiing) was recommended to increase aerobic capacity and cardiorespiratory fitness. Supervised, progressive, individually tailored circuit-type resistance training sessions to improve the functional capacity and strength of the large muscle groups were also offered.

The control group participants were given only general advice about healthy lifestyle at baseline visit to the study clinic. An oral glucose tolerance test was done annually for all participants and if either fasting or 2-hour glucose values reached diabetic levels a confirmatory oral glucose tolerance test was performed. The study endpoint, type 2 diabetes, was only recorded if the second test also reached diabetic levels; otherwise the subjects continued with their randomized treatment.

During the first year of the study, body weight decreased on average 4.5 kg in the intervention group and 1.0 kg in the control group subjects ($p = 0.0001$). Most of the weight reduction was maintained during the second year. Also indicators of central adiposity and fasting glucose and insulin, 2-hour post-challenge glucose and insulin, and HbA1c reduced significantly more in the intervention group than in the control group at both 1-year and 2-year follow-up examinations. At the 1-year and 2-year examinations, intervention group subjects reported significantly more beneficial changes in their dietary and exercise habits, based on dietary and exercise diaries.

By March 2000, a total of 86 incident cases of diabetes had been diagnosed among the 522 subjects with IGT randomized into the DPS trial when the median follow-up duration of the study was three years. Of them 27 occurred in the intervention group and 59 in the control group. The absolute risk of diabetes was 32/1000 person-years in the intervention group and 78/1000 person-years in the control group. The effect of the intervention was rapid: the difference in incidence of diabetes between the groups was statistically significant already after two years: 6% in the intervention group and 14% in the control group. The cumulative incidence of diabetes was 11% (95% CI 6 to 15%) in the intervention group and 23% (95% CI 17 to 29%) in the control group after four years. Based on life-table analysis the risk of diabetes was reduced by 58% ($p < 0.001$) during the trial in the intervention group compared with the control group. The absolute risk of diabetes was 32/1000 person-years in the intervention group and 78/1000 person-years in the control group. Thus the absolute risk reduction was 12% at that point and the number needed to treat (NNT) to prevent one case of type 2 diabetes for three years was 8. Both men and women benefited from lifestyle intervention: the incidence of diabetes was reduced in men by 63% and in women by 54% in the intervention group compared with the control group. Interestingly, none of the people (either in the intervention or control group) who had reached all five lifestyle targets developed diabetes, while approximately one third of the people who did not reach a single one of the targets developed type 2 diabetes. This is a direct empirical proof that the reduction of the diabetes risk was indeed mediated through the lifestyle changes.

An analysis using the data collected during the extended follow-up of the DPS revealed that after a median of 7 years total follow-up a marked reduction in the cumulative incidence of diabetes was sustained. The relative risk reduction during the total follow-up was 43%. More importantly, the effect of intervention on diabetes risk was maintained among those who after the intervention period were without diabetes: after median post-intervention follow-up time of 3 years, the number of incident new cases of type 2 diabetes was 31 in the intervention group among 221 people at risk, and 38 in the control group among 185 people at risk. The corresponding incidence rates were 4.6 and 7.2 per 100 person-years, respectively (log-rank test $p = 0.0401$), that is 36% relative risk reduction. Thus, the absolute risk difference between groups increased slightly during the post-intervention period. There is an important message from the public-health point of view: an intensive lifestyle intervention lasting for a limited time can yield long-term benefits in reducing the risk of type 2 diabetes in high-risk individuals.

The diabetes prevention program [58–60]

The Diabetes Prevention Program (DPP) was a multicenter randomized clinical trial carried out in the United States. It compared the efficacy and safety of three interventions - an intensive lifestyle intervention or standard lifestyle recommendations combined with metformin or placebo. The study focused on high-risk individuals ($n = 3234$) with IGT who also had slightly elevated fasting plasma glucose (>5.5 mmol/l). The original closing date of the study was planned to be in year 2002. However, the study was terminated prematurely soon after the publication of the Finnish DPS results [54] leading to an unscheduled interim data analysis of the DPP. The data safety and monitoring board then advised to close the DPP trial because the results had unequivocally answered the main research questions regarding the reduction in incidence of diabetes. In DPP, intensive lifestyle intervention with a 58% reduction in type 2 diabetes risk compared with the placebo group was also superior to the metformin group where type 2 diabetes risk was reduced by 31% compared with placebo.

The lifestyle intervention in DPP was primarily done by special educators, 'case managers', not regular health personnel, and was quite intense [60]. Thus, the translation of such intervention to a routine primary health care may not be easy. The lifestyle intervention commenced with a 16-session structured core curriculum within the first 24 week after randomization carried out in each. The focus of the dietary intervention was first on reducing total fat intake. Later on the concept of calorie balance was introduced and fat and calorie goals set as means to achieve weight loss goal rather than as a goal in and of itself. The weight loss goal for all participants was a 7% weight reduction and to maintain it throughout the trial. The physical activity goal was approximately 700 kcal per week expenditure from physical activities, which was translated to correspond 150 minutes of moderate physical activity such as brisk walking. Clinical centres also offered supervised activity sessions where attendance was voluntary. Of the DPP participants assigned to intensive lifestyle intervention 74% achieved the study goal of ≥150 minutes of activity per week at 24 weeks. At one-year visit the mean weight loss was 7 kg (about 7%).

The DPP investigators have also attempted to clarify the relative contributions of changes in different components of the lifestyle intervention to the reduction in diabetes incidence in the intensive lifestyle intervention arm of the DPP [61]. Furthermore, they aimed at assessing the contribution of diet and physical activity changes on weight loss.

The main finding was that body weight at baseline and weight reduction during the intervention had the largest effects on diabetes risk. Lower weight (10 kg) at baseline was associated with a 12% lower diabetes incidence even when adjusted for demographics and changes in dietary fat intake and physical activity. For each kilogram lost, the risk of developing diabetes was estimated to be reduced by 16%. In the model assessing one intervention characteristic at a time, energy proportion of fat was a significant predictor of incident diabetes, with a 5% reduction leading to HR of 0.75 (95% CI 0.63 to 0.88). However, in the multivariate models with predictors as continuous variables and with baseline body weight and weight reduction as covariates, neither physical activity nor energy proportion of dietary fat predicted diabetes. Nevertheless, among the participants not meeting the weight loss goal during the first year of the trial, those who achieved the physical activity goal had 44% lower diabetes incidence.

Indian diabetes prevention program (IDPP) [62]

The IDPP reqruited 531 subjects with IGT (mean age 45.9 ± 5.7 years, BMI $25.8 \pm 3.5 \, \text{kg/m}^2$) who were randomized into four groups (control, lifestyle modification, metformin and combined lifestyle modification and metformin). Lifestyle modification included advice on physical activity (30 minutes of brisk walking per day) and reduction in total calories, refined carbohydrates and fats, avoidance of sugar, and inclusion of fibre-rich foods. The intervention included personal sessions at baseline and 6-monthly, and monthly telephonic contacts. The intensity of the intervention thus was lesser than in the DPP and DPS. After median follow-up of 30 months, the relative risk reduction was 28.5% with lifestyle modification, 26.4% with metformin and 28.2% with lifestyle modification and metformin, as compared with the control group. Thus, there was no added benefit from combining the drug and lifestyle interventions. In the control group diabetes incidence was high (55.0% in 3 years) and comparable to the findings from the Chinese study [50].

Japanese prevention trial [63]

The Japanese trial with IGT males included 458 men who were diagnosed with IGT in health screening and allocated randomly to receive either intensive lifestyle intervention ($n = 102$) or standard intervention ($n = 356$). The participants in the intensive intervention group visited hospital every 3–4 months where they were given detailed, repeated advise to reduce body weight if BMI was $\geq 22 \, \text{kg/m}^2$ (otherwise, to maintain present weight) by consuming large amount of vegetables and reducing the total amount of other food by 10%, for example, by using a smaller rice bowl. Intake of fat ($<50 \, \text{g}$ per day) and alcohol ($<50 \, \text{g}$ per day) were limited, as was eating out (no more than once a day) and physical activity recommended (30–40 min per day of walking etc.). The participants in the control group visited hospital every 6 months and were given standard advised to eat smaller meals and increase physical activity.

The cumulative 4-year incidence of diabetes was 3% in the intervention group and 9.3% in the control group, with 67.4% risk reduction ($p < 0.001$). BMI at baseline was 23.8 ± 2.1 in the intervention group and 24.0 ± 2.3 in the control group. Body weight decreased by 2.18 kg in the intervention group and 0.39 kg in the control group during 4 years ($p < 0.001$). There thus was a remarkable reduction in diabetes risk despite the relatively modest weight reduction. Post hoc analyses in the control group revealed that diabetes incidence was positively correlated with change in body weight in this population, however, weight loss apparently was not the sole explanator of diabetes risk reduction.

5.3 Other intervention studies

There are also other interventions that are relevant to the prevention of type 2 diabetes. Promising results on the treatment of obesity come from the Swedish SOS Intervention Study where gastric surgery was used in very obese subjects [64]. The 2-year incidence of diabetes was 30 times lower in surgically treated grossly obese subjects compared to control subjects receiving regular care. The corresponding weight losses were 28 kg vs. 0.5 kg ($p < 0.0001$). These results suggest that severe obesity can and should be treated and that the reduction of obesity results in a marked reduction in the incidence of hypertension, diabetes and some lipid disturbances.

In the SLIM (Study on Lifestyle Intervention and Impaired Tolerance Maastricht) study in the Netherlands 102 men and women were randomized into two groups [65, 66]. Inclusion criteria for all participants were that they are over 40 years old, have a family history of diabetes or BMI 25 kg/m^2 or more, and have impaired glucose tolerance but are not diabetics. In the intervention group, participant received detailed instructions how to regulate diet and increase physical activity aiming at lifestyle recommended by the Dutch Guideline for Healthy Diet. Participants took part in individual follow-up visits every third month. In the control group, participants received only brief information about recommended diet and physical activity. After 1-year follow-up the participants in the intervention group had lost in average 2.8 kg of their weight whereas in the control group the average weight loss was only 0.6 kg (p-value of the difference between the groups <0.01). After 3 years, participants in the intervention group were in average 1.1 kg below their baseline weight and participants in the control group had gained 0.2 kg ($p = 0.011$). A difference was also found in glucose tolerance (-0.8 in the intervention group and $+0.2$ in the control group after first year, p-value of the difference <0.05) but in fasting glucose statistically significant differences were not found between the groups. These results confirm the previous findings that it is possibly to affect BMI and diabetes risk by lifestyle counselling. The participants in this study were leaner (average BMI 29.5 kg/m^2) than in the Finnish DPS (31.2 kg/m^2) or in the DPP (33.9 kg/m^2) studies and show that lifestyle interventions have beneficial effect also in a population where the risk level of type 2 diabetes is lower than in these two previous interventions.

In a intervention study in Italy, 120 menopausal (20–46 years old) obese women (BMI ≥ 30 kg/m^2) were randomly divided into two groups [67]. Women with impaired glucose tolerance or diabetes were excluded. In the intervention group the participants received detailed instructions how to reduce weight by 10% by regulating diet and increasing physical activity. The methods to used included food diaries, personal goal setting, monthly small group sessions, and access to behavioural and psychological counselling. In the control group, women received general information about healthy dieting and physical exercise at baseline and in subsequent monthly visits but not specific individualized programme. The intervention had a beneficial effect on weight, fat distribution, and fasting plasma glucose; after 2-year follow-up these indicators had decreased more in the intervention group (14 kg for weight, 0.08 for waist-to-hip ratio, and 9 mg/dl for plasma glucose) than in the control group (3 kg, 0.04, and 2 mg/dl, respectively). All these differences between these two groups were statistically significant.

In another Italian intervention study, 122 non-insulin-treated type 2 diabetes patients, half of them women, were randomized into two groups [68]. In the intervention group, patients were divided into small groups including nine or ten patients. Educational sessions were held every 3 months including topics about meal planning, burden of overweight, smoke cessation, and physical exercise. In the control group, patients continued individual consultation. After four-year follow-up, statistically significant decrease in body weight was found in the intervention group (2.5 kg, $p < 0.001$) but not in the control group (weight decrease 0.9 kg, NS). Also fasting blood glucose was measured, but it did not show statistically significant change in either of these groups.

Additional evidence for the importance of weight reduction was recently derived from a placebo-controlled multicentre trial called Xendos (Xenical in the Prevention of Diabetes in Obese Subjects) [69]. It used a weight loss agent, orlistat (Xenical) compared with weight reduction with diet alone for the prevention of type 2 diabetes over a period of 4 years. Overweight (BMI $\geq 30 \, \text{kg/m}^2$) subjects aged 30–60 years of whom 21% had IGT at baseline received lifestyle counselling every 2 weeks for the first 6 months of the study and thereafter monthly. They were prescribed a calorie-reduced diet and encouraged to take part in moderate daily physical exercise. At four years mean weight reduction was 4.1 kg in the lifestyle + placebo group and 6.9 kg in the lifestyle + orlistat group. Cumulative incidence of type 2 diabetes was 9.0% in the lifestyle + placebo group and 6.2% in the lifestyle + orlistat group, with a 37% risk reduction in the orlistat group compared with the placebo group. The major problem with this study like with most of other drug intervention studies in type 2 diabetes prevention was a high drop-out rate: only 52% of the lifestyle + orlistat group subjects and 34% of the lifestyle + placebo group subjects completed the four-year treatment phase. Nevertheless, there is no doubt that weight control in obese subjects is an efficient way to prevent the development of type 2 diabetes and there are many ways to reach effective weight reduction in addition to dietary means which obviously is the basis for any weight management in obesity.

In the Fasting Hyperglycemia Study (FHS II) [70] 227 subjects with fasting plasma glucose in the range of 5.5–7.7 mmol l^{-1} on two consecutive tests were randomized to reinforced or basic healthy-living advice and sulfonylurea treatment or control group in a two-by-two factorial design. 201 subjects completed the 1-year follow-up study.

Reinforced advice recommending dietary modification and increased exercise was given every three months, and basic advice was given once at the initial visit. Both the reinforced and basic advice groups had a significant mean reduction in body weight (1.5 kg) at 3 months, although the weight subsequently returned to baseline. After one year, subjects allocated to reinforced advice versus basic advice showed no change in fasting plasma glucose, glucose tolerance, or haemoglobin A1c. Thus, this study was unable to show any effect on the risk of type 2 diabetes of 'healthy-living advice', but it seems that the intervention was not particularly successful since no significant weight change was achieved. Also, compared with other recent trials on type 2 diabetes prevention in high-risk subjects with IGT, this study differed regarding the glucose inclusion criteria that were based on fasting values only. Therefore, while it is clearly shown that type 2 diabetes can be prevented in subjects with IGT, we are still lacking the data on the risk on the reduction of the risk of type 2 diabetes in people screened for high fasting glucose. Prospective studies show that people with high fasting glucose (impaired fasting glycaemia) also have an increased risk of developing type 2 diabetes, even though the risk is lower than that for IGT [71]. Nevertheless, thus far there is no evidence that screening for fasting glucose is a justified strategy for the prevention of type 2 diabetes.

5.4 Conclusions

The results from the major type 2 diabetes prevention trials have provided unequivocal evidence that type 2 diabetes can be prevented, at least in high-risk individuals. It is striking that the two individually randomized trials yielded precisely similar results when the DPP confirmed the 58% relative risk reduction [58] obtained in the Finnish DPS study only a year earlier [54]. Even more striking is that the previous non-randomized Malmö feasibility study had almost identical result, 59% risk reduction [44], and also in 1980 the Malmöhus study showed a 56% risk reduction between the intervention and the control groups [45]. Also the absolute risk reductions were very similar among these studies: a 16–18% reduction in the incidence during 3–6 years' period. The data from the Chinese Da-Qing study [50] were slightly different: while the relative risk reduction was somewhat less, about 40%, the absolute risk reduction was higher, 27% due to the fact that the overall incidence in the Chinese was higher.

   The public health implications of these results are very wide. The primary prevention of type 2 diabetes is possible by a non-pharmacological intervention that can be implemented in the primary health care setting. It has been speculated that there might be differences in the acceptance and compliance with lifestyle modification between different ethnic groups, especially in the United States [72]. The reasoning for this has probably been based on the findings from observational studies suggesting that certain ethnic or socio-economic groups have an increased risk of type 2 diabetes. It may, however, be misleading to imply that an observed disease risk differential between subgroups would also lead to a similar differential in the effect of interventions. On the contrary, one should assume that whenever unhealthy lifestyles are corrected the individual disease risk should reduce regardless the demographic background. The recent trials have now confirmed that lifestyle intervention, once carried out properly, is an efficient way to prevent type 2 diabetes. It is worth noting that the metformin arm of the DPP and other trials [73] have shown that antidiabetic drugs may also prevent worsening of IGT to frank type 2 diabetes, but the pharmacological intervention compared with lifestyle intervention seems inferior. This is not surprising since in the lifestyle intervention causal factors influencing the natural history of type 2 diabetes are modified while antidiabetic drugs have specific and limited modes of action leading to a relative lowering of blood glucose concentration.

In order to prevent the emerging epidemic of type 2 diabetes worldwide it is necessary that the primary prevention of type 2 diabetes will receive more serious attention than it has got in the past. The unfavourable lifestyle patterns are no longer an issue only among adults but also in children and adolescents. As a consequence, the age-at-onset of type 2 diabetes has become younger, not only in special small ethnic groups like Pima Indians but in many societies in both developed and developing countries [74–77]. The effect of these lifestyle patterns is particularly deleterious in those who have born small and thin and who subsequently become heavy already in childhood and adolescence [78]. It is however important to note that in the DPP people aged over 60 years at baseline benefited more from lifestyle intervention than younger ones [58]. Similar results have been observed from the DPS [79]. Thus it is not too late to prevent diabetes in older people with IGT, but the immediate benefits are likely to be even greater than in younger subjects since the absolute risk of type 2 diabetes in a short term is higher in older than in younger people.

While it is useful to accumulate more information from interventions in other populations and cultural environments, the evidence to initiate intensive actions to prevent type 2 diabetes is clearly sufficient. The identification of high-risk subjects for type 2 diabetes is relatively easy; no biochemical or other costly tests are required. It is now recognized that from the prevention point of view, screening for type 2 diabetes is not the same as measuring blood glucose, but one can determine the risk of developing type 2 diabetes using non-invasive data before testing for blood glucose. The Finnish Diabetes Risk Score (FINDRISC) was developed based on the prospective study in Finland, to serve as a fast, cheap and simple screening tool for high risk to develop type 2 diabetes in the future [80].

It is also important to note that most of the high-risk subjects for type 2 diabetes are already regular customers of primary health care services for various reasons. What is needed in the health care system is to determine the future risk of type 2 diabetes using the FINDRISC or other risk screening tool in customers that seem potential candidates of type 2 diabetes, and to target a systematic lifestyle intervention to these individuals regardless their current glucose levels. It is necessary that such an intervention will become a part of routine preventive care in order to reduce the burden of type 2 diabetes that is reaching epidemic proportions in many countries. At the same time, it is also necessary to develop national programmes for the primary prevention of type 2 diabetes that include not only the high risk strategy but also the population strategy, that is to reduce the risk factors for type 2 diabetes such as obesity and physical inactivity in the entire population.

According to the estimates derived from the US third National Health and Nutrition Examination Survey 11% of the US adults aged 40–74 years meet the DPP eligibility criteria [81]. This illustrates the magnitude of the problem well: the number of subjects at high risk of type 2 diabetes who would benefit from lifestyle intervention is large. It will be a major challenge for the health care systems to implement the necessary action to prevent or postpone type 2 diabetes in these people [82]. The interventions on high-risk subjects alone will, however, not be sufficient for the successful prevention of type 2 diabetes in the community. It is necessary to initiate actions based on the population approach, too. These include actions that will assure the shift of the risk factor distribution in the entire population to a lower level without screening for high-risk subjects [55]. Such efforts are likely to be even more important than individual interventions alone, as seen from the prevention of cardiovascular disease in the recent past. The co-ordinated combination of the high-risk approach together with systematic population approach programmes simultaneously will be the most efficient and also necessary strategy to reverse the current increasing trend in the incidence of type 2 diabetes. In such programmes it is necessary to realize that the primary prevention of type 2 diabetes must have a long-term plan and it has to include a range of activities targeted to different age groups from fetal life to the elderly [83].

References

1. Colditz, G.A., Willett, W.C., Stampfer, M.J. *et al.* (1990) Weight as a risk factor for clinical diabetes in women. *American Journal of Epidemiology*, **132**, 501–13.
2. Knowler, W.C., Pettitt, D.J., Savage, P.J. and Bennett, P.H. (1981) Diabetes incidence in Pima Indians: contributions of obesity and parental diabetes. *American Journal of Epidemiology*, **113**, 144–56.
3. Manson, J.E., Nathan, D.M., Krolewski, A.S. *et al.* (1992) A prospective study of exercise and incidence of diabetes among US male physicians. *Journal of the American Medical Association*, **268**, 63–7.
4. DECODE Study Group (2003) Age- and sex-specific prevalences of diabetes and impaired glucose regulation in 13 European cohorts. *Diabetes Care*, **26**, 61–9.
5. Qiao, Q., Hu, G., Tuomilehto, J. *et al.* (2003) Age- and sex-specific prevalence of diabetes and impaired glucose regulation in 11 Asian cohorts. *Diabetes Care*, **26**, 1770–80.
6. Zeggini, E., Scott, L.J., Saxena, R. *et al.* (2008) Meta-analysis of genome-wide association data and large-scale replication identifies additional susceptibility loci for type 2 diabetes. *Nature Genetics*, **40**, 638–40.
7. Boyko, E.J., Fujimoto, W.Y., Leonetti, D.L., and Newell-Morris, L. (2000) Visceral adiposity and risk of type 2 diabetes: a prospective study among Japanese Americans. *Diabetes Care*, **23**, 465–71.
8. Chan, J.M., Rimm, E.B., Colditz, C.A. *et al.* (1994) Obesity, fat distribution, and weight gain as risk factors for clinical diabetes in men. *Diabetes Care*, **17**, 961–9.
9. Despres, J.P. (2001) Health consequences of visceral obesity. *Annals of Medicine*, **33**, 534–41.

10. Bertin, E., Nguyen, P., Guenounou, M. *et al.* (2000) Plasma levels of tumor necrosis factor-alpha (TNF-alpha) are essentially dependent on visceral fat ammount in type 2 diabetic patients. *Diabetes & Metabolism*, **26**, 178–82.

11. Vazquez, G., Duval, S., Jacobs, D., Jr and Silventoinen, K. (2007) Comparison of body mass index, waist circumference, and waist/hip ratio in predicting incident diabetes: a literature-based meta-analysis. *Epidemiologic Reviews*, **29**, 115–28.

12. Popkin, B.M. and Gordon-Larsen, P. (2004) The nutrition transition: worldwide obesity dynamics and their determinants. *International Journal of Obesity and Related Metabolic Disorders*, **28** (Suppl 3), S2–S9.

13. Wild, S., Roglic, G., Green, A. *et al.* (2004) Global prevalence of diabetes: estimates for the year 2000 and projections for 2030. *Diabetes Care*, **27**, 1047–53.

14. Tuomilehto, J. and Lindström, J. (2003) The major diabetes prevention trials. *Current Diabetes Reports*, **3**, 115–22.

15. Bergstrom, R. and Hernell, O. (2001) Obesity and insulin resistance in childhood and adolescence, in *Primary and Secondary Preventive Nutrition* (eds A. Bendich, and R.J. Deckelbaum), Humana Press Inc, Totowa, NJ, pp. 165–83.

16. Maes, H.H., Neale, M.C., and Eaves, L.J. (1997) Genetic and environmental factors in relative body weight and human adiposity. *Behavior Genetics*, **27**, 325–51.

17. Schousboe, K., Willemsen, G., Kyvik, K.O. *et al.* (2003) Sex differences in heritability of BMI: a comparative study of results from twin studies in eight countries. *Twin Research*, **6**, 409–21.

18. Frayling, T.M., Timpson, N.J., Weedon, M.N. *et al.* (2007) A common variant in the FTO gene is associated with body mass index and predisposes to childhood and adult obesity. *Science*, **316**, 889–94.

19. Wardle, J. (2007) Eating behaviour and obesity. *Obesity Reviews*, **8** (Suppl 1), 73–5.

20. Grundy, S.M. (1998) Multifactorial causation of obesity: implications for prevention. *American Journal of Clinical Nutrition*, **67** (suppl 3), 563S–572S.

21. World Health Organization (1998) Preparation and use of food-based diatery guidelines, report of a joint FAO/WHO consultation. Geneva: (WHO Technical Report Series No. 880).

22. Ravussin, E. and Swinburn, B.A. (1992) Pathophysiology of obesity. *Lancet*, **340**, 404–8.

23. Schoeller, D.A. (2001) The importance of clinical research: the role of thermogenesis in human obesity. *American Journal of Clinical Nutrition*, **73**, 511–6.

24. Silventoinen, K., Sans, S., Tolonen, H. *et al.* for the WHO MONICA Project (2004) Trends in obesity and energy supply in the WHO MONICA Project. *International Journal of Obesity*, **28**, 710–8.

25. Lahmann, P.H., Lissner, L., Gullberg, B., and Berglund, G. (2000) Sociodemographic factors associated with long-term weight gain, current body fatness and central adiposity in Swedish women. *International Journal of Obesity*, **24**, 685–94.

26. Martikainen, P.T. and Marmot, M.G. (1999) Socioeconomic differences in weight gain and determinants and consequences of coronary risk factors. *American Journal of Clinical Nutrition*, **69**, 719–26.

27. Flatt, J.P. (1988) Importance of nutrient balance in body weight regulation. *Diabetes Metabolism Review*, **4**, 571–81.

28. Sclafani, A. (1992) Dietary obesity models, in *Obesity* (eds P. Bjorntorp and B.N. Brudoff) JB Lippincott, Philadelphia, pp. 241–8.

29. Shah, M. and Grag, A. (1996) High-fat and high-carbohydrate diets and energy balance. *Diabetes Care*, **19**, 1142–52.

30. Kuczmarski, R.J., Flegal, K.M., Campbell, S.M., and Johnson, C.L. (1994) Increasing prevalence of overweight among US adults. The National Health and Nutrition Examination Surveys, 1960 to 1991. *Journal of the American Medical Association*, **273**, 205–11.

31. Shah, M., Hannan, P.J. and Jeffery, R.W. (1991) Secular trend in body mass index in adult population of three communities from the upper mid-western part of the USA: the Minnesota Heart Health Program. *International Journal of Obesity*, **15**, 499–503.

32. Anon (2004) Trends in intake of energy and macronutrients – United States, 1971–2000. *Morbidity and Mortality Weekly Report*, **53**, 80–2.

33. Mokdad, A.H., Ford, E.S., Bowman, B.A. *et al.* (2000) Diabetes trends in the US: 1990–1998. *Diabetes Care*, **23**, 1278–83.

34. Harnack, L.J., Jeffery, R.W., and Boutelle, K.N. (2000) Temporal trends in energy intake in the United States: an ecologic perspective. *American Journal of Clinical Nutrition*, **71**, 1478–84.

35. Nielsen, S.J., Siega-Riz, A.M., and Popkin, B.M. (2002) Trends in energy intake in US between 1977 and 1999: similar shift seen across age groups. *Obesity Research*, **10**, 370–8.

36. Swinburn, B., Metcalf, P.A., and Ley, S.J. (2001) Long-term (5-year) effects of a reduced fat diet in individuals with glucose intolerance. *Diabetes Care*, **24**, 619–24.

37. Astrup, A., Grunwald, G.K., Melanson, E. *et al.* (2000) The role of low-fat diets in body weight control: a meta-analysis of ad libitum intervention studies. *International Journal of Obesity*, **24**, 1545–52.

38. World Health Organization (2003) 'Diet, nutrition and the prevenion of chronic diseases'. Report of a joint FAO/WHO consultation. World Health Organization, Geneva, pp. 160.

39. World Health Organization (2000) 'Obesity: preventing and managing the global epidemic'. Report of a WHO Consultation WHO Technical Report Series, No 894. World Health Organization, Geneva.

40. James, P.T., Leach, R., Kalamara, E., and Shayeghi, M. (2001) The worldwide obesity epidemic. *Obesity Research*, **9** (suppl 4), 228S–233.

41. Joslin, E. (1921) The prevention of diabetes mellitus. *Journal of the American Medical Association*, **76**, 79–84.

42. World Health Organization Study Group (1994) *Primary prevention of diabetes mellitus*, World Health Organization, Geneva: (Technical Report Series No. 844).

43. Bruce, D.G., Chisholm, D.J., Storlien, L.H., and Kraegen, E.W. (1988) Physiological importance of deficiency in early prandial insulin secretion in non-insulin-dependent diabetes. *Diabetes*, **37**, 736–44.

44. Eriksson, K.F. and Lindgarde, F. (1991) Prevention of type 2 (non-insulin-dependent) diabetes mellitus by diet and physical exercise. The 6-year Malmo feasibility study. *Diabetelogia*, **34**, 891–8.

45. Sartor, G., Schersten, B., Carlstrom, S. *et al.* (1980) Ten-year follow-up of subjects with impaired glucose tolerance: prevention of diabetes by tolbutamide and diet regulation. *Diabetes*, **29**, 41–9.

46. Kahn, C.R., Vicent, D., and Doria, A. (1996) Genetics of non-insulin-dependent (type-II) diabetes mellitus. *Annual Review of Medicine*, **47**, 509–31.

47. Neel, J.V. (1962) Diabetes mellitus: a 'thrifty' genotype rendered detrimental by progress? *American Journal of Human Genetics*, **14**, 353–62.

48. King, H., Aubert, R.E., and Herman, W.H. (1998) Global burden of diabetes, 1995–2025: prevalence, numerical estimates, and projections. *Diabetes Care*, **21**, 1414–31.

49. Hamman, R.F. (2002) *The Evidence Base for Diabetes Care*, John Wiley & Sons, Chichester, pp. 75–176.

50. Eriksson, K.F. and Lindgarde, F. (1998) No excess 12-year mortality in men with impaired glucose tolerance who participated in the Malmo Preventive Trial with diet and exercise. *Diabetologia*, **41**, 1010–16.

51. Pan, X.R., Li, G.W., Hu, Y.H. *et al.* (1997) Effects of diet and exercise in preventing NIDDM in people with impaired glucose tolerance. The Da Qing IGT and Diabetes Study. *Diabetes Care*, **20**, 537–44.

52. Li, G., Zhang, P., Wang, J. *et al.* (2008) The long-term effect of lifestyle interventions to prevent diabetes in the China Da Qing Diabetes Prevention Study: a 20-year follow-up study. *Lancet*, **371**, 1731–3.

53. Eriksson, J., Lindström, J., Valle, T. *et al.* (1999) Prevention of type II diabetes in subjects with impaired glucose tolerance: the Diabetes Prevention Study (DPS) in Finland – study design and 1-year interim report on the feasibility of the lifestyle intervention programme. *Diabetologia*, **42**, 793–801.

54. Tuomilehto, J., Lindström, J., Eriksson, J. *et al.* (2001) Prevention of type 2 diabetes mellitus by changes in lifestyle among subjects with impaired glucose tolerance. *New England Journal of Medicine*, **344**, 1343–50.

55. Uusitupa, M., Louheranta, A., Lindström, J. *et al.* (2000) The Finnish Diabetes Prevention Study. *British Journal of Nutrition*, **83** (suppl 1), S137–S142.

56. Lindström, J., Louheranta, A., Mannelin, M. *et al.* (2003) The Finnish Diabetes Prevention Study (DPS): lifestyle intervention and 3-year results on diet and physical activity. *Diabetes Care*, **26**, 3230–36.

57. Lindström, J., Ilanne-Parikka, P., Peltonen, M. *et al.* (2006) Sustained reduction in the incidence of type 2 diabetes by lifestyle intervention: the follow-up results of the Finnish Diabetes Prevention Study. *Lancet*, **368**, 1673–9.

58. Knowler, W.C., Barrett-Connor, E., Fowler, S.E. *et al.* Diabetes Prevention Program Research Group (2002) Reduction in the incidence of type 2 diabetes with lifestyle intervention or metformin. *New England Journal of Medicine*, **346**, 393–403.

59. The Diabetes Prevention Program Research Group (1999) The Diabetes Prevention Program: design and methods for a clinical trial in the prevention of type 2 diabetes. *Diabetes Care*, **22**, 623–34.

60. The Diabetes Prevention Program Research Group (2002) The Diabetes Prevention Program (DPP): description of lifestyle intervention. *Diabetes Care*, **25**, 2165–72.

61. Hamman, R.F., Wing, R.R., Edelstein, S.L. *et al.* (2006) Effect of weight loss with lifestyle intervention on risk of diabetes. *Diabetes Care*, **29**, 2102–7.

62. Ramachandran, A., Snehalatha, C., Mary, S. *et al.* (2006) The Indian Diabetes Prevention Programme shows that lifestyle modification and metformin prevent type 2 diabetes in Asian Indian subjects with impaired glucose tolerance (IDPP-1). *Diabetologia*, **49**, 289–97.

63. Kosaka, K., Noda, M., and Kuzuya, T. (2005) Prevention of type 2 diabetes by lifestyle intervention: a Japanese trial in IGT males. *Diabetes Research and Clinical Practice*, **67**, 152–62.

64. Sjöström, C.D., Lissner, L., Wedel, H., and Sjöström, L. (1999) Reduction in incidence of diabetes, hypertension and lipid disturbances after intentional weight loss induced by bariatric surgery: the SOS Intervention Study. *Obesity Research*, **7**, 477–84.

65. Mensink, M., Feskens, E.J.M., Saris, W.H.M. *et al.* (2003) Study on Lifestyle Intervention and Impaired Glucose Tolerance Maastricht (SLIM): preliminary results after one year. *International Journal of Obesity*, **27**, 377–84.

66. Roumen, C., Corpeleijn, E., Feskens, E.J.M. *et al.* (2008) Impact of 3-year lifestyle intervention on postprandial glucose metabolism: the SLIM study. *Diabetic Medicine*, **25**, 597–605.

67. Esposito, K., Pontillo, A., Di Palo, C. *et al.* (2003) Effect of weight loss and lifestyle changes on vascular inflammatory markers in obese women: a randomized trial. *Journal of the American Medical Association*, **289**, 1799–1804.

68. Trento, M., Passera, P., Bajardi, M. *et al.* (2002) Lifestyle intervention by group care prevents deterioration of Type II diabetes: a 4-year randomized controlled clinical trial. *Diabetologia*, **45**, 1231–9.

69. Sjöström, L., Torgerson, J.S., Hauptman, J., and Boldrin, M. (2002) 'XENDOS (XENical in the prevention f Diabetes in the Obese Subjects): a landmark study', Sao Paulo, Brazil.

70. Dyson, P.A., Hammersley, M.S., Morris, R.J. *et al.* (1997) The Fasting Hyperglycaemia Study: II randomized controlled trial of reinforced healthy-living advice in subjects with increased but not diabetic fasting plasma glucose. *Metabolism: Clinical and Experimental*, **46** (suppl 1), 50–5.

71. Shaw, J.E., Zimmet, P.Z., de Courten, M. *et al.* (1999) Impaired fasting glucose or impaired glucose tolerance. What best predicts future diabetes in Mauritius? *Diabetes Care*, **22**, 399–402.

72. Tataranni, P.A. and Bogardus, C. (2001) Changing habits to delay diabetes. *New England Journal of Medicine*, **344**, 1390–92.

73. Chiasson, J.L., Josse, R.G., Gomis, R. *et al.* STOP-NIDDM Trail Research Group (2002) Acarbose for prevention of type 2 diabetes mellitus: the STOP-NIDDM randomised trial. *Lancet*, **369**, 2072–7.

74. Dabelea, D., Hanson, R.L., Bennett, P.H. *et al.* (1998) Increasing prevalence of type II diabetes in American Indian children. *Diabetologia*, **41**, 904–10.

75. Ehtisham, S., Barrett, T.G., and Shaw, N.J. (2000) Type 2 diabetes in UK children – an emerging problem. *Diabetes Medicine*, **17**, 867–71.

76. Sinha, R., Fisch, G., Teague, B. *et al.* (2002) Prevalence of impaired glucose tolerance among children and adolescents with marked obesity. *New England Journal of Medicine*, **346**, 802–10.

77. Lammi, N., Taskinen, O., Moltchanova, E. *et al.* (2007) A high incidence of type 1 diabetes and an alarming increase in the incidence of type 2 diabetes among young adults in Finland between 1992 and 1996. *Diabetologia*, **50**, 1393–400.

78. Dabelea, D., Pettitt, D.J., Hanson, R.L. *et al.* (1999) Birth weight, type 2 diabetes, and insulin resistance in Pima Indian children and young adults. *Diabetes Care*, **22**, 944–50.

79. Lindström, J., Peltonen, M., Eriksson, J. *et al.* (2008) Determinants for the effectiveness of lifestyle intervention in the Finnish Diabetes Prevention Study. *Diabetes Care*, **31**, 857–62.

80. Lindström, J. and Tuomilehto, J. (2003) The Diabetes Risk Score: a practical tool to predict type 2 diabetes risk. *Diabetes Care*, **26**, 725–31.

81. Benjamin, S.M., Valdez, R., Geiss, L.S. *et al.* (2003) Estimated number of adults with prediabetes in the US in 2000: opportunities for prevention. *Diabetes Care*, **26**, 645–9.

82. Saydah, S.H., Byrd-Holt, D., and Harris, M.I. (2002) Projected impact of implementing the results of the diabetes prevention program in the US population. *Diabetes Care*, **25**, 1940–5.

83. Eriksson, J., Lindström, J., and Tuomilehto, J. (2001) Potential for the prevention of type 2 diabetes. *British Medical Bulletin*, **60**, 183–99.

6

Diet and food-based therapies for obesity in diabetic patients

Catherine Rolland and Iain Broom
The Robert Gordon University, Aberdeen, UK

6.1 Introduction

The strategies for delivering diet based therapies for the management of obesity may differ in type 1 (insulin-dependent) and type 2 (insulin-independent) diabetes mellitus. The role of diet, however, in the management of type 1 diabetes mellitus is primarily in minimising the short-term fluctuations in plasma glucose, specifically hypoglycaemia and to reduce the risks of long-term complications (micro- and macrovascular).

Despite approaches in the past where emphasis was placed on eating less carbohydrate in type 1 diabetes mellitus, this possibly leading to increased atherogenesis in this group, the general nutritional requirements of the diabetic patient are now deemed to be no different from that of the non-diabetic population. Thus dietary recommendations are no different from the general population (Table 6.1). The same is also true for type 2 diabetes mellitus but other approaches may be adopted in treating obesity associated with type 2 diabetes mellitus, which is resistant to standard dietary approaches (see below).

6.2 Type 2 diabetes

Obesity is the main aetiological factor in the development of type 2 diabetes mellitus with 70–80% of type 2 diabetes patients presenting with obesity (BMI $>30\,\text{kg/m}^2$). This obese phenotype is associated with insulin-resistance and thus differs metabolically from type 1 diabetes, which is an insulin-deficient state. Thus, in general, obesity management in diabetes is primarily a problem of type 2 diabetes and further discussion will be centred around the management of the type 2 diabetic patient.

Obesity and Diabetes, Second Edition   Edited by Anthony H. Barnett and Sudhesh Kumar
© 2009 John Wiley & Sons, Ltd

Table 6.1   General principles for the management of diabetic patients

Energy intake[a]	Recommendations for diabetes mellitus to approach and maintain BMI of 25
Carbohydrate	>55% of total energy
Fat	<30–35% of total energy[b] (Saturated fat ≤10%)
Protein	10–15% of total energy
Salt	<6 g daily (<3 g if hypertensive)
Sucrose (added)	<25 g per day
Dietary fibre	>30 g per day
'Diabetic foods' (as labelled)	None

BMI = body mass index ([weight in kg]/[height in m]^2).
[a]Dependent on sex, age and activity.
[b]A higher total fat intake is allowed if monosaturated fatty acids form a major component of the diet for example olive oil.

6.3   Patterns of weight loss in diabetes

The obese diabetic patient provides a particular challenge in terms of achieving sustainable weight loss. In all studies, when compared to the non-diabetic patient, weight loss achieved at 1 year is approximately 50% [1,2] when the best diet and lifestyle advice and support is given (Figure 6.1). Thus, the presence of type 2 diabetes gives the patient increased problems in achieving clinically significant weight loss. As an added confounder the natural history of weight alteration in the diabetic patient is for this to slowly increase, the rate of increase being dependent on drug therapy used [3], both insulin and sulfonylurea increasing the rate of weight gain.

On achieving sustainable weight loss and maintenance, it is important to take notice of the above and to relay this informtion to the patient to allow his/her better

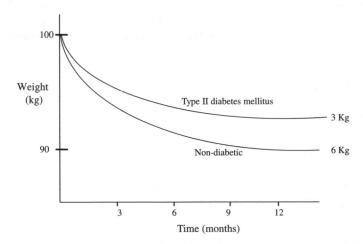

Figure 6.1   Weight loss in type 2 diabetes mellitus compared to non-diabetics

understanding of energy metabolism. Clear and frank discussion with patients in respect of difficulties in achieving and maintaining weight loss is essential. The approach to the patient by the whole healthcare delivery team as to the role of diet and lifestyle alteration needs to send the same message. It is also important that non-verbal communication to patients from the diabetic management team re-enforces the verbal statements. Contradictory messages will lead to patient confusion, lack of confidence, and ultimate failure in achieving weight reduction and hence failure to achieve improved glycaemic control, blood pressure and/or lipid parameters.

6.4 Target setting

Goal-setting is a pre-requisite prior to the initialization of diet therapy. It is essential to set a realistic target of weight loss in a fixed period of time for example 5–10% of body weight in six months. Patients should be advised that achieving an 'ideal weight' for height that is to give a BMI of <25 kg/m^2 may not be an achievable target, and that not achieving such an ideal weight should not be seen as failure. Other targets to discuss with the patient are achievable changes in food intake, increased activity and decreased inactivity. It is not appropriate in attempting to alter diet and lifestyle to institute absolute negative attitudes towards certain foodstuffs, or current lifestyle, but to slowly change attitudes to both, with positive, as opposed to negative, reinforcement. Such target setting may allow small but sustainable weight losses that are clinically significant and allow patients to stabilize at a new lower weight, with consequent improvement in glycaemic control and other outcomes, prior to attempting further weight reduction measures at a later date (Figure 6.2).

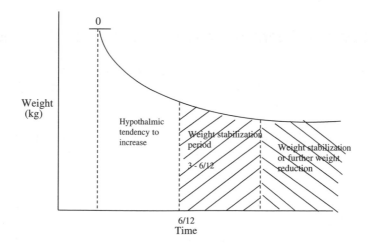

Figure 6.2 Weight loss and maintenance including the influence of hypothalamic control. Weight loss programmes should be carried out in 6 monthly stages with periods of weight stabilization

6.5 Dietary and lifestyle alterations

It is important to address alterations in diet and lifestyle simultaneously and diet alone should not be targeted in an attempt to achieve sustainable weight loss [2,4–6]. In addition the use of cognitive behaviour therapy has clearly shown to add benefits to sustainable weight loss when used in conjunction with diet and lifestyle changes. It is therefore appropriate to use an holistic approach when dealing with weight loss and maintenance in obese individuals be they diabetic or non-diabetic [2].

It is important to understand, however, dietary intake cannot be reliably estimated in the overweight patient as they consistently understate their food intake by the order of 20% [7]. The energy intake required to maintain body weight is best estimated by using standard formulae derived from metabolic rate measurements and appropriate reductions in intake advised by altering proportions of foodstuffs in the diet.

Currently Diabetes UK recommends energy intake prescriptions for diabetes patients to be that required to maintain a BMI of $25 \, \text{kg/m}^2$ [8]. In the obese diabetes patient this may be too strict an energy deficit to allow longer-term adherence, with consequent patient and treatment failure. It is more appropriate to induce small changes in energy intake to allow an approximate deficit of 500–600 kcal/day [9].

This standard approach to BMI of $25 \, \text{kg/m}^2$ is reasonable for Caucasian populations, although rarely attainable in practice. In Asian populations the susceptibility to type 2 diabetes and metabolic syndrome increases dramatically at a lower BMI ($23 \, \text{kg/m}^2$). Certainly in disease prevention such targets should be considered as maximal desirable within the relevant populations.

The subsequent discussion will be restricted to diet and food-based treatment only. The independent effects of exercise on weight loss and maintenance, improved insulin sensitivity and well-being will be discussed elsewhere, as will the effects of cognitive behavioural therapy (see Chapters 7 and 8).

6.6 Dietary nutrient composition in type 2 diabetes

There is considerable evidence in support of high fat, relatively low carbohydrate (but high sugar), low fibre diets of Western societies being a major aetiological factor in susceptible individuals. Excess dietary fat is more easily converted to adipose tissue lipid stores than carbohydrate [10]; diet-induced thermogenesis is less with fat than carbohydrates or protein thus inducing lower metabolic rates with high fat diets [11,12]; dietary fat has minimal effects on both appetite and satiety [13]; hyperinsulinaemia has been associated with high fat intakes possibly through components of the hormonal enteroinsular axis [14]. The associated hyperinsulinaemia will favour further fat deposition and aggravate the insulin resistance of type 2 diabetes increasing associated metabolic dysregulation for example dyslipidaemia (Figure 6.3).

In addition, in the obese individual, dietary-induced thermogenesis is lower than in the non-obese and hence further weight increase is more likely with energy dense diets [15].

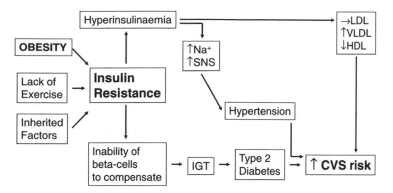

Figure 6.3   Metabolic syndrome. LDL, low density lipoprotein; VLDL, very low density lipoprotein; HDL, high density lipoprotein; SNS, sympathetic nervous system; IGT, impaired glucose tolerance; CVS, cardiovascular system

For the majority of type 2 diabetes patients therefore, diets based on reduced fat-intake and higher unrefined carbohydrates are recommended (Table 6.2). Such approaches in association with mild energy restriction should lead to weight reduction and maintenance of this reduced weight.

Changing to such a diet is frequently sufficient to induce weight loss without the need for energy restriction, especially in males.

It is clear, therefore, that specific dietary recommendations in type 2 diabetes do not differ from dietary recommendations in the non-diabetic population [8,16,17]. If, however, in the overweight (90%) or obese (60–70%) type 2 diabetes patients there is no reduction in weight, or indeed an increase in weight, then additional dietary energy restriction has to be instituted. Overweight type 2 diabetes patients will need reassurance from the *whole* diabetes management team that such alterations in diet are

Table 6.2   Advantages of high carbohydrate versus high fat intake in achieving and maintaining weight loss in type 2 diabetes mellitus

Dietary intake	
High carbohydrate	High fat
Low energy density	High energy density
Appetite suppression (inclusive of bulk effect of fibre)	Low appetite suppression
Increased satiety	No satiety effects
Reduced food intake	Increased food intake
Reduced hyperinsulinaemia	Tendency to hyperinsulinaemia
Increased diet-induced thermogenesis	Decreased diet-induced thermogenesis
Increased intake: reduced tendency to fat deposition	Increased intake: tendency to fat deposition
Reduction in metabolic dysregulation	Increased metabolic dysregulation
↓ Atherogenic effects ↑	

effective both in controlling their disease but also in achieving small but sustainable weight loss. It is also important that consistent messages are given to these patients that diet (and lifestyle) are the major factors involved in achieving adequate diabetes control and that weight loss in the overweight/obese is a prerequisite to this improved control.

6.7   The approach to dietary prescription

The initial approach to the patient and the initial emphasis on diet and dietary alterations are of extreme importance. This may be the only advice the patient remembers and first approaches to dietary intervention are liable to provide the best outcomes relative to both improved control and weight loss in the overweight/obese diabetic. The restriction of single nutrients such as sugar is not advised but dietary habits in general should be discussed, as well as the modification and reduction or increase in specific food groups, for example reduction in overall fat and increase in complex carbohydrate.

Simple guidelines for dietary manipulation, suitable for the primary care health team to provide at the time of diagnosis, are preferable until, and if, fuller advice is given by the community and hospital dietician. It is well recognized, however, that weight loss and maintenance in the overweight/obese diabetic is more difficult than in the non-diabetic, generally speaking about half that expected in the non-diabetic [1,2,18]. This will therefore require the re-emphasis of diet and weight loss in achieving optimum control and the setting of achievable targets for patients in both the short and longer term. It is better and easier to bring weight down in stages with intervening periods of weight stabilization than to attempt more major weight reductions in the obese type 2 diabetic.

6.8   Failure of therapy

Because of the reduced rate of weight loss seen in type 2 diabetes when compared with the non-diabetic population and indeed the general failure with lifestyle advice to achieve sustainable weight loss over the longer term (most individuals returning to initial weight by 5 years) [19], 'failure' is seen as inevitable. Failure is, however, a relative term and the explanation to patients of patterns of weight loss and gain are essential. The importance of small amounts of weight lost relative to improvements in disease outcomes should be emphasized and the importance of maintaining good control by dietary means alone without the need for pharmacotherapy also stressed [20].

It is equally important for the clinician and the healthcare workers to understand patterns of weight loss and gain and for such individuals to provide continual encouragement. It is particularly unhelpful to continually castigate the patient about his/her 'failure to comply' with diet adherence. Indeed such attitudes often have the opposite effect and increase the rate of weight gain, and alienate the patient towards further therapeutic approaches based on lifestyle modification.

Again in the 'failing patient' it is important to emphasize the positive effects of achieving further modest reductions in weight without dwelling on the negative. Here patient motivation is important and changing his/her attitudes towards weight loss paramount. Lastly, failure in patients is frequently not that, but one of treatment withdrawal after short-term 3–6 months' intensive support. Weight loss and maintenance require long-term input and support by both healthcare workers and the family unit.

6.9   Fat or carbohydrate

For the majority of patients (diabetic and non-diabetic) who have a problem with weight maintenance, targeting fat in the diet is appropriate for the reasons outlined above. This is also the sensible option for Government to adopt as far as population targets are concerned. It must be realized, however, that high carbohydrate intakes can also lead to marked obesity and consequently increase the likelihood of the development of type 2 diabetes. Individual patient therapy may therefore differ from that applied to population or generally applied to achieve weight reduction. Where increased carbohydrate is identified as the main dietary energy substrate involved in the aetiology of obesity in an individual, strategies to reduce weight based on increased carbohydrate intake are likely to fail. Cognisance must therefore be taken of other approaches to reduce weight and optimize metabolic control.

There is considerable controversy over the use of low carbohydrate, high protein diets especially in type 2 diabetes. The most common of these is the Atkins Diet [21] although there are a number of such diet treatments based on switching energy substrate metabolism from a carbohydrate base to a fat base, involving ketogenesis and ketone body utilization by brain and peripheral tissues. The appropriate utilization of fat as an energy substrate by the brain takes time to develop (Figure 6.4) but once this occurs there is marked appetite suppression. It is interesting that William Banting described the first low-carbohydrate diet to achieve popular success in the 1860s and claimed that on this diet he was never hungry [22].

Numerous professional bodies have, however, at the least cautioned against the use of low-carbohydrate diets. They have suggested that such diets have serious medical consequences particularly for patients with known cardiovascular disease, type 2 diabetes, dyslipidaemia or hypertension. It should be said that such statements have been made without good evidence. A meta-analysis and systematic review of such dietary treatment by Bravata *et al.* [23] and by Nordman *et al.* [24] stated that there is insufficient evidence to make such recommendations against the use of such dietary therapy. In the Nordman review, the conclusion about the use of high protein diets indicated that there were improvements in triacylglycerol and high density cholesterol but unfavourable changes in low density lipoprotein cholesterol when a low-carbohydrate approach is used to achieve weight loss. However, the review by Nordman *et al.* [24] failed to include a study by Sharman *et al.* [25] which demonstrated that the increase in low-density cholesterol was accompanied by a change in low-density

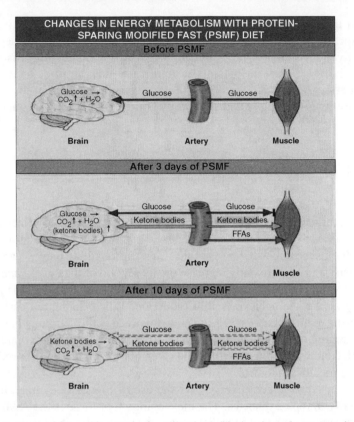

Figure 6.4   Patterns of fat and ketone body utilization with time in patients on reduced carbohydrate intake

cholesterol particle size resulting in a less atherogenic profile. Kirk and colleagues [26] demonstrated an increase in high-density lipoproteins (HDL) but not in low-density lipoproteins (LDL) in diabetics, but it was unclear if the particle density and therefore progression of atherosclerosis were affected by a low-carbohydrate diet in type 2 diabetes patients. Indeed, the dyslipidaemia associated with type 2 diabetes and metabolic syndrome reduced circulating levels of HDL and raised triacylglycerols. There is no difference in serum LDL concentrations between the diabetic and non-diabetic populations. Previously, Reaven and colleagues [27] suggested that a high-carbohydrate diet increased glucose and insulin levels resulting in greater cardiovascular risk. In addition, data analysed by McKeown *et al.* [28] looking at 2834 subjects from the Framingham Offspring study established that a higher glycaemic index and higher glycaemic load of the diet resulted in an association with the development of insulin resistance and metabolic syndrome.

A recent meta-analysis of restricted carbohydrate diets in patients with type 2 diabetes [26] further supported the use of lower-carbohydrate diets in the treatment of type 2 diabetes. The results of the meta-analysis suggested that even moderate

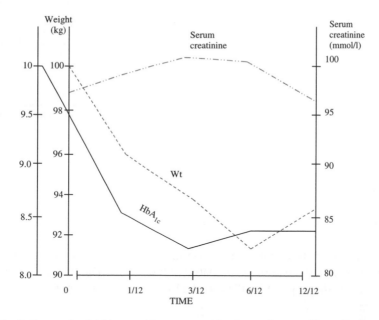

Figure 6.5 Patterns of weight loss and improvement in glycaemic control in patients treated with low carbohydrate, high protein diets

decreases in carbohydrate intake improved fasting glucose, HbA1c and triacylglycerols in type 2 diabetics.

The jury is therefore out as to the efficacy and longer-term safety of such approaches. Part of the reason for this confusion is due to the variability between study design, subjects, measurements, attrition rates, medication and conditions under which the research up to date has been carried out. It is clear, however, that patients in general do not adopt this dietary approach for longer than 6 months with both weight loss and fall in HbA1c being maximal at this time period [29] (Figure 6.5).

This study also demonstrated no adverse effects on renal function with time and this was reiterated in a review of low carbohydrate diets by Kennedy *et al.* [30]. With the associated high protein intake there is also a rise in serum urea concentration as would be expected.

In general these diets are classified as high in fat. This is the case when fat is expressed as percentage of energy consumed, but in absolute terms the amount of fat consumed is low and the tendency to overeat suppressed by the action of such diets on control mechanisms affecting appetite and satiety (Table 6.3).

Such diets can use standard food components with protein comprising at least 120 g per day or may be constituted in powder format. These latter act as meal replacement therapy.

Approaches based on low-carbohydrate intake are usually supplemented with additional vitamins or trace elements. Calcium is also frequently added as loss of bone mineral mass has been suggested to accompany such high protein intakes although

Table 6.3   Nutrient content of high protein low-carbohydrate diets (1000 kcal intake)

Nutrient	Weight (g)	%Energy	Absolute energy (kcal)
Protein	120	41	408
Carbohydrate	40	16	160
Fat[a]	43	43	432

[a]Absolute amount of fat in standard healthy eating – 600 kcal (Diabetes UK) is 51–59 g based on 1600 kcal intake that is 30–35% total energy

again evidence for this is lacking [23]. In fact, evidence from Baba *et al.* [31] demonstrated that overall calcium balance remained the same in patients consuming a high protein diet where the higher content of calcium in a high-protein diet offset urinary losses.

Lastly, evidence in the literature suggests that, overall, there is a lower attrition rate in the low carbohydrate/high protein compared to the low fat/healthy eating intervention groups, giving further support for the use of a low-carbohydrate approach (Figure 6.6).

6.10   Meal replacement therapy

Many companies offer meal replacement techniques in an effort to reduce weight. Such therapies can be based on standard low energy intakes but nutrient complete (e.g. Slimfast) or are based on low-carbohydrate intakes (e.g. Modifast, Cambridge Diet, LighterLife, etc.).

The success of such treatments remains to be confirmed and appropriate trials in this area are sadly lacking, especially in the management of type 2 diabetes. The BBC programme *Diet Trials* examined in detail meal replacement therapies and found these

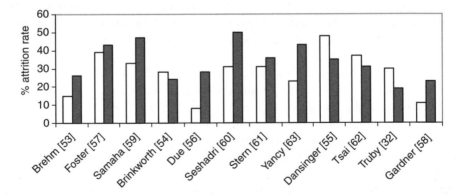

Figure 6.6   Percentage attrition rate in low-carbohydrate (white) and low fat diets (black) reported in the literature

to be as good as but no better than other weight loss strategies when compared to no therapeutic approach in healthy obese subjects [32]. However, several meal replacement studies carried out in patients with type 2 diabetes demonstrated significantly greater weight loss [33] and improved glycaemic control and blood lipids in the short term [34] and less regain after 1 year of maintenance diet than standard diets [35]. Other studies have also demonstrated that soy [36] and whole grain based [37] meal replacements can be effective for weight loss and metabolic risk factors in type 2 diabetics.

6.11 Very low calorie diets

A very low calorie diet (VLCD) is defined as a diet of <800 kcal/day [17]. A variety of synthetic and food based formula diets are available which give energy intakes of 300–400 kcal/day designed to achieve weight loss while maintaining lean body mass by providing high levels of protein supplemented with vitamins, minerals, electrolytes and fatty acids [38]. Such diets appear to be safe in the short to medium term, although a number of side effects have been reported [39]. Certainly, in the short term, VLCDs produce excellent weight loss [38,40,41] but this appears not to be sustained at 1 year when they confer no advantage over standard approaches [2]. In the short term, patients with type 2 diabetes do show an improvement in fasting glucose, HbA1c, insulin sensitivity and inflammation [42–46]. Interestingly, the evaluations of short-term VLCDs in obese patients with type 2 diabetes demonstrated a sustained improvement in various parameters at 12 and 18 months [38,47]. Based on their results, Dhindsa *et al.* [38] suggested giving greater consideration in the use of VLCDs in the treatment of the 'difficult-to-manage and symptomatic patient group'. There is also evidence that short-term and possibly long-term use of VLCDs may be a safe and effective treatment for pediatric patients with type 2 diabetes [48].

There has been evidence to suggest that diabetic patients are likely to regain weight more rapidly than non-diabetic patients following an 'intensive' period of weight loss [49]; however, Dhindsa *et al.* [18] suggest that the time course and extent of weight regain may have been overestimated. Furthermore, evidence from Jazet *et al.* [47] demonstrated that 18 months after a 1 month VLCD, despite weight regain, patients using insulin had a better cardiovascular risk profile than before the dietary intervention. There is to date only one case study reporting the use of a VLCD for a 12 month period in type 2 diabetic patients. The results suggest that a VLCD can be used safely and effectively for a period of 12 months in some obese type 2 diabetic patients, but that patients should remain under close medical supervision [50].

Modern VLCDs must be distinguished from those used in the 1960s and 1970s to effect weight reduction. These latter dietary approaches were associated with sudden death syndrome, thought to be due to electrolyte and micronutrient deficiencies. Modern VLCDs do not induce such deficiencies. It is clear that short-term use of VLCDs produces improvements in glycaemic control, blood pressure and lipids. Longer-term effects both on weight and other outcomes remain to be investigated.

6.12   Conclusions

There are currently no robust data on the effectiveness of the dietary treatment of type 2 diabetes [51]. Yet, dietary modification remains the cornerstone in the management of the obese type 2 diabetic and the best long-term outcomes are achieved when optimal control is achieved by this means. There remains considerable research to determine the best way of delivering such therapy to achieve long-term weight reduction and optimum metabolic control. Identification of patient-specific dietary therapy remains the ideal goal. It is clear that no one approach to diet and food-based therapies is applicable to all patients. At this stage, there is evidence to suggest that the use of lower carbohydrate diets, meal replacements and VLCDs improve cardiovascular risk in type 2 diabetics and broaden patient choice as they provide an alternative to the standard dietary interventions. However, there is still a lack of evidence for the use of these approaches in the longer term. There is a vital need for better designed studies [26,51,52]. Further work is therefore needed to identify patient-matched diet treatment for long-term sustained weight loss, possibly in association with drug-based therapies.

References

1. Hollander, P.A., Elbein, S.C., Hirsch, I.B. *et al.* (1998) Role of orlistat in the treatment of obese patients with type 2 diabetes. A 1-year randomized double-blind study. *Diabetes Care*, **21**, 1288–94.
2. Avenell, A., Broom, J., Brown, T.J. *et al.* (2003) Systematic review of the long-term outcomes of the treatments for obesity and implications for health improvement and the economic consequences for the National Health Service. *Health Technology Assessment*, **8**, 1–458.
3. UK Prospective Diabetes Study Group (1998) Effect of intensive blood glucose control with metformin on complications in overweight patients with type 2 diabetes. *Lancet*, **352**, 854–6.
4. Uusitupa, M. (1996) Early lifestyle intervention in patients with non-insulin-dependent diabetes mellitus and impaired glucose tolerance. *Annals of medicine*, **28**, 445–9.
5. Torjesen, P.A., Birkeland, K.I., Anderssen, S.A. *et al.* (1997) Lifestyle changes may reverse development of the insulin resistance syndrome. The Oslo Diet and Exercise Study: a randomized trial. *Diabetes Care*, **20**, 26–31.
6. Eriksson, J., Lindstrom, J., Valle, T. *et al.* (1999) Prevention of Type II diabetes in subjects with impaired glucose tolerance: the Diabetes Prevention Study (DPS) in Finland. Study design and 1-year interim report on the feasibility of the lifestyle intervention programme. *Diabetologia*, **42**, 793–801.
7. Prentice, A.M., Black, A.E. and Loward, W.A. (1986) High levels of energy expenditure in obesity. *British Medical Journal*, **242**, 83–7.
8. Connor, H., Annan, F., Bunn, E. *et al.* Nutrition Subcommittee of the Diabetes Care Advisory Committee of Diabetes UK (2003) The implementation of nutritional advice for people with diabetes. *Diabetic Medicine*, **20**, 786–807.
9. Lean, M.J. and James, W.P.T. (1986) Prescription of diabetic diets in the 1980s. *Lancet*, **1**, 723–5.
10. Flatt, J.P. (1985) Energetics of intermediary metabolism, in *Substrate and Energy Metabolism* (eds J.S. Garrow, D. Halliday), J. Libbey, London, pp. 58–69.

11. Lean, M.E. and James, W.P. (1988) Metabolic effects of isoenergetic nutrient exchange over 24 hours in relation to obesity in women. *International Journal of Obesity*, **12**, 15–27.

12. Lean, M.J., James, W.P.T. and Garthwaite, P.H. (1989) Obesity without overeating, in Obesity in Europe 88. (eds P. Bjortorp, and S. Rossner,), J. Libbey, London, pp. 281–6.

13. Caterson, I.D. and Broom, J. (2001) *Pocket Picture Guide Obesity*, Harcourt Health Communications, London.

14. Grey, N. and Kipnes, D.M. (1971) Effect of diet composition on the hyperinsulinaemia of obesity. *New England Journal of Medicine*, **285**, 827–31.

15. Bruce, A.C., McNurlan, M.A., McHardy, K.C. *et al.* (1990) Protein synthesis in human tumour and muscle is enhanced more by TPN than by solutions enriched with branched-chain amino acids. *Clinical Nutrition*, (Suppl 21), 21–2.

16. DHSS-COMA (1984) *Diet and Cardiovascular Disease. Report on Health and Social Subjects*, HMSO, London.

17. National Task Force on the Prevention and Treatment of Obesity (1993) Very-low-calorie diets. *Journal of the American Medical Association*, **270**, 967–74.

18. Broom, I., Wilding, J., Stott, P., Myers, N. UK Multimorbidity Study Group (2002) Randomised trial of the effect of orlistat on body weight and cardiovascular disease risk profile in obese patients: UK Multimorbidity Study. *International Journal of Clinical Practice*, **56**, 494–9.

19. Lean, M.J. (1998) *Clinical Handbook of Weight Management*. Dunitz IV, London.

20. Nutrition and Diabetes Study Group of the European Association for the Study of Diabetes (1988) Nutritional recommendations and principles for individuals with diabetes mellitus. *Diabetes Nutrition and Metabolism*, **1**, 145–9.

21. Atkins, R.C. (1998) *Dr Atkins New Diet Revolutions*, Avon Books, New York, NY.

22. Banting, W. (1863) *Letter on Corpulence, Addressed to the Public*, 2nd edn, Harrison and Sons, London.

23. Bravata, D.M., Sanders, L., Huang, J. *et al.* (2003) Efficacy and safety of low-carbohydrate diets: a systematic review. *Journal of the American Medical Association*, **289**, 1837–50.

24. Nordmann, A.J., Nordmann, A., Briel, M. *et al.* (2006) Effects of low-carbohydrate vs low-fat diets on weight loss and cardiovascular risk factors: a meta-analysis of randomized controlled trials. *Archives of Internal Medicine*, **166**, 285–93.

25. Sharman, M.J., Kraemer, W.J., Love, D.M. *et al.* (2002) A ketogenic diet favorably affects serum biomarkers for cardiovascular disease in normal-weight men. *Journal of Nutrition*, **132**, 1879–85.

26. Kirk, J.K., Graves, D.E., Craven, T.E. *et al.* (2008) Restricted-carbohydrate diets in patients with type 2 diabetes: a meta-analysis. *Journal of the American Dietetic Association*, **108**, 91–100.

27. Reaven, G., Strom, T.K. and Fox, B. (2001) *Syndrome X, The Silent Killer: The New Heart Disease Risk*, Simon & Schuster, New York.

28. McKeown, N.M., Meigs, J.B., Liu, S. *et al.* (2004) Carbohydrate nutrition, insulin resistance, and the prevalence of the metabolic syndrome in the Framingham Offspring Cohort. *Diabetes Care*, **27**, 538–46.

29. Robertson, A.M., Broom, J., McRobbie, L.J. and MacLennan, G.S. (2002) Low carbohydrate diets in treatment resistant overweight patients with type 2 diabetes. *Diabetic Medicine*, **19**, S24.

30. Kennedy, R.L., Chokkalingam, K. and Farshchi, H.R. (2005) Nutrition in patients with type 2 diabetes: are low-carbohydrate diets effective, safe or desirable? *Diabetic medicine: a journal of the British Diabetic Association*, **22**, 821–32.

31. Baba, N.H., Sawaya, S., Torbay, N. *et al.* (1999) High protein vs high carbohydrate hypoenergetic diet for the treatment of obese hyperinsulinemic subjects. *International Journal of Obesity and Related Metabolic Disorders*, **23**, 1202–06.

32. Truby, H., Baic, S., deLooy, A. *et al.* (2006) Randomised controlled trial of four commercial weight loss programmes in the UK: initial findings from the BBC 'diet trials'. *BMJ (Clinical Research Ed.)*, **332**, 1309–14.

33. Ditschuneit, H.H. (2006) Do meal replacement drinks have a role in diabetes management? *Nestle Nutrition Workshop Series. Clinical & Performance Programme*, **11**, 171–9, discussion 179–81.

34. Harder, H., Dinesen, B. and Astrup, A. (2004) The effect of a rapid weight loss on lipid profile and glycemic control in obese type 2 diabetic patients. *International Journal of Obesity and Related Metabolic Disorders*, **28**, 180–2.

35. Cheskin, L.J., Mitchell, A.M., Jhaveri, A.D. *et al.* (2008) Efficacy of meal replacements versus a standard food-based diet for weight loss in type 2 diabetes: a controlled clinical trial. *The Diabetes Educator*, **34**, 118–27.

36. Li, Z., Hong, K., Saltsman, P. *et al.* (2005) Long-term efficacy of soy-based meal replacements vs an individualized diet plan in obese type II DM patients: relative effects on weight loss, metabolic parameters, and C-reactive protein. *European Journal of Clinical Nutrition*, **59**, 411–18.

37. Rave, K., Roggen, K., Dellweg, S. *et al.* (2007) Improvement of insulin resistance after diet with a whole-grain based dietary product: results of a randomized, controlled cross-over study in obese subjects with elevated fasting blood glucose. *British Journal of Nutrition*, **98**, 929–36.

38. Dhindsa, P., Scott, A.R. and Donnelly, R. (2003) Metabolic and cardiovascular effects of very-low-calorie diet therapy in obese patients with Type 2 diabetes in secondary failure: outcomes after 1 year. *Diabetic Medicine*, **20**, 319–24.

39. Hanefield, M. and Weck, M. (1989) Very low calorie diet therapy in obese non-insulin dependent diabetes patients. *International Journal of Obesity*, **13** (Suppl 2), 33–7.

40. Capstick, F., Brooks, B.A., Burns, C.M. *et al.* (1997) Very low calorie diet (VLCD): a useful alternative in the treatment of the obese NIDDM patient. *Diabetes Research and Clinical Practice*, **36**, 105–11.

41. Williams, K.V., Mullen, M.L., Kelley, D.E. and Wing, R.R. (1998) The effect of short periods of caloric restriction on weight loss and glycemic control in type 2 diabetes. *Diabetes Care*, **21**, 2–8.

42. Allick, G., Bisschop, P.H., Ackermans, M.T. *et al.* (2004) A low-carbohydrate/high-fat diet improves glucoregulation in type 2 diabetes mellitus by reducing postabsorptive glycogenolysis. *Journal of Clinical Endocrinology and Metabolism*, **89** (12), 6193–7.

43. Gannon, M.C. and Nuttall, F.Q. (2004) Effect of a high-protein, low-carbohydrate diet on blood glucose control in people with type 2 diabetes. *Diabetes*, **53**, 2375–82.

44. Sharman, M.J. and Volek, J.S. (2004) Weight loss leads to reductions in inflammatory biomarkers after a very-low-carbohydrate diet and a low-fat diet in overweight men. *Clinical Science (London)*, **107**, 365–9.

45. Boden, G., Sargrad, K., Homko, C. *et al.* (2005) Effect of a low-carbohydrate diet on appetite, blood glucose levels, and insulin resistance in obese patients with type 2 diabetes. *Annals of Internal Medicine*, **142**, 403–11.

46. O'Brien, K.D., Brehm, B.J., Seeley, R.J. *et al.* (2005) Diet-induced weight loss is associated with decreases in plasma serum amyloid a and C-reactive protein independent of dietary macronutrient composition in obese subjects. *Journal of Clinical Endocrinology and Metabolism*, **90**, 2244–9.

47. Jazet, I.M., de Craen, A.J., van Schie, E.M. and Meinders, A.E. (2007) Sustained beneficial metabolic effects 18 months after a 30-day very low calorie diet in severely obese, insulin-treated patients with type 2 diabetes. *Diabetes Research and Clinical Practice*, **77**, 70–6.

48. Willi, S.M., Martin, K., Datko, F.M. and Brant, B.P. (2004) Treatment of type 2 diabetes in childhood using a very-low-calorie diet. *Diabetes Care*, **27**, 348–53.

49. Guare, J.C., Wing, R.R. and Grant, A. (1995) Comparison of obese NIDDM and nondiabetic women: short- and long-term weight loss. *Obesity Research*, **3**, 329–35.
50. Sumithran, P. and Proietto, J. (2008) Safe year-long use of a very-low-calorie diet for the treatment of severe obesity. *Medical Journal of Australia*, **188**, 366–68.
51. Nield, L., Moore, H.J., Hooper, L. *et al.* (2007) Dietary advice for treatment of type 2 diabetes mellitus in adults. *Cochrane Database of Systematic Reviews*, **3**, CD004097.
52. Avenell, A., Brown, T.J., McGee, M.A. *et al.* (2004) What are the long-term benefits of weight reducing diets in adults? A systematic review of randomized controlled trials. *Journal of Human Nutrition and Dietetics*, **17** (4), 317–35.

7
Behaviour change components of obesity treatment

Brent Van Dorsten

Department of Physical Medicine and Rehabilitation, University of Colorado Health Sciences Center, Aurora, CO USA

7.1   Introduction

While often considered a specific treatment, behaviour modification is best conceptualized as the application of a set of behaviour change strategies derived from the experimental analysis of human behaviour [1]. These strategies can be applied in various combinations to create adaptive desirable behaviours, strengthen and sustain their performance, and promote long-term durability of these behaviours. Brownell *et al.* [2] proposed three phases of behaviour change including exacting commitment and motivation for change, initial change, and maintenance of change. Behaviour change techniques can be applied to observable behaviours, cognitions or thoughts, and affect or mood. They are ubiquitously applied in weight management to modify environmental stimuli, behaviours and thoughts influencing food intake and physical activity. A fundamental assumption in applying behavioural strategies to weight loss is that the balance between behaviours controlling food intake and energy expenditure is tipped in the direction of excessive intake, and that these behaviours are learned and thus can be modified to produce a shift in this balance towards energy expenditure [3].

Persons with body mass index (BMI) of $25.0–29.9\,kg/m^2$ who have two or more health risk factors are encouraged to consume a low-calorie diet and increase physical activity consistent with the United States Surgeon General's recommendation for 30 minutes or more per day most days of the week [4,5]. This amount of activity has been shown effective in reducing risk of cardiovascular problems or diabetes [6], however has been shown to be less effective than studies achieving >150 minutes per week in producing weight loss [7]. To successfully maintain weight loss, a considerable amount

Obesity and Diabetes, Second Edition   Edited by Anthony H. Barnett and Sudhesh Kumar
© 2009 John Wiley & Sons, Ltd

of recent literature supports the use of even greater durations (e.g. $\geq$200–300 minutes per day) of exercise [8,9]. The need to increase energy expenditure for successful weight maintenance has been emphasized by multiple studies [10–13].

Behavioural lifestyle modification has comprised the fundamental cornerstone of weight loss and diabetes treatment for decades, and typically involves group-led weekly meetings focusing on dietary change, activity increase and instruction in behaviour change techniques. Treatment programme lengths have doubled from an average of 20 to over 40 weeks in the past two decades [14,15], with the active instructional phases typically lasting 16–26 weeks and follow-ups extended to one or more years. Dietary recommendations include limiting calories to 1000–1800 kcal/day with no more than 20–30% of calories from fat. Behaviour change strategies include improving food choices and decreasing portion sizes, and modifying the environments, cognitions, or emotions associated with maladaptive health patterns. For improving cardiovascular fitness and decreasing health risk, exercise prescriptions typically entail brisk walking some 30–40 minutes per day most days per week (e.g. $\geq$150 minutes of moderate intensity walking per week). In a study by Manson *et al.* [16], moderate intensity walking produced similar cardioprotective benefits as vigorous exercise for post-menopausal women while controlling for baseline age, race and BMI. Further, cumulative short bouts of exercise (i.e. 10 minutes) throughout the day have been associated with improved adherence and health benefits, and availability of home exercise equipment may also enhance outcomes [12,17]. While of limited value in producing weight loss, exercise appears to strongly contribute to improving weight maintenance [13,18–20].

7.2   The 'toxic environment'

The rapid escalation of overweight and obesity across genders, ages and ethnicities strongly implicates etiological factors that supercede genetics alone [21,22]. The term 'toxic environment' [23,24] has been coined to denote the rapid global changes shared by developed and developing countries. For years, overweight and obesity was pejoratively attributed to personality characteristics and this stance allowed environmental factors to escape close empirical investigation. Perceptions that obesity somehow signifies personal weakness or failure, and a public proclivity to blame or hold individuals with emotional or physical problems responsible for their circumstance [25] have been difficult to overcome. In fact, several published surveys of clinicians, nurses and researchers have identified a significant perpetuation of anti-obesity biases and stereotypes even among informed professionals [26–29]. Considering current population demographics the 'average' person in the population is overweight and gaining quickly.

It is beyond debate that prominent environmental obstacles to weight loss exist. Multiple dietary challenges exist including ready access to inexpensive, nutrient rich foods, drive-thru and food delivery, buffet dining, television advertising of unhealthy products, school contracts with soft drink companies, and availability of fast food outlets on school properties. The increase in the sedentary nature of the population reflects the 'double-edged sword' of technological advances that require less energy expenditure via physical labor and transportation, increased leisure time with abundant access to computers, the internet and games consoles, increased television viewing, decreased emphasis on physical education classes in schools, and ever-increasing safety concerns that restrict access to walking, playgrounds and other outdoor pursuits. King *et al.* [30] reported that living within 20 minutes of a park, walking trail or retail stores produced increases in walking in neighborhood residents suggesting the importance of community convenience as a factor.

Sedentary behaviour is a primary contributor to the increase in body weight and prevalence of diabetes. Sedentary activity has been shown to associate with a doubled risk of all-cause cardiovascular mortality [31,32], and the cardiovascular risks associated with sedentary activity may exceed the cardiac risk attributed to chronic disease processes like diabetes mellitus [33]. Van Dorsten [34] emphasized the need to address both decreasing sedentary activity *and* increasing physical activity in behavioural programmes designed to improve weight loss and overall health. In an increasingly technological world, sitting at one's desk and watching television after work increasingly compose the majority of daily activities for many adults. In fact, it has been reported that the average US adult spends 30 or more hours per week watching television [35], and television viewing has been shown to independently associate with obesity and diabetes risk. The television viewing estimates discussed above more than double the risk of type 2 diabetes for both men and women [36,37]. Hu *et al.* [37] estimated a 23% increased obesity risk and a 14% type 2 diabetes risk for each two hour per day increment that females watch television. In contrast, these authors reported that one hour per day of brisk walking produced a 24% reduction in obesity risk and 34% reduction in diabetes risk. As such, while the health benefits of consistent moderate intensity exercise are well known, the significant challenge to motivate and sustain behaviour change efforts against these environmental barriers is apparent [38].

7.3   Motivational readiness

Behavioural lifestyle modification strategies can be applied in weight management *before* a person begins increasing activity or makes their first intentional dietary change. Determining readiness to attempt behavioural change has been suggested as a useful factor in predicting sustained health behaviour change efforts [39], and has been specifically applied to readiness for behaviour change associated with weight loss [40–42].

In assessing readiness for change, obesity treatment providers frequently use motivational interviewing techniques [43] to assist patients in identifying personal motivations to attempt weight loss and to validate and analyze feelings of ambivalence they may feel about committing to weight loss. Motivational interviewing (MI) is designed to elucidate specific obstacles that might be encountered during behaviour change and mobilize personal resources to address these obstacles. MI techniques have been successfully applied to adherence with behavioural weight control and dietary change efforts in both adults and children [44,45]. In a comprehensive review of the MI and weight loss literature, Van Dorsten [46] concluded that literature supports the efficacy of MI adaptations for weight loss, weight loss maintenance, and increasing exercise behaviours and regimen adherence. In a meta-analysis of 72 clinical trials involving the application of MI techniques across a number of health behaviours [47], Hettema *et al.* concluded promising initial results for various MI applications in exercise, diet and eating disorder treatment. Motivational interview strategies have successfully been used in combination with other behavioural interventions to increase reported physical exercise [48–50], and studies utilizing MI in obesity treatment with various diet and exercise strategies have reported improved treatment adherence [44,51].

7.4 Patient expectations for treatment

A 5–10% reduction in body weight is considered sufficient to improve health risk factors and to increase the probability for weight loss maintenance. However, previous research has obviated the need to explicitly identify patient goals for weight loss treatments. Foster *et al.* [52] assessed the 'dream weight', 'happy weight', 'goal weight', acceptable weight' and disappointing weight' of 60 obese women prior to beginning a 48 week behavioural weight loss treatment programme. Surprisingly, this group identified a 32% reduction in total body weight as their average weight loss goal. Nearly half of the 45 women who completed the 48 week treatment did not achieve even a 'disappointing' weight loss goal, despite losing an average 16 kg during the programme. This 16 kg loss – a 16% total body weight reduction - was approximately one-half of the desired loss, and none of the participants reached their 'dream' weight. Foster *et al.* [53] reported similarly unreasonable weight loss goals for patients seeking weight loss via either behavioural interventions or surgery, with the heaviest of participants desiring the greatest absolute weight losses to meet their satisfaction. Unrealistic weight loss expectations were also identified in persons seeking pharmacological treatment for obesity as subjective pretreatment weight loss goals were nearly 25% of total body weight [54]. Of significant clinical interest, Wadden *et al.* [53] reported that provision of both explicit verbal and written information regarding what participants might reasonably expect for weight loss with one year of sibutramine use (5–15% of total body weight) had little impact on the continued unreasonable expectations of participants throughout weight loss treatment.

7.5 Behavioural modification strategies in obesity treatment

There are multiple published articles describing the commonly employed behavioural modification strategies for dietary change, exercise adoption, and relapse prevention [56–59]. Useful techniques in modifying behaviours associated with weight loss are: establishing reasonable, specific short- and long-term goals; daily self-monitoring of dietary intake and exercise behaviours; modifying the environment to support adaptive changes; using stimulus control techniques to modify environmental and intrapersonal factors that precede and cue food intake; cognitive restructuring to address maladaptive thoughts impacting behaviour change; problem-solving environmental, emotional, or motivational challenges to change efforts; enlisting social support resources, and relapse prevention training. Several examples of how the primary behavioural modifications strategies might be incorporated into the weight loss process are provided in Table 7.1.

Table 7.1 Examples of applications of behavioral modification strategies in weight loss

Behavioral technique	General purpose(s)	Potential targets/examples

Goal setting	Specify realistic, measurable, obtainable incremental goals for target behaviours	Gradual weight loss
		    0.5–1 kg per week weight loss
		    Daily calorie range goal
		    Daily fat gram goal
		Activity increase
		    Minutes per day/week
		    Number of steps on pedometer
		    Number of days per week

Self-monitoring	Increase awareness of behaviour patterns Increase accuracy of behaviour estimates Reinforce changes in target behaviours	Dietary intake (fat, calories) Eating patterns (time, portions) Activity minutes/Pedometer steps Factors influencing food intake Mood, social events Medication adherence Self-monitoring BG

Stimulus control/cues	Prompt occurrence of target behaviours	Keep walking shoes in sight
		
		Electronic calendar prompts
		Colour dots to prompt behaviours
		    BG checks
		    Medication intake
		    Exercise initiation
		    Reminder of calorie goals

Changing the environment	Making changes in the home and social environments to encourage behaviour change	Modify shopping habits to increase Availability of desired food choices Pre-packaged foods or meal supplements available for use Making exercise shoes/clothes conveniently available for use

(*continued*)

Table 7.1 (*Continued*)

Behavioral technique	General purpose(s)	Potential targets/examples
		Increase exposure to social others with similar behavior change goals or involve friends in family in efforts to lose weight for support
Problem solving	Provide step-wise structure to modify challenges to consistent efforts at behaviour change	Obstacles to exercise adherence
		Adverse weather
		Minor injury
		Social pressure to limit
		Obstacles to healthy food intake
		Holidays/social parties
		Eating in restaurants
		Skipping meals
		Social pressure to eat
Cognitive restructuring	Identify and modify negative or self-defeating thoughts and increase rewarding thoughts to encourage change efforts	Challenge maladaptive self-perceptions
		'Slow metabolism' problem
		Lazy, weak, failure
		Lack will-power
		Encouraging thoughts
		Will succeed in the long run
		Little changes will help
		A lapse is not a crisis
		Proud of myself for trying

Goal setting

Considering the important potential divergence of treatment goals between providers and treatment seekers, the development of realistic attainable goals prior to beginning weight loss is critical to facilitating personal acceptance and maintenance of losses actually achieved. Behaviour change goals in obesity treatment may include targeting a specific number of pounds to lose (as opposed to a more obscure goal of 'losing some weight'), specific metabolic or psychosocial improvements, or potential changes in medication intake or insulin requirements for co-morbid conditions. Potential decreases in oral medication requirements for co-morbid health conditions are often a salient motivation for individuals to begin and maintain behavioural lifestyle changes. Behavioural weight loss goals of 8–10% total body weight are attainable and can produce important health risk reductions. Further, establishing moderate weight loss goals may be associated with more successful achievement and long-term maintenance of these goals [60]. An overall weight loss goal can be subdivided into weekly goals for 0.5–0.75 kg (1–1.5 lb) losses with precise identification of the incremental behaviour changes necessary to produce this outcome. These incremental changes may include restricting calorie and fat intake and increasing minutes of physical activity. Explicit behavioural commitments or contracts between an individual and a counsellor or group can assist in clarifying the frequency, intensity and duration of activities the person will perform to attain these weekly or monthly goals. These behaviour change contracts, often publicly signed by others witnessing the commitment, can be important strategies in motivating patients to maintaining efforts over time [61,62]. Behavioural contracts should clearly specify the contingencies under which the person will reward themselves for the efforts they have made to change behaviour. Since weight itself is not a behaviour, but rather an *artifact* of several behaviours, rewards must be contingent upon behavioural effort (i.e. number of times walked or number of minutes accumulated) and not outcome (i.e. number of pounds lost).

Self-monitoring

Self-monitoring describes the systematic recording of a behaviour that is targeted for change. In weight loss, calories or fat grams consumed, minutes of daily walking, number of steps taken, and even emotional factors influencing food intake can be quantified via self-monitoring. Self-recording may serve many purposes including establishing baseline values of a behaviour, increasing awareness of personal patterns, improving accuracy of unstructured behaviour estimates, and providing feedback and reinforcement for changes in a target behaviour. Ensuring accurate base rates of targeted behaviours is critical as the published error in unstructured estimates of caloric intake and energy expenditure may reach 50% [63–65]. Consistent and accurate self-monitoring has been identified as an important component in maintaining long-term weight loss [66], and successfully maintaining weight during shorter 'high-risk for regain' periods such as the holidays [67,68]. Wadden *et al.* [69] reported that weight loss subjects who more frequently recorded their food intake during weight loss actually lost more than twice the weight than those who did so infrequently.

Stimulus control

Stimulus control is the term applied to the behaviour change strategy designed to identify and modify environmental cues associated with food or activity patterns. Environmental cues which prompt overeating or sedentary behaviours may be modified to those which more adaptively prompt and support improved eating habits or physical activity [70]. For example, cues (e.g. colour dots) may be intentionally placed in a person's home to prompt medication adherence, walking shoes can be placed in visible sight to cue increased walking, and snack foods may be removed from the home to remove a cue for eating undesirable foods. Considering the media bombardment of cues that promote food intake and inactivity, the utilization of personal environmental cues can be immensely helpful in 'reminding' patients of behaviour change goals and agreements in the interim between group or counselor visits. While a 167: 1 ratio may be considered weak in mathematical terms, this ratio may represent the 'best case scenario' in weight loss treatment. Specifically, if a counselor were to meet with a weight loss client every week for 1 hour, this person would have 167 hours in this same week to independently attempt to implement changes. Utilizing additional 'prompts' to cue the occurrence of new behaviours and motivate daily efforts may increase long-term success.

Changing the environment

Any of several combinations of the behavioural strategies discussed can be used to alter one's environment from one that tolerates or promotes inactivity and poor dietary habits to one that prompts and supports change efforts. Altering shopping habits to increase the ready availability of positive food choices, prearranging snacks, and ridding pantries of undesirable foods can all contribute to improving food choices and promoting decreased calorie intake. Arranging exercise equipment near televisions or windows increases availability and convenience and provides an important visual prompt to exercise. Packing several sets of exercise clothes and shoes to be kept in one's home, office and car may further increase the ease of initiating exercise sessions. Rearranging home, meal and work schedules to include and account for activity periods can raise the probability that exercise will occur. Surveying one's neighborhood for available parks, sidewalks, malls or exercise facilities that can be incorporated into a physical activity regimen is critical. Changing one's environment might also including modifying the social environment to increase exposure to others who are similarly attempting behaviour change or to increase contact with those who support and encourage weight loss efforts to improve health.

Problem solving

In prolonged obesity treatment, few patients might accurately anticipate the number and intensity of obstacles they might encounter as they strive to initiate and sustain diet and activity changes across time and settings. As such, a valuable component of behavioural skill instruction is providing individuals with a framework for identifying, defining and problem solving physical, environmental, or psychosocial challenges to sustained performance. Problem-solving strategies compose five steps including:

1. identification and detailed definition of a specific challenge;

2. brainstorming potential alternatives;

3. weighing the relative benefits and disadvantages of each option;

4. selecting and implementing the option that holds the highest probability for rectifying the circumstance;

5. evaluating efficacy after implementation.

These strategies can be flexibly applied to any number of challenges including time management or schedule conflicts, employment or transportation issues, adverse weather, minor physical injuries, holidays or restaurant eating, or mood or negative self-talk challenges. As most active treatment programmes are time limited, problem-solving training can provide individuals with a systematic framework to define and solve unforeseen challenges to attaining their weight loss goals. Perri *et al.* [71] reported that the inclusion of problem-solving significantly improved weight loss maintenance.

Cognitive restructuring

Emotional factors can have considerable impact on a person's dedication to weight change and may be a strong antecedent to overeating or abandoning activity. Negative affect and self-defeating cognitions regarding one's ability to succeed at weight loss may hamper efforts. Most obese persons have endured many unsuccessful weight loss attempts and this history can fuel maladaptive expectations of future failure if not addressed as a part of comprehensive cognitive behavioural treatment. Negative self-attributions associated with failure to lose weight (e.g. 'can't do it', 'weak', or 'don't have the willpower') or inaccurate physical attributions such as having a resistant or 'slow metabolism' are frequently encountered in weight treatment. While the latter may seem desirable as a potential explanation for failure to achieve weight loss despite repeated efforts, one recent study rejected this phenomenon as a primary explanation for failure to lose weight [65].

Based upon with work of Beck and colleagues, cognitive–behavioural theory suggests that cognition and behaviour are in part determined by perceptions of self and the factors believed to control one's world. Tailored cognitive restructuring involves teaching individuals to become aware of maladaptive cognitive perceptions or 'distortions' [72], and to explicitly describe and actively challenge maladaptive self-perceptions. A variety of behavioural change strategies may be combined to increase awareness (e.g. self-monitoring of cognitions), devise a change plan (e.g. problem-solving alternatives to negative self-talk), and reinforcing efforts to challenge the validity of these perceptions. In an impressive report of the potential influence of addressing weight related thoughts and beliefs, Stahre *et al.* [73] reported significantly greater weight losses at 10 weeks and 18 months for women subjects assigned to a cognitive therapy group than for those assigned to a behavioural programme. These results reiterated findings by Stahre and Hallstrom [74] who reported 10.4 kg weight loss for subjects who completed a 10 week manual-led cognitive treatment designed to target self-control, self-esteem related to weight and weight change, and stress expression.

Social support

Just as weight gain in one's familial and social network has been shown to have significant influence on a given individual's likelihood of weight gain [75], increasing social support and influential others' awareness of behaviour change efforts can positively affect long-term motivation and results. Existing data suggests that those who perceive greater social support, attend weight loss groups, and who involve family or friends in weight loss efforts may more successfully lose weight, increase physical activity, and sustain efforts for a longer period of time [76–82].

Behavioural weight loss is typically conducted in closed groups as peer familiarity, validation of struggles, modelling coping and incremental success, encouragement and group accountability to meet goals all add important dimensions to the weight loss process. In order to promote real-world adoption of behavioural changes, primary social support may be transitioned from weight loss counsellors or the weight loss group to resources in the person's social circle. The frequency of group meetings is typically faded over time and participants are taught to engender personal social support resources to maintain their efforts. These personal social supports may include family, friends, physicians, community support groups, or electronic contacts (e.g. diet-related web sites, chat rooms).

Relapse prevention

The most commonly identified problem in obesity treatment is long-term maintenance of weight loss [77,83,84]. A primary factor known to contribute to adherence with behaviour change strategies and maintenance of weight loss is maintaining episodic long-term contact with treatment providers and/or peers [85–87]. These follow-up contacts can be accomplished via face-to-face meetings, telephone or email [88–90]. The optimal frequency of maintenance contacts is largely unknown, but should be devised in response to attendance and weight maintenance data. Restart programmes which give patients the opportunity to re-engage in an active intervention strategy for a short period of time (e.g. exercise groups or meal replacements for 6 weeks) may be offered to re-establish the benefits and behavioural patterns of the active intervention. It should be noted however that Smith and Wing [91] found that repeated diets produced lower levels of programme adherence and less weight loss than was achieved during an original intervention period. Alternatively, provision of personal trainers and monetary incentives [13,92], and group-contingent work site competitions [62,93] have been successfully used to achieve ongoing participation with weight loss programmes.

Many unique insights regarding successful maintenance of weight loss have been gained from the members of the National Weight Control Registry (NWCR), a roster of several thousand people who have lost at least 13 kg (30 lb) and maintained this loss for at least 1 year [66]. In fact, the average weight loss of Registry members is 30 kg (67 lb) with an average successful maintenance period of over 5 years. While registry members endorsed using several dietary strategies to lose weight, three primary strategies have been utilized in their efforts to maintain losses. Consistent self-monitoring of intake, frequent weighing, and increasing physical activity beyond that required to produce initial weight loss remain strong recommendations.

On a positive note, NWCR members have reported that as time since original weight loss increases, maintenance requires fewer strategies and becomes more pleasurable [94]. Considering the importance of sustained physical exercise to weight maintenance, it is somewhat encouraging that studies have reported that participants who exercised in the convenience of their homes, as compared to exercising at a weight loss clinic or health club, demonstrated increased adherence, weight maintenance, and in some cases continued weight reduction [95–97]. This finding, coupled with the evidence supporting the benefits of accumulating short bouts of activity, provides promise for achieving the increased activity levels necessary for weight maintenance.

7.6 Efficacy of combination treatments

It is difficult to succinctly evaluate the efficacy of 'behavioural management' of obesity since the term generally encompasses all facets of treatment aside from surgery. Considering the multiple variations of diet, physical activity and behavioural modification strategies – and adding adherence techniques, relapse prevention, meal replacements, motivational interviewing adaptations, and medication to this matrix – an exponential number of combinations exist against which to assess the success of treatment packages. A brief review of the relative contribution of these components to obesity treatment follows.

Behavioural treatments

Behavioural treatments for weight loss are designed to produce a 0.5–1.0 kg average weekly weight reduction, or an approximate 8.5–9.0 kg decrease (8–10% of total body weight) from pre- to post-treatment, with attrition rates generally under 20% [15,98,99].

In an early report of the efficacy of behavioural-based treatment, Bjorvell and Rossner [100] assigned 107 obese subjects (basal BMI women 40.5, men 42.9) to receive a 6-week clinic-based intervention consisting of twice weekly group behavioural therapy, a supervised 600 kcal/day clinic diet plus nutritional advice on low-fat cooking, and therapist-led exercise three times per week. This programme also provided a remarkable 4-year maintenance programme with optional weekly weighing and nutritional 'booster sessions'. Those who did not attend boosters were frequently contacted via telephone or letter, and those who relapsed were provided short-term 'refresher courses'. Mean weight losses for women and men at 6 weeks, 1 year, and 4 years were 10.0/12.2 kg, 15.0/30.9 kg, and 11.5/18.4 kg respectively. Study attrition at four years was 31%. A follow-up of this study indicated average weight losses maintained at 10–12 year follow-up equalled 9.5 kg for women, and 17.5 kg for men [101]. While the authors demonstrated that a comprehensive behavioural modification programme could produce positive long-term weight loss results, the findings are difficult to compare with current studies given the comprehensiveness and duration of the intervention.

Few recent studies have specifically compared different combinations of diet and exercise versus diet alone, and some studies surprisingly fail to support the benefits of combining strategies. Skender *et al.* [102] reported marginal but non-significant differences in diet plus exercise versus diet alone, in a study whose conclusions were limited by attrition. Wadden *et al.* [103] reported the 1 year follow-up of a clinical trial which compared four conditions including diet alone, diet plus either aerobic or strength training, or combination of all. All participants received similar diets and a 48-week group behavioural programme. At week 48, participants across all groups averaged a 15.1 kg weight loss, and no significant difference was noted between groups. Weight losses were well maintained, but no group differences were found at one-year follow-up. Wing [15] suggests that these studies may fail to support combining strategies as participants struggled to maintain sufficient long-term exercise adherence to adequately assess the potential effect in each. A host of additional articles support the superiority of diet plus exercise interventions in producing weight loss and long-term weight loss maintenance [104–106]. Several large-scale national studies have provided further evidence that standard behavioural recommendations for weight loss including reduced caloric diet and increased physical activity can produce moderate sustained weight loss and decreased health risks in overweight or obese adults with type 2 diabetes, and prevent or delay onset of type 2 diabetes in those at high risk for up to 3 years [16,107,108].

Both the provision of food products and structured meal plans has been reported to improve weight loss results. Jeffrey *et al.* [109] found that patients who were prescribed standard reduced calorie diets, and were provided most of the food for this diet, lost significantly more weight after 6 and 18 months of treatment than did patients who were randomized to a self-selected decreased calorie diet. Wing *et al.* [110] expanded these results by reporting that the provision of structured meal plans (i.e. what to eat for specific meals) produced similar results without providing food.

Very low calorie diets (VLCD)

Very-low-calorie diets typically provide less than 800 kcal/d (as compared with low-calorie-diets ([LCD] 800–1500 kcal/day), but include sufficient amounts of protein (i.e. lean meat, fowl, or liquid formula) to minimize loss of lean muscle mass during weight loss. Several studies in the past two decades have confirmed the capacity of VLCD to produce superior weight loss [111–113]. The common features of these studies include stringent dietary intake restrictions, with or without behavioural counselling, and follow up of 1–8 years [111,112,114]. Aggregate results suggest that VLCD typically produces weight reductions of 15–25% of baseline body weight within 8–16 weeks of treatment [115]. While this weight loss is significant in comparison to the low calorie self-selected food diets, rapid regain is common with VLCD diets and non-significant differences in weight loss are common between the two dietary approaches at one-year post treatment [113,116]. The addition of behaviour therapy in addition to VLCD alone appears to marginally improve weight loss maintenance.

As before, the efficacy of behavioural weight loss approaches is diminished by the disappointing durability of changes. Problems with weight regain are well known, with most patients regaining at least 30–40% of initial weight loss at 1 year, and more than half regaining all weight lost within 3–5 years [117]. These results must be viewed however in light of epidemiological observations that without treatment most obese individuals naturalistically gain 0.5–1 kg per year [118,119].

Liquid meal replacements

Despite their historical public popularity, liquid meal replacements have received relatively little empirical attention until the recent past. Ditschuneit *et al.* [120] conducted a study in which 100 patients received nutrition consultation and random assignment for three months to either a 1200–1500 kcal/day self-selected diet or an isoenergetic diet in which two meals and two snacks per day were replaced liquid meal replacements. After three-months of treatment, both groups were prescribed a similar energy-restricted 1200–1500 kcal/day diet with one meal and one snack replacement for an additional 2 years. Three month results indicated mean weight losses of 1.5 and 7.8 kg for the respective groups, with increased weight losses to 3.2 and 8.4 kg per respective group approximately four-years after treatment initiation [121].

In an interesting minimal contact, community-based intervention, Rothacker [118] replaced two meals per day with liquid meal replacements for 3 months for 141 overweight adults, then 1–2 per day until reaching an unspecified weight goal. If regain of more than 1–2 kg occurred at any point in the following 5 years, patients were encouraged to return to the twice daily replacements. After weekly weighing at a local facility for the first 12 weeks, patients were then seen twice yearly for maintenance with no other treatment provided. Data for this treatment group was compared against age- and weight-matched no treatment controls who simply provided weights in 1992 and 1997. In the initial 3-month treatment phase, weight loss for treatment males and females were 7.4 and 6.4 kg, with losses of 5.9 and 4.2 kg maintained at 5 years. Control males and females *gained* 6.7 and 6.5 kg respectively over the 5 year period. This investigation suggests that meal replacements, with even minimal additional contact, may be capable of producing modest weight losses. A number of additional studies suggest that meal replacement strategies may produce larger initial weight losses and improved maintenance of losses versus standard dietary changes alone [122–124], and meal replacements have been incorporated into the dietary intervention in the multi-centre, multi-year Look Ahead study (2007) [107].

Behavioural modification plus pharmacotherapy

Published guidelines from a National Institutes of Health (NIH) expert panel on obesity recommend that pharmacological interventions are appropriate for persons with BMI $\geq$ 30.0 kg/m^2, BMI $\geq$ 27 kg/m^2 with co-morbid health conditions, or for those who have not achieved weight reduction with repeated conservative efforts [4]. A history of adverse events has plagued pharmacological attempts at weight management [125,126], and despite the five years since the initial publishing of this book, there remain only two US Federal Drug Administration (FDA) approved medications for obesity treatment. Sibutramine (Meridia) is a central nervous system agent that inhibits the reuptake of norepinephrine and serotonin, and functions by reducing appetite and energy intake [127]. This medication has been shown to produce both initial and sustained weight loss with and without the addition of behavioural therapy [127,128]. In contrast, orlistat (Xenical) does not act on the central nervous system, but functions as a lipase inhibitor blocking the absorption of about one-third of consumed fat. Orlistat may also modify food preference via aversive conditioning and the unpleasant gastrointestinal symptoms commonly experienced after high fat intake. Both medications are typically prescribed as an adjunct to diet, exercise and behaviour modification to produce greater initial losses, while receiving the reduction in health risks associated with healthy lifestyle.

Phelan and Wadden [129] provided a comprehensive review of published double-blind, placebo controlled trials of both orlistat and sibutramine and lifestyle modification for obesity. Similar to behavioural treatment, obesity medications typically produce losses of 8–10% of initial weight for up to 2 years with continued use [115,126], and the combination of strategies appears to enhance both initial weight losses and maintenance. Wadden *et al.* [54] reported significantly greater weight losses and patient satisfaction at one year when behavioural care was added to sibutramine treatment alone. In a comprehensive study comparing sibutramine (15 mg per day) alone, Sibutramine plus brief primary care physician counseling, lifestyle modification counselling alone, or lifestyle counseling plus sibutramine, Wadden *et al.* [69] reported that subjects receiving drug plus a lifestyle modification programme lost significantly more weight than all other conditions. All subjects in this study received similar dietary and exercise recommendations.

Similarly, two studies reported significantly greater losses and 1 year maintenance with orlistat and behavioural care versus placebo and behavioural care [130,131]. Orlistat has been shown to produce losses of 5–13% of initial weight, with 2-year maintenance of the majority of weight lost [129]. Hoping to combine mechanisms of action, Wadden *et al.* [132] found no additional benefit of adding orlistat to patients who had lost weight during 1 year of treatment with sibutramine plus lifestyle. Nonetheless, continued investigation of the optimal combinations of medications, doses and behavioural packages appears strongly indicated.

7.7   Conclusions and future work

Despite advances in the treatment of obesity in the past 20 years, practitioners have been unable to turn back the obesity epidemic. Significant environmental challenges to behaviour change exist and substantiate the need to continue to refine and improve treatments. Dunn *et al.* [88] reported that many positive study results have had little demonstrated impact on the magnitude of the global obesity problem as most studies have employed time and resource demanding individual or small group intervention strategies. These authors suggested strategies to reach larger numbers of individuals via work-site programmes, computer-based programmes or web-based behaviour change programmes. Wing [133] similarly encouraged the development of large-scale interventions including improved community development to increase activity convenience (e.g. sidewalks, improved lighting) and community programme development (e.g. walking programmes) to address the broad need to increase the general public's physical activity.

Obesity treatment programmes must necessarily be designed to provide extended provider contact, and flexibly combine cognitive and behavioural, meal replacement and perhaps pharmacological treatment strategies. Combination treatment packages appear more promising in achieving long-term weight loss than single treatments, and multidisciplinary provider teams may improve adherence, initial losses and maintenance. Treatment programmes should include both community-based and in-home resources for increasing physical activity whenever possible. Obesity must be conceptualized as a chronic health condition similar to diabetes or hypertension, and physicians using pharmacotherapy must be prepared to provide long-term management [130]. Given the limited number and availability of behaviourally-trained professionals to confront this problem, non-behavioural community providers (e.g. physicians, physician assistants, nurses) must be trained to competently utilize behavioural modification strategies with their patients on a daily basis, since until more treatment resources arrive, the bulk of the responsibility for weight change may continue to reside with the individual and their primary care providers.

References

1. Miltenberger, R.G. (1997) *Behavior Modification: Principles and Procedures*, Brooks/Cole Publishing Company, Pacific Grove, CA.
2. Brownell, K.D., Marlatt, G.A., Lichtenstein, E. and Wilson, G.T. (1986) Understanding and preventing relapse. *American Psychologist*, **41**, 765–82.
3. Jeffery, R.W., Epstein, L.H., Wilson, G.T. *et al.* (2000) Long-term maintenance of weight loss: Current status. *Health Psychology*, **19** (1 Suppl), 5S–16S.
4. National Heart, Lung, and Blood Institute (NHLBI) & North American Association for the Study of Obesity (NAASO) (2000) *Practical Guide to the Identification, Evaluation, and Treatment of Overweight and Obesity in Adults*, National Institutes of Health, Bethesda, MD.
5. United States Department of Health and Human Services (1996) *Physical Activity and Health: A Report of the Surgeon General*, Centers for Disease Control, Atlanta, GA.
6. Diabetes Prevention Program Research Group (2002) Reduction in the incidence of type 2 diabetes with lifestyle intervention and metformin. *New England Journal of Medicine*, **346** (6), 393–403.
7. Paffenberger, R.S., Wing, A.L. and Hyde, R.T. (1978) Physical activity as an index of heart attack risk in college alumni. *American Journal of Epidemiology*, **108**, 161–75.
8. American College of Sports Medicine (2001) Appropriate intervention strategies for weight loss and prevention of weight regain for adults. *Medicine and Science in Sports and, Exercise*, **33**, 2145–56.

9. Jakicic, J.M. and Otto, A.D. (2005) Physical activity considerations for the treatment and prevention of obesity. *American Journal of Clinical Nutrition*, **82**, S226–S229.

10. Jakicic, J. (2002) The role of physical activity in prevention and treatment of body weight gain in adults. *Journal of Nutrition*, **132**, S3826–S3829.

11. Jakicic, J.M., Wing, R.R. and Winters-Hart, C. (2002) Relationship of physical activity to eating behaviors and weight loss in women. *Medicine and Science in Sports and Exercise*, **34**, 1635–9.

12. Jakicic, J., Winters, C., Lang, W. and Wing, R.R. (1999) Effects of intermittent exercise and use of home exercise equipment on adherence, weight loss, and fitness in overweight women. *Journal of the American Medical Association*, **282**, 1554–60.

13. Jeffrey, R.W., Wing, R.R., Thorson, C. and Burton, L.R. (1998) Use of personal trainers and financial incentives to increase exercise in a behavioral weight loss program. *Journal of Consulting and Clinical, Psychology*, **66** (5), 777–83.

14. Perri, M.G., Nezu, A.M., Patti, E.T. and McCann, K.L. (1989) Effect of length of treatment on weight loss. *Journal of Consulting and Clinical, Psychology*, **57**, 450–2.

15. Wing, R.R. (2002) Behavioral weight control, in *Handbook of Obesity Treatment* (eds T.A. Wadden and A.J. Stunkard), Guilford Press, New York, pp. 301–16.

16. Manson, J.E., Greenland, P., LaCroix, A.Z. *et al.* (2002) Walking compared with vigorous exercise for the prevention of cardiovascular events in women. *New England Journal of Medicine*, **347**, 716–25.

17. DeBusk, R.F., Stenestrand, U., Sheehan, M. and Haskell, W.L. (1990) Training effects of long versus short bouts of exercise in healthy subjects. *American Journal of Cardiology*, **65**, 1010–3.

18. Grilo, C.M. (1995) The role of physical activity in weight loss and weight loss management. *Medicine, Exercise, Nutrition and Health*, **4**, 60–76.

19. Pronk, N.P. and Wing, R.R. (1994) Physical activity and long-term maintenance of weight loss. *Obesity Research*, **2**, 587–99.

20. Wing, R.R. (1999) Physical activity in the treatment of adulthood overweight and obesity: current evidence and research issues. *Medicine and Science in Sports and, Exercise*, **31**, S547–S552.

21. Hill, J.O. and Peters, J.R. (1998) Environmental contributions to the obesity epidemic. *Science*, **280**, 1371–4.

22. Popkin, B.M. and Doak, C.M. (1998) The obesity epidemic is a worldwide phenomenon. *Nutrition Reviews*, **56**, 106–14.

23. Battle-Horgen, K. and Brownell, K.D. (2002) Confronting the toxic environment: environmental and public health actions in a world crisis, in *Handbook of Obesity Treatment* (eds T.A. Wadden and A.J. Stunkard), Guilford Press, New York, pp. 95–107.

24. Wadden, T.A., Brownell, K.D. and Foster, G.D. (2002) Obesity: responding to the global epidemic. *Journal of Consulting and Clinical Psychology*, **70** (3), 510–25.

25. Wortman, C.B. and Silver, R.C. (1989) The myths of coping with loss. *Journal of Consulting and Clinical Psychology*, **57** (3), 349–57.

26. Bagley, C.R., Conklin, D.N., Isherwood, R.T. *et al.* (1989) Attitudes of nurses toward obesity and obese patients. *Perceptual and Motor Skills*, **68**, 954.

27. Brown, I. (2006) Nurses' attitudes towards adult patients who are obese: literature review. *Journal of Advanced Nursing*, **53**, 221–32.

28. Maroney, D. and Golub, S. (1992) Nurses' attitudes toward obese persons and certain ethnic groups. *Perceptual and Motor Skills*, **75**, 387–91.

29. Schwartz, M.B., O'Neal Chambliss, H., Brownell, K.D. *et al.* (2003) Weight bias among health professionals specializing in obesity. *Obesity Research*, **11** (9), 1033–9.

30. King, A.C., Brach, J.S., Belle, S. *et al.* (2003) The relationship between convenience of destinations and walking levels in older women. *American Journal of Public Health*, **18**, 74–82.

31. Blair, S.N., Kohl, H.W., Paffenbarger, R.S. *et al.* (1989) Physical fitness and all-cause mortality: A prospective study of healthy men and women. *Journal of the American Medical Association*, **262**, 2395–401.

32. Kujala, U.M., Kaprio, J., Sarna, S. and Koskenvuo, M. (1998) Relationship of leisure-time physical activity and mortality. *Journal of the American Medical Association*, **276**, 440–4.

33. Blair, S.N., Kampert, J.B., Kohl, H.W. *et al.* (1996) Influences of cardiorespiratory fitness and other precursors on cardiovascular disease and all-cause mortality in men and women. *Journal of the American Medical Association*, **276**, 205–10.

34. Van Dorsten, B. *Behavior Change Strategies for Increasing Exercise in Diabetes*, Humana Press, Totowa, NJ.

35. Nielsen Report on Television (1998) New York: Nielsen Media Research.

36. Hu, F.B., Leitzmann, M.F., Stampfler, M.J. *et al.* (2001) Physical activity and television watching in relation to risk of type 2 diabetes in men. *Archives of Internal Medicine*, **1612**, 1542–8.

37. Hu, F.B., Li, T.Y., Colditz, G.A. *et al.* (2003) Television watching and other sedentary behaviors in relation to risk of obesity and type 2 diabetes mellitus in women. *Journal of the American Medical Association*, **289**, 1785–91.

38. Dubbert, P.M. (2002) Physical activity and exercise: recent advances and current challenges. *Journal of Consulting and Clinical Psychology*, **70** (3), 526–36.

39. Prochaska, J.L., DiClemente, C.C. and Norcross, J.C. (1992) In search of how people change: applications to addictive behaviors. *American Psychologist*, **47**, 1102–14.

40. Clark, M.M., Pera, V., Goldstein, M.G. *et al.* (1996) Counseling strategies for obese patients. *American Journal of Preventive Medicine*, **12**, 266–70.

41. Curry, S.J., Kristal, A.R. and Bowen, D.J. (1992) An application of the stage model of behavior change to dietary fat reduction. *Health Education Research*, **7**, 97–105.

42. Greene, G.W., Rossi, S.R., Rossi, J.S. *et al.* (1999) Dietary applications of the stages of change model. *Journal of the American Dietetic Association*, **99** (6), 673–8.

43. Miller, W.R. and Rollnick, S. (2002) *Motivational Interviewing: Preparing People for Change*, Guilford Press, New York.

44. Smith, D., Heckemeyer, C., Kratt, P. and Mason, D. (1997) Motivational interviewing to improve adherence to a behavioral weight-control program for older obese women with NIDDM. *Diabetes Care*, **20** (1), 52–8.

45. Berg-Smith, S.M., Stevens, J.J., Brown, K.M. *et al.* (1999) A brief motivational intervention to improve dietary adherence in adolescents. *Health Education Research*, **14** (3), 399–410.

46. Van Dorsten, B. (2007) The use of motivational interviewing in weight loss. *Current Diabetes Reports*, **7**, 386–90.

47. Hettema, J., Steele, J. and Miller, W.R. (2005). Motivational interviewing. *Annual Review of Clinical Psychology*, **1**, 91–111.

48. Brodie, D.A. and Inoue, A. (2005) Motivational interviewing to promote physical activity for people with chronic heart failure. *Journal of Advanced Nursing*, **50**, 518–27.

49. Jones, K.D., Burchhardt, C.S. and Bennett, J.A. (2004) Motivational interviewing may encourage exercise in persons with fibromyalgia by enhancing self efficacy. *Arthritis and Rheumatism*, **51**, 864–7.

50. Scales, R. and Miller, J.H. (2003) Motivational techniques for improving compliance with an exercise program: Skills for primary care physicians. *Current Sports Medicine Reports*, **2**, 166–72.

51. DiLillo, V., Siegfried, N.J. and Smith-West, D. (2003) Incorporating motivational interviewing into behavioral obesity treatment. *Cognitive Behavioral Practice*, **10**, 120–30.

52. Foster, G.D., Wadden, T.A., Vogt, R.A. and Brewer, G. (1997) What is reasonable weight loss? Patient's expectations and evaluations of obesity treatment outcomes. *Journal of Consulting and Clinical Psychology*, **65** (1), 79–85.

53. Foster, G.D., Wadden, T.A., Phelan, S. *et al.* (2001) Obese patient's perceptions of treatment outcomes and the factors that influence them. *Archives of Internal Medicine*, **161** (17), 2133–9.

54. Wadden, T.A., Berkowitz, R.I., Sarwer, D.B. *et al.* (2001) Benefits of lifestyle modification in the pharmacological treatment of obesity. *Archives of Internal Medicine*, **161**, 218–27.

55. Wadden, T.A., Womble, L.G., Sarwer, D.B. *et al.* (2003) Great expectations: 'I'm losing 25% of my weight no matter what you say.' *Journal of Consulting and Clinical Psychology*, **71** (6), 1084–9.

56. Brownell, K.D. (2000) *The LEARN Program for Weight Management 2000*, American Health, Dallas, TX.

57. Foreyt, J.P. and Poston, W.S.C. (1998) What is the role of cognitive-behavioral therapy in patient management? *Obesity Research*, **6** (Suppl), 18S–22S.

58. Poston, W.S.C. and Foreyt, J.P. (2000) Successful management of the obese patient. *American Family Physician*, **61**, 3615–22.

59. Wing, R.R. (1998) Behavioral approaches to the treatment of obesity, in *Handbook of Obesity* (eds G. Bray, C. Bouchard and W.P.T. James), Marcel Dekker, New York, pp. 855–73.

60. Jeffrey, R.W., Wing, R.R. and Mayer, R.R. (1998) Are smaller weight losses or more achievable weight loss goals better in the long term for obese patients? *Journal of Consulting and Clinical Psychology*, **66** (4), 641–5.

61. Ureda, J.R. (1980) The effect of contract witnessing on motivation and weight loss in a weight control program. *Health Education Quarterly*, **7**, 163–84.

62. Zandee, G.L. and Oermann, M.H. (1996) Effectiveness of contingency contracting. *American Association of Occupational Health Nursing Journal*, **44**, 183–8.

63. Bandini, L.G., Schoeller, D.A., Cyr, H.N. and Dietz, W.H. (1990) Validity of reported energy intake in obese and non-obese adolescents. *American Journal of Clinical Nutrition*, **52**, 421–5.

64. Irwin, M.L., Ainsworth, B.E. and Conway, J.M. (2001) Estimation of energy expenditure from physical activity measures: determinants of accuracy. *Obesity Research*, **9**, 517–25.

65. Lichtman, S.W., Pisarska, K., Berman, E.R. *et al.* (1992) Discrepancy between self-reported and actual caloric intake and exercise in obese subjects. *New England Journal of Medicine*, **327**, 1893–8.

66. Klem, M.L., Wing, R.R., McGuire, M.T. *et al.* (1997) A descriptive study of individuals successful at long-term maintenance of substantial weight loss. *American Journal of Clinical Nutrition*, **66**, 239–46.

67. Boutelle, K.N. and Kirschenbaum, D.S. (1998) Further support for consistent self-monitoring as a vital component of successful weight control. *Obesity Research*, **6** (3), 219–24.

68. Boutelle, K.N., Kirschenbaum, D.S., Baker, R.C. and Mitchell, E.M. (1999) How can obese weight controllers minimize weight gain during the high risk holiday season? By self-monitoring very consistently. *Health Psychology*, **18** (4), 364–8.

69. Wadden, T.A., Berkowitz, R.I., Womble, L.G. *et al.* (2005) Randomized trial of lifestyle modification and pharmacotherapy for obesity. *New England Journal of Medicine*, **353**, 2111–20.

70. Foreyt, J.P. and Goodrick, G.K. (1993) Evidence for success of behavioral modification in weight loss and control. *Annals of Internal Medicine*, **119**, 698–701.

71. Perri, M.G., Nezu, A.M., McKelvey, W.F. *et al.* (2001) Relapse prevention training and problem-solving therapy in the long-term management of obesity. *Journal of Consulting and Clinical Psychology*, **69**, 722–6.

72. Beck, A.T. and Weishar, M. (1989) Cognitive therapy, in *Comprehensive Handbook of Cognitive Therapy* (eds A. Freeman, K.M. Simon, L.E. Beutler and H. Arkowitz), Plenum Publishing Company, New York.

73. Stahre, L., Tarnell, B., Hakanson, C.E. and Hallstrom, T. (2007) A randomized controlled trial of two weight reducing short-term group treatment programs for obesity with an 18 month follow-up. *International Journal of Behavioral Medicine*, **14**, 48–55.

74. Stahre, L. and Hallstrom, T. (2005) A new short-term cognitive treatment program gives substantial weight reduction up to 18 months from the end of treatment: A randomized controlled trial. *Journal of Eating and Weight Disorders*, **10**, 51–8.

75. Christakis, N.A. and Fowler, J.H. (2007) The spread of obesity in a large social network over 32 years. *New England Journal of Medicine*, **357**, 370–9.

76. Brekke, H.K., Jansson, P.A., Mansson, J.E. and Lenner, R.A. (2003) Lifestyle changes can be achieved through counseling and follow-up in first degree relatives of patients with type 2 diabetes. *Journal of the American Dietetic Association*, **103**, 835–43.

77. Foreyt, J.P. and Goodrick, G.K. (1991) Factors common to successful therapy for the obese patient. *Medicine and Science in Sports and Exercise*, **23** (3), 292–7.

78. Foreyt, J.P. and Goodrick, G.K. (1994) Attributes of successful approaches to weight loss and control. *Applied and Prevention Psychology*, **3**, 209–15.

79. Orth, W.S., Madan, A.K., Taddeucci, R.J. *et al.* (2008) Support group meeting attendance is associated with better weight loss. *Obesity Research*, **18**, 391–4.

80. Renjilian, D.A., Perri, M.G., Nezu, A.M. *et al.* (2001) Effects of matching participants to their treatment preference. *Journal of Consulting and Clinical Psychology*, **69**, 717–21.

81. Wallace, J.P., Raglin, J.S. and Jastremski, C.A. (1995) Twelve month adherence of adults who joined a fitness program with a spouse vs without a spouse. *Journal of Sports Medicine and Physical Fitness*, **35**, 206–13.

82. Wing, R.R. and Jeffrey, R.M. (1999) Benefits of recruiting participants with friends and increasing social support for weight loss maintenance. *Journal of Consulting and Clinical Psychology*, **67** (1), 132–8.

83. DePue, J.D., Clark, M.M., Ruggiero, L. *et al.* (1995) Maintenance of weight loss: a needs assessment. *Obesity Research*, **3**, 241–7.

84. Perri, M.G. (1998) The maintenance of treatment effects in the long-term management of obesity. *Clinical Psychology: Science and Practice*, **5**, 526–43.

85. Perri, M.G., McAdoo, W.G., McAllister, D.A. *et al.* (1987) Effects of peer support and therapist contact on long term weight loss. *Journal of Consulting and Clinical Psychology*, **55** (4), 615–7.

86. Perri, M.G., McAdoo, W.G., McAllister, D.A. *et al.* (1986) Enhancing the efficacy of behavior therapy for obesity: Effects of aerobic exercise and a multicomponent maintenance program. *Journal of Consulting and Clinical Psychology*, **54**, 670–5.

87. Perri, M.G., McAdoo, W.G., Spevak, P.A. and Newlin, D.B. (1984) Effect of a multicomponent maintenance program on long-term weight loss. *Journal of Consulting and Clinical Psychology*, **52**, 480–1.

88. Dunn, A.L., Anderson, R.E. and Jakicic, J.M. (1998) Lifestyle physical activity interventions: history, short and long-term effects and recommendations. *American Journal of Preventive Medicine*, **15**, 398–412.

89. Tate, D.F., Jackvony, E.H. and Wing, R.R. (2003) Effects of internet behavioral counseling on weight loss in adults at risk for type 2 diabetes. *Journal of the American Medical Association*, **289**, 1833–6.

90. Lindstrom, L.L., Balch, P. and Reese, S. (1976). In person versus telephone treatment for obesity. *Journal of Behavior Therapy and Experimental Psychiatry*, **7**, 367–9.

91. Smith, D.E. and Wing, R.R. (1991) Diminished weight loss and behavioral compliance during repeated diets in obese patients with type II diabetes. *Health Psychology*, **10**, 378–83.

92. Jeffrey, R.W., Bjornson-Benson, W.M., Rosenthal, B.S. *et al.* (1984) Effectiveness of monetary contracts with two repayment schedules on weight reduction in men and women from self-referred and population samples. *Behavior Therapy*, **15**, 273–9.

93. Brownell, K.D., Yopp-Cohen, R., Stunkard, A.J. *et al.* (1984) Weight loss competitions at the work site: Impact on weight, morale, and cost-effectiveness. *American Journal of Public Health*, **74**, 1283–5.

94. Klem, M.L., Wing, R.R., Lang, W. *et al.* (2000) Does weight loss maintenance become easier over time? *Obesity Research*, **8**, 438–44.

95. King, A.C., Keirnan, M., Oman, R.F. *et al.* (1997) Can we identify who will adhere to long-term physical activity? Signal detection methodology as a potential aid to clinical decision making. *Health Psychology*, **16** (4), 380–9.

96. Leermarkers, E.A., Jakicic, J.M., Viteri, J. and Wing, R.R. (1998) Clinic-based vs. home-based interventions for preventing weight gain in men. *Obesity Research*, **6** (5), 346–52.

97. Perri, M.G., Martin, A.D., Leermarkers, E.A. *et al.* (1997) Effects of group versus home-based exercise in the treatment of obesity. *Journal of Consulting and Clinical Psychology*, **65** (2), 278–85.

98. Poston, W.S.C., Foreyt, J.P., Borrell, L. and Haddock, C.K. (1998) Challenges in obesity management. *Southern Medical Journal*, **91**, 710–20.

99. Perri, M.G. and Corsica, J.A. (2002) Improving the maintenance of weight lost in behavioral treatment of obesity, in *Handbook of Obesity Treatment*, (eds T.A. Wadden and A.J. Stunkard), Guilford Press, New York, pp. 357–79.

100. Bjorvell, H. and Rossner, S. (1985) Long-term treatment of severe obesity: four year follow-up of results of combined behavioral modification programme. *British Medical Journal*, **291**, 379–82.

101. Bjorvell, H. and Rossner, S. (1992) A ten year follow-up of weight change in severely obese subjects treated in a behavior modification programme. *International Journal of Obesity*, **16**, 623–5.

102. Skender, M.S., Goodrick, G.K., Del Jungo, D.J. *et al.* (1996) Comparison of 2-year weight loss trends in behavioral treatments of obesity: diet, exercise and combination interventions. *Journal of the American Dietetic Association*, **96**, 342–6.

103. Wadden, T.A., Vogt, R.A., Foster, G.D. and Anderson, D.A. (1998) Exercise and maintenance of weight loss: 1-year follow-up of a controlled clinic trial. *Journal of Consulting and Clinical Psychology*, **66**, 429–33.

104. Miller, W.C., Koceja, D.M. and Hamilton, E.J. (1997) A meta-analysis of the past 25 years of weight loss research using diet, exercise or diet plus exercise intervention. *International Journal of Obesity*, **21**, 941–7.

105. Volek, J.S., VanHeest, J.L. and Forsythe, C.E. (2005) Diet and exercise for weight loss: a review of current issues. *Sports Medicine*, **35**, 1–9.

106. Votruba, S.B., Horvitz, M.A. and Schoeller, D.A. (2000) The role of exercise in the treatment of obesity. *Nutrition*, **16**, 179–88.

107. Look AHEAD Research Group (2007) Reduction in weight and cardiovascular disease risk factors in individuals with type 2 diabetes: one year results of the LookAHEAD trial. *Diabetes Care*, **30**, 1374–83.

108. Tuohimehto, J., Lindstrom, J., Eriksson, J.G. *et al.* (2001) Prevention of type 2 diabetes mellitus by changes in lifestyle among subjects with impaired glucose tolerance. *New England Journal of Medicine*, **344** (18), 1343–9.

109. Jeffrey, R.W., Wing, R.R., Thorson, C. *et al.* (1993) Strengthening behavioral interventions for weight loss: A randomized trial of food provision and monetary incentives. *Journal of Consulting and Clinical, Psychology*, **61**, 1038–45.

110. Wing, R.R., Jeffrey, R.M., Burton, L.R. *et al.* (1996) Food provisions vs. structured meal plans in the behavioral treatment of obesity. *International Journal of Obesity*, **20**, 56–62.

111. Wadden, T.A., Sternberg, J.A., Letizia, K.A. *et al.* (1989) Treatment of obesity by very low calorie diet:, behavior therapy, and their combination: a five year perspective. *International Journal of Obesity*, **13**, 39–46.

112. Wadden, T.A., Stunkard, A.J. and Liebschutz, J. (1988) Three-year follow-up of the treatment of obesity by very low calorie diet, behavior therapy, and their combination. *Journal of Consulting and Clinical Psychology*, **56**, 925–8.

113. Wing, R.R., Blair, E.H., Marcus, M.D. *et al.* (1994) Year-long weight loss treatment for obese patients with type 2 diabetes: does including an intermittent very-low-calorie diet improve outcome? *American Journal of Medicine*, **97**, 354–62.

114. Kirschner, M.A., Schneider, G., Ertel, N.H. and Gorman, J. (1988) An eight year experience with a very-low-calorie formula diet for control of major obesity. *International Journal of Obesity*, **12**, 69–80.

115. Wadden, T.A. and Osei, S. (2002) The treatment of obesity: An overview, in *Handbook of Obesity Treatment* (eds T.A. Wadden and A.J. Stunkard), Guilford Press, New York, pp. 229–48.

116. Wadden, T.A., Foster, G.D. and Letizia, K.A. (1994) One-year behavioral treatment of obesity: comparison of moderate and severe caloric restriction and the effects of maintenance therapy. *Journal of Consulting and Clinical Psychology*, **62**, 165–71.

117. Institute of Medicine (1995) *Weighing the Options: Criteria for Evaluating Weight Management Programs*, National Academy Press, Washington DC.

118. Rothacker, D.Q. (2000) Five-year self-management of weight using meal replacements: Comparison with matched controls in rural Wisconsin. *Nutrition*, **16**, 344–8.

119. Williamson, D.F. (1993) Descriptive epidemiology of body weight and weight changes in US adults. *Annals of Internal Medicine*, **119**, 646–9.

120. Ditschuneit, H.H., Flechtner-Mors, M., Johnson, T.D. and Adler, G. (1999) Metabolic and weight loss effects of long-term dietary intervention in obese patients. *American Journal of Clinical Nutrition*, **69**, 198–204.

121. Flechtner-Mors, M., Ditschuneit, H.H., Johnson, T.D. *et al.* (2000) Metabolic and weight loss effects of long-term dietary intervention in obese patients: four-year results. *Obesity Research*, **8**, 399–402.

122. Ashley, J.M., St. Jeor, S.T., Perumean-Chaney, S. *et al.* (2001) Meal replacements in weight intervention. *Obesity Research*, **9**, S312–S320.

123. Heymsfield, S.B., van Mierlo, C.A., van der Knapp, H.C. *et al.* (2003) Weight management using a meal replacement strategy: meta and pooling analysis from six studies. *International Journal of Obesity and Related Metabolic Disorders*, **5**, 537–49.

124. Keogh, J.B. and Clifton, P.M. (2005) The role of meal replacements in obesity treatment. *Obesity Reviews*, **6**, 229–34.

125. Bray, G.A. (1998) Drug treatment of obesity: don't throw the baby out with the bath water. *American Journal of Clinical Nutrition*, **67**, 1–2.

126. Bray, G.A. (2002) Drug treatment of obesity, in *Handbook of Obesity Treatment* (eds T.A. Wadden and A.J. Stunkard), Guilford Press, New York, pp. 317–38.

127. Rolls, B.J., Shide, D.J., Thorwart, M.L. and Ulbrecht, J.S. (1998) Sibutramine reduces food intake in non-dieting women with obesity. *Obesity Research*, **6**, 1–11.

128. Lean, M.E.J. (1997) Sibutramine – A review of clinical efficacy. *International Journal of Obesity*, **21** (Suppl), 30–6.

129. Phelan, S. and Wadden, T.A. (2002) Combining behavioral and pharmacological treatments for obesity. *Obesity Research*, **10**, 560–74.

130. Miles, J.M., Leiter, L., Hollander, P. *et al.* (2002) Effect of orlistat in overweight and obese patients with type 2 diabetes treated with metformin. *Diabetes Care*, **25**, 1123–8.

131. Lindgarde, F. (2000) The effect of orlistat on body weight and coronary heart disease risk profile in obese patients: the Swedish Multimorbidity Study. *Journal of Internal Medicine*, **248**, 245–54.

132. Wadden, T.A., Berkowitz, R.I., Womble, L.G. *et al.* (2000) Effects of sibutramine plus orlistat in obese women following 1 year of treatment by sibutramine alone: a placebo-controlled trial. *Obesity Research*, **8**, 431–7.

133. Wing, R.R. (2002). Behavioral weight control, in *Handbook of Obesity Treatment*. (eds T.A. Wadden, and A.J. Stunkard), Guilford Press, New York, pp. 301–16.

8

Physical activity, obesity and type 2 diabetes

Carlton B. Cooke and Paul J. Gately

Carnegie Research Institute, Leeds Metropolitan University, Leeds, UK

8.1   Introduction

As a consequence of obesity many people experience reduced glucose tolerance from an increase in insulin resistance, which causes excessive insulin output (hyperinsulinaemia). For such individuals, many of whom will develop type 2 diabetes, regular physical activity or exercise can reduce resting plasma insulin levels and lower insulin output during fasted oral glucose tolerance tests, thereby indicating improved insulin sensitivity. There is no doubt that regular physical activity and exercise can provide an important contribution to the prevention and treatment of both obesity and type 2 diabetes. This chapter evaluates the research evidence regarding the role that physical activity can play in the prevention and treatment of obesity and type 2 diabetes. It also offers guidance on how physical activity can be increased in the lives of those who are obese and/or type 2 diabetic.

8.2   Physical activity and exercise, what is the difference?

Physical activity is defined as any bodily movement produced by skeletal muscles that results in energy expenditure, whereas exercise is planned, and repetitive bodily movement done to improve or maintain one or more of the components of fitness [1,2]. Exercise may include training, sports participation or going to some form of regular exercise class. Physical activity is therefore the umbrella term with types of exercise, sport and physical recreation forming subsets of physical activity. Physical activity can therefore take many forms, as a means of transport, occupational requirements, daily

Obesity and Diabetes, Second Edition   Edited by Anthony H. Barnett and Sudhesh Kumar
© 2009 John Wiley & Sons, Ltd

living activity and leisure time activity. It is important to realize that most individuals do not discriminate between physical activity, exercise and sport. If you ask people how active they are, evidence suggests that they will probably interpret the question as to how much sport or exercise they do. According to the National Fitness Survey [3] 75% of the participants knew that exercise is good for your health, but many people do not recognize that they can look to their everyday life to find ways to be more active without the need to engage in formal exercise if they do not wish to. Working from an understanding of the perspective and lifestyle of the obese or type 2 diabetic individual is therefore important in supporting their efforts to increase their physical activity. This is especially important since they will commonly view exercise and sport participation as unattainable and not desirable.

8.3   Current physical activity behaviour and guidelines

The Department of Health [4] highlighted that 70% of the adult population was not undertaking sufficient physical activity to benefit their health. The Health Survey for England (2002) showed that 30% of boys and 40% of girls were not undertaking sufficient physical activity to benefit their health [5], although the commonly accepted level required to confer health benefits has only a limited scientific basis [6,7].

The Department of Health [4] suggest the following recommended physical activity levels:

- Adults should undertake at least 30 minutes of at least moderate intensity physical activity on five or more days of the week.

- Children and young people should undertake at least 1 hour of at least moderate intensity physical activity on each day of the week. At least twice a week this should include activities that develop bone health, muscle strength and flexibility.

- Older people should undertake the physical activity recommendations for adults. However, older people should be careful to keep moving and retain their mobility through daily activity. They should participate in specific activities that develop strength, co-ordination and balance.

- Specific medical conditions such as obesity prevention, adults should undertake 45–60 minutes of moderate intensity physical activity on each day of the week.

- Weight management and obesity: achieving the recommendation of at least 30 minutes of at least moderate intensity physical activity on 5 or more days a week (a total of 150 minutes) will represent a significant increase in energy expenditure for most people, and will contribute substantially to their weight management. However, in many people and in the absence of a reduction in energy intake, 45–60 minutes of activity each day may be needed in order to prevent the development of obesity. People who have been obese and who have lost weight may need to do 60–90 minutes of activity a day in order to maintain their weight loss.

- Type 2 diabetes: regular moderate intensity physical activity carried out three times a week can produce small but significant improvements in blood glucose control. Both aerobic and resistance exercise programmes produce similar benefits. Higher levels of intensity of physical activity produce greater benefits. Moderate to high levels of physical fitness appear to reduce the risk of all-cause mortality in patients with type 2 diabetes.

- The daily-recommended level of physical activity can be achieved in one session or through several shorter sessions of activity lasting 10 minutes or more.

More recent adult recommendations, which are similar, have been published by the American College of Sports Medicine (ACSM) and American Heart Association (AHA) [8]. Nelson *et al.* [9] also published recommendations for older adults (over the age of 65) on behalf of the ACSM and the American Heart Association. The recommendations for older adults are relevant for the obese or type 2 diabetic, with an emphasis on aerobic exercise that is appropriate for the level of fitness of the individual, muscle-strengthening activity, reducing sedentary behaviour, and risk management.

It is important that sedentary adults, including the obese or type 2 diabetic, build up gently towards participating in sufficient moderate physical activity to meet or exceed the guidelines. Moderate physical activities are defined as those that raise the heart rate sufficiently to leave you warm and slightly out of breath and include brisk walking, climbing stairs, swimming, social dancing and heavy DIY, gardening and housework.

For most adults who are not regularly active but are able to walk comfortably, walking can become a good way to establish an active lifestyle. It is important to build up activity and fitness gradually and for most inactive adults taking longer walks more often and more briskly is an excellent way to improve activity and health.

Adults can also make the most of other opportunities to be active in their everyday life by walking up stairs instead of taking the lift, walking to the shops or work rather than taking the car or bus (or getting off to walk part of the way if public transport is necessary because of the distance of the journey) playing with the children or being active as a family. Adults should consider taking up a sport or physical recreation activity as exercising with others is more sociable and you do not need to be a 'sporty person' to have fun and enjoyment in the many different indoor and outdoor activities available. The emphasis on fun and enjoyment in physical activity, be it play or sport, is also crucial to keep young people participating in an active lifestyle.

Any person who has been diagnosed as a type 2 diabetic or is chronically obese should consult their GP or consultant before starting regular physical activity. Most individuals who are obese and/or type 2 diabetic will have most probably led a very sedentary existence for a number of years. Such individuals will have impaired exercise tolerance and may have a number of co-morbidities that require clinical treatment or monitoring in order that physical activity may be undertaken safely.

In the case of obese individuals weight-bearing exercise may be difficult and painful to sustain for any period of time that will have a significant impact on calorific expenditure. In such cases individuals may need to undertake exercise where their body mass is supported during the activity, such as in swimming, the use of seated or recumbent cycle ergometers or resistance training. Such forms of exercise are unlikely to be sustainable over long periods of time for many sedentary overweight people, especially children, as they may well find them boring and unsatisfying, even though some members of the population do exercise regularly in this way. When engaging individuals in physical activity it is important to establish their likes and dislikes and work with them in terms of behaviour management to set achievable short-term goals. In our experience this approach may move some adults from non-weight-bearing exercise to a mixture of active transport and active leisure and some children into recreational or competitive sport.

In terms of tracking physical activity through childhood and into adulthood there is a moderate relationship between the amount and type of physical activity in childhood with that in youth, but low levels of tracking from youth into adulthood. However, in specific groups such as overweight and obese children the persistence of obesity is high, as shown by Freedman *et al.* [10], where 77% of obese children remained obese at 17 years follow up.

8.4 The importance of physical activity to health

There is now a strong evidence base demonstrating the numerous health benefits associated with regular physical activity, including beneficial effects on up to 20 chronic diseases or disorders [3,4,11–15].

Although obesity and type 2 diabetes are the major focus of this chapter, they are both closely related to the metabolic syndrome, where responses to physical activity or exercise are beneficial to improved metabolic and haematological control, fat loss, and an increase in muscle mass.

Physical activity and type 2 diabetes

The ACSM position stand on exercise and type 2 diabetes states that 'physical activity is an under-utilized mode of therapy for type 2 diabetes, often due to a lack of understanding' [16]. The role of physical activity in the care of type 2 diabetics is summarised in the American Diabetic Association's most recent position statement on standards of medical care in diabetes [17], based on Sigal *et al.* [18].

The specific benefits of physical activity to improved glucose tolerance and control are associated with regular bouts of exercise that repeatedly provoke the acute effects of a single bout. These and other improvements in metabolic control associated with physical activity are not only important to those with type 2 diabetes but also to the sedentary and overweight, and those who have the metabolic syndrome. Significant improvements in metabolic fitness have been associated with increased physical activity that may not be sufficient in intensity to increase the more traditional measures of fitness such as maximal oxygen uptake ($\dot{V}O_{2max}$, the maximum rate at which an individual can take up and utilize oxygen while breathing air at sea level [19]). However, sustained changes in activity levels are required for the benefits of exercise or physical activity to positively affect insulin action [16,20,21]. According to Albright *et al.* [16] favourable changes in glucose tolerance and insulin sensitivity usually deteriorate within 72 hours of the last exercise session. Therefore sustained changes in daily physical activity are required to ensure the repeated stimulus associated with the acute effects of exercise.

Several long-term studies have shown improvements in glycaemic control [22,23]. These improvements in carbohydrate metabolism and insulin sensitivity were also shown to be maintained for at least 5 years in those patients that continued to participate in physical activity and exercise. Improvements in HbA1c were around 10–20% compared to baseline. The improvements in glycaemic control were greatest in those patients with mild type 2 diabetes, and those who were likely to be most insulin resistant [24–26]. The mechanisms of this improved control are poorly understood, what is known is that exercise increases the number of glucose transporter proteins (GLUT4) in the plasma membrane. Although Chipkin *et al.* [27] also highlighted that in poorly controlled diabetic patients, the ability of exercise to stimulate GLUT4 transporters is decreased.

In addition to the independent benefit of physical activity to cardiovascular health, the combined benefits to blood lipid profile, haematological profile and blood pressure further support the use of physical activity and exercise for the type 2 diabetic patient [28–30].

A number of reviews have shown that programmes that include a prescription of exercise involving 60–85% $\dot{V}O_{2max}$ lasting 30–60 minutes three to four times per week for 6–12 weeks achieve significant improvements in $\dot{V}O_{2max}$ [27,53]. Other studies have also shown that diabetic patients have lower aerobic fitness than sedentary non-diabetic individuals, which would increase the magnitude of improvement in fitness with regular physical activity or exercise, but will require a gentle progression in exercise intensity, duration and frequency from the sedentary state.

Physical activity and obesity

Exercise is the most variable component of energy expenditure, it is therefore clear to see why exercise has been adopted as a component to treat overweight and obesity. Indeed, exercise or physical activity is promoted within a range of guidelines for the prevention and treatment of overweight and obesity [4,15,31]. Understanding the impact of physical activity and exercise on obesity and associated variables is important, as an increase in physical activity not only has significant positive effects on body mass and body fat mass, but also on a range of other variables associated with health [11]. Physical activity has been suggested to have favourable effects on: weight loss, decreased fat percentage, decreased skinfold thickness, android disease, decreased risk of coronary heart disease (CHD), improved glucose metabolism, increased basal metabolic rate (BMR), prevention of loss of fat free mass (FFM), increased dietary thermogenesis, reduced blood pressure, improved cardiovascular fitness and benefits to psychosocial health [11–15].

Table 8.1 Relative risk by categories of percentage body fat for fit and unfit groups of men

Lean (<17% body fat)	Fit = 1.0	Unfit = 3.16 (1.12–8.92)
Normal (17–25%body fat)	Fit = 1.43 (0.77–2.67)	Unfit = 2.94 (1.48–5.83)
Obese (>25% body fat)	Fit = 1.35 (0.66–2.76)	Unfit = 4.11 (2.20–7.68)

Adapted from [32].

A review by Blair and Brodney [11] suggested that the negative health consequences of obesity are more associated with low physical fitness (maximal exercise treadmill test, a proxy measure of physical activity) than obesity per se (based on body mass index (BMI) and % body fat). Blair and Brodney [11] showed that the risk of CHD in active overweight or obese males (fat but fit individuals) was the same as normal-weight active control subjects, while the risk associated with the sedentary normal weight controls was greater. Further evidence from the same group of researchers [32] supported these findings with a study of 21 925 men aged 30–83 years conducted between 1971 and 1989, which showed that the relative risk (RR) of Cardiovascular disease mortality was not significantly different for fit and lean, normal and fit or obese and fit, whereas for the same percentage body fat categories the unfit had significantly higher relative risk (Table 8.1).

8.5 Energy expenditure

Energy expenditure associated with physical activity is quantified in the literature in various forms using energy units such as the kilocalorie or the Joule (SI unit) and other dimensionless quantities which are multiples of BMR (the PAL or the MET). Although the Joule is the SI unit of energy the kilocalorie is still in common use. A MET is defined as the energy requirement for BMR, PAL stands for physical activity level and is also a multiple of BMR, where in both cases 1 MET and a PAL of 1 are both equivalent to the energy requirement of BMR.

Ainsworth *et al.* [33] have presented a comprehensive compendium of physical activities classified in terms of intensity according to the number of METS of energy required. Total energy expenditure expressed as $kcal.day^{-1}$ is divided by BMR to determine the value for PAL. PALs therefore express the proportion of total energy expenditure that is expended in physical activity, including energy expended in the thermic response to food. BMR increases with size, but the PALs of heavier individuals may not differ significantly in weight bearing exercise to those of normal weight individuals because the energy cost of movement also increases with size. A sedentary person would have a PAL of about 1.4, while an individual engaged in a lot of physical activity would have a PAL of about 2, whereas endurance trained athletes may have a PAL in excess of 4 [34]. The fact that the PAL is body size dependent means that it may be flawed when used for estimating energy expenditure [35]. Values for energy expenditure are also expressed in absolute terms (kcal, J) or relative to time ($kcal.min^{-1}$ W) or time and body mass ($kcal.kg.^{-1}min^{-1}$, $W.kg.^{-1}min^{-1}$). McArdle *et al.* [36] provide estimates of energy expenditure values for a range of activities in $kcal.kg.^{-1}min^{-1}$.

Physical activity is the most variable component of daily energy expenditure. Ravussin and Swinburn [37] suggested that physical activity typically represents between 20 and 40% of daily energy expenditure. Other studies assessing the energy expenditure of individuals in a respiratory chamber have shown there are large differences in individuals with respect to spontaneous physical activity (SPA), which range from 100 to 800 kcal.day^{-1} [38].

A major feature of current recommendations for adults and children in the UK and in the USA is the emphasis that is placed on moderate intensity exercise, although vigorous exercise has now reappeared for those capable of regular comfortable moderate intensity physical activity. In the recommendations outlined above examples of moderate exercise are given which can be easily understood by members of the public and health professionals. The use of qualitative descriptors in describing energy expenditure associated with physical activity can be confusing given the range of intensities of physical activity described as moderate exercise [2]. Moderate intensity exercise is typically defined as 3–6 METS, which is equated to the energy requirements of walking at 3 and 4 mph respectively. Light activities are described as requiring <3 METS and heavy or vigorous activities are those requiring >6 METS. This is not the case for all studies so it is important to look for definitions of such qualitative descriptors when assessing research literature concerned with physical activity interventions.

Prescribing exercise using relative exercise intensity

To add to the confusion the same qualitative descriptors of light, moderate and vigorous are often used to describe relative exercise intensity, that is the exercise intensity relative to maximal heart rate predicted for age or predicted maximal oxygen consumption (or directly measured, but not normally for obese or type 2 diabetics). For example, two individuals can be exercising at the same absolute energy expenditure, say walking together at a speed of 3 mph (4.8 km.h^{-1}, 3 METS). The least fit obese person may be working at a vigorous exercise intensity relative to their aerobic fitness (defined as >60% of $\dot{V}O_{2max}$, [2]), whilst the fitter individual may be working at a light exercise intensity relative to their aerobic fitness (<40% of $\dot{V}O_2$). Table 8.2 shows a comparison of absolute and different relative exercise intensities that are used together with qualitative descriptors, but these are not consistently applied in the physical activity literature (Table 8.3).

$\dot{V}O_{2max}$ is the maximum rate at which an individual can take up and utilise oxygen while breathing air at sea level [19]. It has traditionally been used as the criterion standard of cardiorespiratory fitness. The sensitivity of $\dot{V}O_{2max}$ to the establishment of regular physical activity is strongly related to the degree of development that may ultimately be realised, which reflects a combination of endowment and habitual physical activity. Individual $\dot{V}O_{2max}$ values are used to provide one form of relative exercise intensity (Table 8.2) where absolute exercise intensity in the form of oxygen uptake is expressed as a percentage of the individual's $\dot{V}O_{2max}$, as in the example of the two individuals walking together at the same walking speed.

Table 8.2 Examples of absolute and relative exercise intensity (based on [41])

Qualitative descriptor	Relative exercise intensity			Absolute exercise intensity	
	% $\dot{V}O_{2max}$ or %HRR	% HR_{max}	RPE (6–20 scale)	METs	
				20–39 yr	40–64 yr
Light	40	63	10	4.2	4.0
Moderate	50	69	11	5.5	5.0
Moderate	60	76	12	7.2	6.0
Hard	70	82	14	8.4	7.0
Hard	80	89	15	9.5	8.0
Very Hard	85	92	16	10.2	8.5
Very Hard	90	95	18	10.8	9.0
Maximal	100	100	20	12.0	10.0

Table 8.3 Examples of activities that expend 150 kcal for an average 70 kg adult

Descriptor of intensity	Activity	Approximate duration (minutes)
Light	Typing	85–90
Light	Sitting playing with child	50–60
Light	Washing and polishing a car	45–60
Light	Washing windows or floors	45–60
Light	Playing volleyball	45
Light	General gardening	30–45
Light	Volleyball (non-competitive)	43
Light	Wheeling a wheelchair	30–40
Light	Walking 1.75 miles at 3 mph	35
Moderate	Basketball (Shooting Baskets)	30
Moderate	Cycling 5 miles at 10 mph	30
Moderate	Dancing fast (social)	30
Moderate	Pushing a pushchair 1.5 miles	30
Moderate	Raking leaves	30
Moderate	Water aerobics	30
Moderate	Swimming lengths	20
Moderate	Wheelchair basketball	20
Moderate	Game of basketball	15–20
Moderate	Cycling 4 miles at 16 mph	15
Moderate	Skipping	15
Moderate	Running 1.5 miles at 6 mph	15
Moderate	Shovelling snow	15
Moderate	Climbing stairs	15
Hard	Jogging at 5 mph	18
Hard	Field hockey (game)	16

Adapted from Clinical Guidelines, NIH [31] and Surgeon General's Report [51].

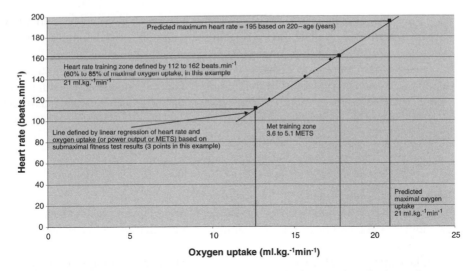

Figure 8.1   Heart rate training zone defined by results from a submaximal exercise test

Heart rate is a common method used for setting relative exercise intensity. There are three ways in which this can be done, but all are based on the assumption that heart rate is a linear function of exercise intensity, which it is throughout most of the submaximal range, but not necessarily at very low or high exercise intensities [19]. Using data from a progressive, incremental steady state exercise test, heart rate at the end of each stage can be plotted against oxygen uptake or MET values (Figure 8.1). Maximum heart rate can be predicted by using 220 – age (years), but this can be in error by ± 10 beats.min^{-1}. $\dot{V}O_{2max}$ can then be predicted by either extrapolation of the heart rate oxygen uptake line to predicted maximum heart rate [39] or a nomogram can be used to estimate it [40]. It should be noted that the standard error of predicting maximal oxygen uptake using the nomogram is up to 15% in moderately trained individuals of different ages [19]. Indeed, the authors concluded that this drawback holds true for any submaximal cardiorespiratory test. $\dot{V}O_{2max}$ can be measured directly but this procedure requires maximal exercise to volitional exhaustion. It is not recommended as a positive experience for obese or type 2 diabetics and will often be so symptom limited in terms of effort and discomfort that the measurement will not represent a valid assessment of $\dot{V}O_{2max}$.

The $\dot{V}O_{2max}$ and maximum heart rate values are then used to calculate the training zone for aerobic exercise known to promote a training response in terms of increasing cardiorespiratory fitness (60–85% of $\dot{V}O_{2max}$, [41]). For example, given a predicted $\dot{V}O_{2max}$ of 21 ml.kg.$^{-1}$min^{-1} (which is equivalent to 6 METS, 1 MET is approximately equivalent to 3.5 ml.kg.$^{-1}$min^{-1} of oxygen uptake) and a maximum heart rate of 195 beats.min^{-1} (age 25 years) the target heart rate zone or MET zone would be 112–162 beats.min^{-1} or 3.6 to 5.1 METS respectively (Figure 8.1). It is important to note that heart rate response to exercise is dependent on the mode of exercise. Therefore if exercise testing is undertaken partly for the purpose of setting relative exercise intensity for training the same mode of exercise should be used in both where possible. Readers interested in more detail on exercise testing and prescription are directed to Heyward [41] and Cooke [42].

The second of the common procedures for determining target heart rates for training is to use the Karvonen percentage of heart rate range. This method uses the resting heart rate (HR_{rest}) and the heart rate range (HRR), which is the difference between maximum (HR_{max}) and resting heart rate. Maximum heart rate must therefore be predicted by use of a formula such as $220 - age$.

$$\text{Target heart rate} = (\%HRR/100) \times (HR_{max} - HR_{rest} \text{ rest}) + HR_{rest}$$

The ACSM [43] recommends using 50–85% HRR.

Using the 25-year-old individual as an example again and given a resting heart rate of 72 beats.min^{-1}, the target heart rate for training at 50%HRR would be given by:

$$\text{Target heart rate} = (50/100) \times (195 - 72) + 72, \text{ which gives a target heart rate of } 134 \text{ beats.}min^{-1}.$$

Comparing this value with the target heart rate zone in Figure 8.1 shows this value to be in the middle of the heart rate zone. Given the comments already made regarding the typical sedentary nature of the lifestyle of the obese or type 2 diabetic, it is always better to start off at very low exercise intensities and then progress according to the principle of progressive overload. As the individual adapts their functional capacity to cope easily with the exercise challenge, so the exercise challenge is extended slightly.

The third common procedure for estimating target heart rates for setting relative exercise intensity is to use percentage of predicted maximal heart rate (again using the formula 220-age). This method makes use of the strong linear relationship between percentage heart rate max and percentage $\dot{V}O_{2max}$ (Table 8.2). The ACSM [43] recommends prescribing target heart rates between 60 and 90% of HR_{max}, depending on the fitness of the individual. Returning to our 25-year-old individual and selecting 60% of HR_{max}, the target heart rate is given by:

$$\text{Target heart rate} = (\%HR_{max}/100) \times HR_{max}, \text{ which gives } 117 \text{ beats.}min^{-1}.$$

This method produces a target heart rate close to the bottom of the target heart rate zone. Compared to the Karvonen method the %HR_{max} method produces a lower target heart rate when the same relative exercise intensity is used. However, this method therefore has advantages for use with obese and type 2 diabetics as it provides a conservative estimate of the target heart rate using a simple procedure without the need for exercise testing.

An alternative to using heart rate for setting and monitoring exercise intensity is rating of perceived exertion (RPE). RPE scales (Table 8.2) are reported as valid and reliable for assessing the level of exertion during aerobic exercise [44–46]. Dunbar *et al.* [46] suggest that RPEs of 11 and 16 closely approximate 50 and 85% HRR. Heyward [41] suggests the use of MET values corresponding to RPEs of 12 (somewhat hard) and 16 (hard) to set the minimum and maximum training intensities for aerobic exercise.

Even if some forms of heart rate training zone or values are estimated they must not form the sole focus of monitoring relative exercise intensity. How the individual is feeling and how hard they perceive the effort to be is more important. It is better to start off with short periods of enjoyable and achievable exercise when working with previously sedentary individuals, but especially with the obese or type 2 diabetic. Use of heart rate or RPE values for the obese or type 2 diabetic should be at the lowest recommended values to start with. This is recognised as important by the ACSM [43] as they state that poorly conditioned individuals may be able to exercise at a low intensity (40% $\dot{V}O_{2max}$) for only about 10 minutes (see the next section for exercise tolerance values for obese adults and children). The obese or type 2 diabetic person may therefore need to perform short bouts of exercise throughout the day to accumulate half an hour of regular habitual physical activity. The exercise intensity, duration and frequency can then be progressively increased as the functional capacity of the individual increases, building up to achieving the general recommendations for physical activity and beyond.

The combination of a lack of valid methods of assessment and the complex interactions between physical activity, energy intake and energy balance, complicate the accurate determination of energy balance in obesity [37,47–49].

8.6   Exercise tolerance and cardiorespiratory fitness in overweight and obese adults and children

There is very little data published on the exercise tolerance of obese adults. We tested 19 obese adults (4 males and 15 females aged 40.3 ± 13.5 years) for exercise tolerance [50]. Mean body mass and BMI of the group was 112.6 ± 18.9 kg and 37.9 ± 10.6 kg.m^{-2} respectively. Exercise tolerance was assessed using the treadmill walking test protocol developed for the National Fitness Survey [3]. Exercise tolerance was low as identified by a symptom limited mean peak $\dot{V}O_2$ of 2.05 ± 0.51 l.min^{-1} or 19.62 ± 5.45 ml.kg.$^{-1}$min^{-1} for the females and 2.15 ± 1.06 l.min^{-1} or 16.28 ± 8.56 ml.kg.$^{-1}$min^{-1} for males respectively. Average values for the Allied Dunbar National Fitness Survey (ADNFS) for females and males aged 35–44 years were 34.8 and 45.5 ml.kg.$^{-1}$min^{-1} respectively. Even comparing the values with the fifth percentile from the ADNFS (24.5 ml.kg.$^{-1}$min^{-1} for the females and 34.2 ml.kg.$^{-1}$min^{-1} for the males respectively) the values for the obese are significantly lower (20% and 54% for the females and males respectively). This comparison demonstrates that the obese or type 2 diabetic adult is likely to be starting from a position of extremely limited exercise tolerance, especially when considering the challenge of weight bearing exercise such as walking.

The criterion for defining the endpoint of the walking test is normally the achievement of 85% of age related maximum heart rate. However, all participants stopped walking before the target heart rate was achieved. Most gave the reason of pain in the lower legs, normally in the calves, as the reason for stopping the test. Overall, these data illustrate that exercise tolerance is severely restricted in these obese subjects. They required greater than 50% of their peak $\dot{V}O_2$ (60% HR_{max}) to be able to walk at $4.8\,km.h^1$ on the flat. Walking therefore constitutes a major exercise challenge for these participants, illustrating the need for specialist prescription of exercise for the chronically obese, sedentary type 2 diabetic population involving non-weight-bearing activity in the early stages. Walking as a form of physical activity to meet the recommendations for weekly moderate physical activity is therefore not likely to be an immediate or short-term goal for such adults, but one they might aspire to as a medium term objective. Different forms of non-weight-bearing exercise such as swimming (although this has obvious problems regarding use of public swimming pools in terms of psychological and emotional stress for many obese individuals), recumbent or seated cycle ergometry or resistance training may be required in combination with simple physical activity challenges around the home, before many individuals can begin to work towards regular sustained walking as a daily physical activity. It is important to ensure that the physical activity suggested is acceptable and achievable for the individual, hopefully in a setting where they have appropriate social support and encouragement and can get a sense of achievement, satisfaction and enjoyment from their hard work.

Our data on overweight and obese children (OWC) tested with the same treadmill walking test shows that they also have impaired exercise tolerance. We tested 65 OWC (28 males and 37 females aged 14.04 ± 2.06 years, body mass $87.9 \pm 27.6\,kg$) and found significantly ($p < 0.001$) lower (39%) levels of relative submaximal aerobic fitness compared to sixty three normal weight children (NWC)(30 males and 33 females aged 14.22 ± 1.07 years, body mass $55.03 \pm 11.43\,kg$). Peak VO_2 at 85% HR_{max} was $23.28 \pm 5.84\,ml.kg.^{-1}min^{-1}$ for the OWC group compared with $38.26 \pm 9.32\,ml. kg.^{-1}min^{-1}$ for the NWC. As with the adult's data, consideration of these findings is important when prescribing exercise for overweight and obese children.

8.7 Guidelines for exercise and activity prescription (including practical issues of clinical management for diabetics and the obese)

There is a concern that sedentary people engaging in physical activity may increase their risk of sudden cardiac death [51]. However, Albert *et al.* [52] concluded that there is a transient increase in risk but that habitual vigorous exercise had a low risk (1 sudden death per 1.51 million episodes of exertion). These data are supported by the ACSM and the AHA recommendations for physical activity (2007).

Evaluation of the type 2 diabetic patient prior to physical activity prescription

Prior to exercise prescription a detailed medical history and assessment of a range of physical factors, which includes the heart, blood vessels, eyes, kidneys, nervous system and feet, should be undertaken. The age of the patient, duration of diabetes and extent of co-morbidity will affect the appropriate choice of prescription options. A joint position statement by the ACSM/American Diabetes Association [53] suggested that a graded exercise test may be helpful prior to beginning an exercise programme if a patients is at high risk of cardiovascular disease, based on the following criteria:

- Age >35 years

- Type 2 diabetes >10 years duration

- Presence of any additional risk factor for coronary artery disease

- Presence of microvascular disease (retinopathy or nephropathy, including microalburminuria)

- Peripheral vascular disease

- Autonomic neuropathy.

Further tests with imaging techniques may also be appropriate for some patients. The position statement also suggests that for patients embarking on low intensity forms of exercise (<60% of maximal heart rate) the general practitioner/physician should use clinical judgment in deciding whether to recommend an exercise stress test [53]. The following factors should be considered during the prescription of exercise for the type 2 diabetic and are covered in more detail in the recent American Diabetes Association position statement [17].

Acute control of blood glucose

Hypoglycaemia is a potential complication for the exercising diabetic. The risk of hypoglycaemia is highest when insulin levels reach a peak at the same time as activity is undertaken, as well as glucose availability from food intake during exercise. A number of considerations are important in order to prevent hypoglycaemia during exercise, these include the form and the location of the insulin administration. Regular physical activity participation would promote better glycemic control to prevent hypoglycaemia, as the patient will be more able, through improved experience, to achieve glycaemic control. Chipkin *et al.* [27] suggested that the following should be undertaken by the exercising diabetic: blood glucose levels should be measured before, during and after exercise, easily absorbable carbohydrates should be available during exercise, extra carbohydrate should be taken for unplanned exercise and insulin dosages should be decreased by 50% for planned exercise.

Minimising foot trauma

It is essential to consider the health of the feet of the patient prior to engaging in exercise or physical activity, this is especially important for patients with peripheral neuropathy. Appropriate footwear, socks and care of feet before and after the exercise bout is important. Daily visual checks by the patient and regular checks by a health professional are also important [16,21,27]. Furthermore, weight bearing exercise may not be appropriate for some patients with severe peripheral neuropathy.

Nephropathy
According to Chipkin *et al.* [27] little is known about the effects of exercise on long-term renal function. In addition, dialysis limits exercise capacity, although some researchers have successfully provided suitable exercise programmes [54].

Autonomic neuropathy
Sudden death and painless myocardial ischaemia have been observed in both type 1 and type 2 diabetic patients [53]. In addition, patients with autonomic neuropathy have lower stroke volumes and decreased ejection fractions during exercise. Hypo- or hypertension are also possible in patients with autonomic neuropathy following vigorous exercise, particularly when they are at the start of an exercise programme.

8.8   Research evidence on the role of physical activity in the prevention and treatment of obesity and type 2 diabetes

Physical activity and the prevention of weight gain

Schulz and Schoeller [55] examined the relationship between % body fat and non-basal energy expenditure and proposed that a PAL of 1.75–1.80 should be a threshold target for the population as a whole. Black *et al.* [56] using data on 574 free-living individuals stated that their modal PAL was between 1.55 and 1.65 for both men and women. Thus, to raise the PALs of these individuals to a value that would prevent unhealthy weight gain would require an increase of 0.3 PAL, which relates to moderate exercise lasting between 30 and 60 minutes four to five times per week.

Although such findings are useful, studies using such levels of physical activity prescription have been limited in their ability to achieve weight management. Seidell [57] has shown, based on crude estimates, that the increased prevalence of obesity in the Netherlands related to approximately 1 kg gain over a 10 year period (i.e. 2 kcal/day). The requirement for such a small amount of daily energy imbalance to make a difference in preventing weight gain or providing weight maintenance, demonstrates the challenge of making small but sustainable changes in behaviour.

Three prospective cohort studies have highlighted the positive impact of physical activity on preventing weight gain in adults [58–60]. However, the effects of physical activity on prevention of weight gain are not that well established in the research literature. More recently, Wareham *et al.* [61] identified six interventions to increase physical activity with the aim of preventing weight gain. Four of the interventions showed a significant but small effect size. The lack of evidence on trials aimed at preventing weight gain leads to the conclusion that we do not yet know which approaches will prevent weight gain.

Physical activity and the treatment of overweight and obesity

There have been a number of review articles that have demonstrated greater success with the inclusion of physical activity in the treatment of overweight and obesity [62–64]. It is clear from a variety of intervention studies that acute treatments lead to significant weight loss [62–64] but weight loss maintenance tends to be limited [65,66].

Studies comparing the outcomes of diet only versus exercise only interventions, show that the ability of exercise only interventions to achieve weight loss is very limited [62,67].

However, encouraging data from the National Weight Control Registry (United States) [68] shows that inclusion of physical activity is particularly important in promoting weight loss maintenance compared to dietary restriction alone. Despite long histories of overweight and obesity, the 629 women and 155 men in the registry lost an average of 30 kg and maintained a required minimum weight loss of 13.6 kg for 5 years. Just over half lost weight through formal programmes, the remainder lost weight on their own. Both groups reported using diet and physical activity to lose weight. It is important to note that almost 77% of the sample reported that a triggering event in their lives had preceded their weight loss. Current physical activity was reported to be very high relative to current population guidelines in both the United States and the United Kingdom, at 404 kcal.day^{-1}. Klem *et al.* [68] were surprised that 42% of the sample reported that maintaining their weight loss was less difficult than losing the weight.

A meta-analysis by Anderson *et al.* [69] based on 29 studies with a 5 year follow up of structured weight loss programmes showed that an average weight loss of 3.0 kg or 23% of initial weight loss was maintained. They also reported that weight loss maintenance was significantly greater when participants exercised more.

Dunn *et al.* [70] compared a lifestyle physical activity programme with a structured exercise programme in adults ($n = 235$), at six months both groups had increased their energy expenditure (mean $\pm$ SE) 1.53 ± 0.19 kcal.kg.$^{-1}$day^{-1} for the lifestyle group and 1.53 ± 0.19 kcal.kg.$^{-1}$day^{-1} structured exercise group. Both groups had a significant increase in cardiorespiratory fitness (maximal treadmill test) but the increase in the structured group was significantly ($p < 0.01$) greater, 3.64 ± 0.33 ml.kg.$^{-1}$min^{-1} and 1.58 ± 0.33 ml.kg.$^{-1}$min^{-1} for the structured and lifestyle groups respectively. Dunn *et al.* [70] suggested that the key outcome was the emphasis on behavioural skill building rather than exercise prescription, as for the lifestyle group this was equally as effective at achieving increases in physical activity.

Physical activity and obesity treatment in children

A review by Epstein and Goldfield [71] has outlined the important elements of intervention programmes for overweight and obese children. The only area where there was a sufficient number of studies to make a quantitative analysis led to the conclusion that diet plus exercise programmes achieved greater weight loss. Two studies have shown that subjects involved in a diet only intervention were less successful than subjects involved in diet plus exercise (Epstein *et al.* [72] (−3.8 kg diet only versus −6.8 kg diet and exercise) and Hills and Parker [73] (−2.6 kg diet only versus −5.5 kg diet and exercise)). Gutin *et al.* [74] has shown that exercise only interventions can produce improvements in a range of variables such as body composition, fitness and biochemical profiles, although body mass increased (1.1 kg).

Several researchers have promoted the use of strategies to decrease sedentary behaviours or lifestyle activities (such as limiting access to TV and computer games) [75–77]. Epstein *et al.* [76] has suggested that one possible explanation for the greater success of reducing sedentary behaviour is that the children are provided with choice and control. Choice and control are powerful psychological variables that have been shown to influence exercise adherence. Epstein and Myers [64] concluded that for children increased physical activity is critical to long term success in weight control.

Physical activity and the prevention of type 2 diabetes

Two randomized trials have showed that lifestyle interventions including 150 min.week^{-1} of physical activity and diet-induced weight loss of 5–7% reduced the risk of progression from impaired glucose tolerance (IGT) to type 2 diabetes by 58% [78,79].

The Diabetes Prevention Program Research Group [78] also included a metformin (850 mg twice daily) intervention group that produced a significant reduction of 31%, and a placebo group during the 2.8 year period of treatment. Both forms of treatment were concluded to be highly effective means of delaying or preventing type 2 diabetes. Tuomilehto *et al.* [79] showed similar results in the incidence of diabetes in a sample of 522 middle aged overweight subjects treated with a lifestyle intervention programme (5% weight loss, total intake of fat <30% of energy consumed, intake of saturated fat to <10% of energy consumed, and increase in fibre intake to at least 15 g per 1000 kcal and at least 30 min of moderate exercise each day). The risk of diabetes was also reduced by 58% in the intervention group.

A cluster-randomized trial found that diet alone, exercise alone, and combined diet and exercise were equally effective in reducing the progression from IGT to diabetes [80]. These studies provide good evidence that programmes of increased physical activity and modest weight loss are effective in reducing the incidence of type 2 diabetes in individuals with impaired glucose tolerance.

Several studies published in the 1990s provided strong evidence in support of the role of physical activity as an important factor in the prevention of type 2 diabetes [81–84].

Physical activity in the treatment of type 2 diabetes

Boulé *et al.* [85] undertook a meta-analysis of structured exercise interventions in clinical trials of 8 weeks duration on HbA1c (A1C) and body mass in type 2 diabetes.

Post intervention A1C was significantly lower in exercise than control groups (7.65 vs. 8.31%, weighted mean difference ($0.66\%; p = 0.001$)). Whereas, post intervention body mass was no different for the exercise and control groups. The study confirmed that the beneficial effect of exercise on A1C was independent of any effect on body mass and that exercise programmes had a significant beneficial effect on glycemic control. A more recent meta-analysis by Boulé *et al.* [86] showed that exercise intensity was a better predictor of post intervention differences in A1C ($r = 0.91$, $p = 0.002$) than exercise volume ($r = 0.46, p = 0.26$). Type 2 diabetic individuals who are already exercising comfortably at moderate intensity should therefore consider increasing the intensity of their exercise to obtain additional benefits in both aerobic fitness and glycemic control.

Several large cohort studies have showed that higher levels of habitual aerobic fitness and/or physical activity are associated with significantly lower subsequent cardiovascular and overall mortality in type 2 diabetics, than could be explained by glucose lowering alone [87–89].

A meta-analysis by Brown *et al.* [90] involving 89 studies and 1800 subjects, examined the outcomes of strategies to achieve weight loss and improved metabolic control (change in glycosylated haemoglobin) in obese diabetic patients. In this analysis diet alone achieved the greatest weight loss and improvement in metabolic control [−9 kg (−20 lb) and −2.7% glycosylated haemoglobin)], behavioural programmes alone also achieved significant improvements [−3 kg (−6.4 lb) and −1.5%]. Exercise studies also achieved improvements but they were not statistically significant [−1.5 kg (−3.4 lb) and −0.8%]. Behaviour and diet therapies achieved statistically significant improvements [−3.7 kg (−8.5 lb) and −1.6%] but these changes were not as high as diet only programmes. However, as with most of the reviews on weight loss maintenance in the obese, the author concluded that most of the studies were limited with a general lack of reported data on long-term follow up.

Although relatively little research has been conducted on the impact of intensity of intervention on treatment outcomes, McAuley *et al.* [91] compared a modest treatment (similar to current standard treatment programmes) and a more intensive treatment programme. The more intensive treatment programme produced a more significant improvement in insulin sensitivity (23%, $p = 0.006$ (intensive intervention group) versus 9% $p = 0.23$ (modest/standard intervention group and for aerobic fitness (11% increase in intensive group, $p = 0.02$ versus 1% in the modest group, $p = 0.94$). The differences in response of these groups and the lack of improvement in insulin sensitivity for standard treatment shown in this study highlight the significant challenge ahead with the increasing prevalence of type 2 diabetes.

According to the ACSM/American Diabetes Association [53] position statement, all patients with diabetes can use resistance training, although as with general training recommendations the resistance training programme should relate to the ability, experience and fitness of the diabetic patient. Two clinical trials provide the strongest evidence for the efficacy of resistance training in type 2 diabetes [92,93]. In both studies the resistance-training programme involved multiple exercises at high intensity (three sets, three times per week), and HbA1c declined 1.1–1.2% in resistance-training subjects compared with no significant change in the controls. Other studies of resistance exercise in type 2 diabetics have used less intense programmes, but have generally showed smaller beneficial effects.

8.9   Physical activity and the behavioural treatment of obesity

The behavioural treatment of obesity refers to a set of principles and techniques designed to help overweight and obese individuals reverse their maladaptive eating, activity and thinking habits [94].

A number of important factors that effect physical activity behaviour change have been highlighted by researchers, these include:

- Personal and environmental factors – (e.g. [95,96]).

- Choice – (e.g. [97]).

- Social support – (e.g. [96]).

- Safety and the environment – (e.g. [96]).

- Psychological comorbidties – (e.g. [98,99]).

- Personal factors – (e.g. [100]).

- Reasons for participation in physical activity [101–105].

For a thorough consideration of the role of behavioural approaches in the treatment of obesity the reader is referred to the preceding chapter and a number of reviews of this subject [94,106,107].

8.10   Linking research and practice

Our team has developed the Carnegie International Camp, a summer residential 'fun type' skill-based intervention programme that combines physical activity, diet and behaviour modification [108]. We are also now running successful weekend and weekday evening interventions. The programmes have been developed during our 12 years evaluative research of residential treatment programmes for children [108,109] and our further research on translating our success to other forms of intervention. Our programmes are based on the principle that in order to engage children in persistent behaviour change, children should be given positive experiences of physical activity and healthy eating. It is our view that most treatment programmes do not adopt such an approach, but rather they prioritize the determination of the dietary restriction and physical activity levels to achieve a specific energy imbalance. Few studies consider the elements of the process of behaviour change for overweight and obese people engaged in weight loss strategies. We believe that understanding the process of intervention is critical to the successful treatment of this disease. There are some common principles in successful weight loss intervention but they need to be flexible and enable the intervention to be tailored to the individual. General advice and guidelines will therefore not work for many people. Our experience supports the work of McAuley *et al.* [91] that showed that more intensive treatments produced better outcomes than so called standard treatments for type 2 diabetes. Clearly, more research is required in order to determine how different interventions can be applied efficaciously in different settings for different target groups, but research seems to suggest that more resources are needed to offer more intensive treatment and support to deal with both obesity and type 2 diabetes. Readers interested in more information on our various intervention programmes and associated research are directed to www.carnegieweightmanagement. com.

8.11 Summary

Physical activity, obesity and type 2 diabetes

- Physical activity is an important component in both the prevention and treatment of obesity and type 2 diabetes.

- Achievement of current guidelines for physical activity will make a significant contribution to energy balance and metabolic control in the obese and type 2 diabetic populations.

- Physical activity and fitness are important for decreasing the risk profile and improving health status independently of weight loss, although also decreasing excess body fat is still preferable.

- Any increase in physical activity is to be encouraged and positively reinforced in the sedentary population.

Physical activity in the treatment of obesity and type 2 diabetes

- Physical activity is most effective as a treatment intervention when applied together with improvements in eating behaviour set in the framework of sustainable behaviour modification of lifestyle.

- Physical activity helps maintain fat free mass during calorific restriction.

- Physical activity can increase basal metabolic rate through increasing muscle mass.

- Increasing physical activity will produce functional adaptations in the body that improve the risk profile and health status of the participant in terms of overweight, obesity and type 2 diabetes.

- Achievement of current population guidelines for physical activity may represent a relatively long term goal for the chronically obese and long-term sedentary type 2 diabetic due to their severely limited exercise tolerance.

- Non-weight-bearing physical activity in short bouts of a few minutes regularly throughout the day will be needed in the most sedentary and obese due to poor exercise tolerance.

- The chronically obese and type 2 diabetics should be evaluated and monitored by their clinicians both before embarking on and during regular habitual physical activity.

- Most obese and type 2 diabetics will have led a sedentary existence for some considerable time, often many years, therefore treatments incorporating physical activity must be realistic in setting and managing expectations in participants.

- Substantial and sustained weight loss is often triggered by a key event so it will not work in all cases.

- Substantial weight loss and sustained weight maintenance are commonly associated with a sustainable increase in daily habitual physical activity.

- Many overweight and obese people like physical activity and sport, but not all do. Individual needs, lifestyle and enjoyment must be considered when attempting to increase physical activity in a sustainable way.

Physical activity in the prevention of obesity and type 2 diabetes

- Achievement of the general current physical activity recommendations will not be sufficient in energy expenditure terms to offset the energy intake of many individuals, the result of which is seen in the continued increase in prevalence of overweight and obesity.

- Increasing physical activity must be achievable within the lives of the participants in such a way that they can enjoy it and see it as sustainable.

- Increasing physically activity must be targeted to the needs of the individual with appropriate support and guidance, simply telling people to eat less and take more exercise does not work.

- Barriers and determinants of a physically active lifestyle will vary from person to person. Addressing the issues of enjoyment, physical competence in terms of improved skills, choice, opportunity, empowerment, social and emotional support are more likely to lead to sustainable lifestyle change, including increased activity.

References

1. Casperson, C.J., Powell, K.E. and Christenson, G.M. (1985) Physical activity, exercise and fitness. *Public Health Report*, **100**, 125–31.
2. American College of Sports Medicine (1998) *Resource Manual for Guidelines for Exercise Testing and Prescription*, 3rd edn, Williams & Wilkins, Baltimore.
3. Activity and Health Research (1992) Allied Dunbar National Fitness Survey: Main Findings. Health Education Authority and Sports Council.
4. Department of Health (2004) *At Least Five a Week: Evidence on the impact of physical activity and its relationship to health*, Department of Health, London.
5. Sproston, K. and Primatesta, P. (2003) *Health Survey for England 2002. The Health of Children and Young People*, The Stationery Office, London.
6. Biddle, S., Sallis, J. and Cavill, N. (1998) Young and Active? in *Young People and Health-Enhancing Physical Activity – Evidence and Implications*, Health Education Authority, London.
7. Twisk, J. (2001) Physical activity guidelines for children and adolescents. A critical review. *Sports Medicine*, **31**, 617–27.
8. Amercian College of Sports Medicine and American Heart Association (2007) Physical Activity and Public Health: updated recommendations for adults from the American College of Sports Medicine and the American Heart Association. *Circulation*, **116**, 1081–93.
9. Nelson, M.E., Rejeski, W.J., Blair, S.N. *et al.* (2007) Physical activity and public health in older adults: recommendation from the American College of Sports Medicine and the American Heart Association. *Medicine and Science in Sports and Exercise*, **39**, 1435–45.
10. Freedman, D.S., Khan, L.K., Dietz, W.H. *et al.* (2001) Relationship of childhood obesity to coronary heart disease risk factors in adulthood: the Bogalusa Heart Study. *Pediatrics*, **108** (3), 712–8.
11. Blair, S.N. and Brodney, S. (1999) Effects of physical inactivity and obesity on morbidity and mortality: current evidence and research issues. *Medicine and Science in Sports and Exercise*, **31**, S646–S662.
12. Bouchard, C. and Blair, S.N. (1999) Roundtable introduction, introductory comments for the consensus on physical activity and obestiy. *Medicine and Science in Sports and Exercise*, **31**, S498–S501.
13. Rissanen, A. and Fogelholm, M. (1999) Physical activity in the prevention and treatment of other morbid conditions and impairments associated with obesity: current evidence and research issues. *Medicine and Science in Sports and Exercise*, **31**, S635–S645.
14. Ross, R. and Janssen, I. (1999) Is abdominal fat preferentially reduced in response to exercise-induced weight loss? *Medicine and Science in Sports and Exercise*, **31**, S568–S572.
15. World Health Organization (1997) Obesity: preventing and managing the global epidemic. Report of a WHO consultation on obesity. Geneva. Switzerland.
16. Albright, A., Franz, M., Hornsby, G. *et al.* (2000) American College of Sports Medicine. Position stand on exercise and type 2 diabetes. *Medicine and Science in Sports and Exercise*, **32**, 1345–60.

17. American Diabetes Association (2008) Standards of medical care in diabetes – 2008. *Diabetes Care*, **31**(Supplement 1), S1–S54.

18. Sigal, R.J., Kenny, G.P., Wasserman, D.H. *et al.* (2006) Physical activity/exercise and type 2 diabetes: a consensus statement from the American Diabetes Association. *Diabetes Care*, **29**, 1433–8.

19. Astrand, P.O., Rodahl, K., Dahl, H.A. and Stromme, S.B. (2003) *Textbook of Work Physiology, Physiological Bases of Exercise*, 4th edn, Human Kinetics, Champaign, IL.

20. Ivy, J.L., Zderic, T.W. and Fogt, D.L. (1999) Prevention and treatment of non-insulin-dependant diabetes mellitus. *Exercise and Sport Sciences Reviews*, **47**, 37–44.

21. American Diabetes Association (2002) The prevention or delay of type 2 diabetes. *Diabetes Care*, **25**, 742–9.

22. Heath, G.W., Wilson, R.H., Smith, J. and Leonard, B.E. (1991) Community based exercise and weight control: diabetes risk reduction and glycemic control in Zuni Indians. *American Journal of Clinical Nutrition*, **53**, S1642–S1646.

23. Vanninen, E., Uusitupa, M. and Siitonen, O. (1992) Habitual physical activity, aerobic capacity, and metabolic control in patients with newly diagnosed type 2 diabetes mellitus: Effect of a 1 year diet and exercise intervention. *Diabetologia*, **35**, 340–6.

24. Ruderman, N.B., Ganada, O.P. and Johansen, K. (1979) The effect of physical training on glucose tolerance and plasma lipids in maturity-onset diabetes. *Diabetes*, **28**, 89–94.

25. Saltin, B., Lindfarde, F., Houston, M. *et al.* (1979) Physical training and glucose tolerance in middle-aged men with chemical diabetes. *Diabetes*, **28**, 30–79.

26. Schneider, S.H., Khachadurian, A.K., Amorosa, L.F. *et al.* (1992) Ten-year experience with an exercise-based outpatient lifestyle modification program in the treatment of diabetes mellitus. *Diabetes Care*, **15**, 1800–10.

27. Chipkin, S.R., Klugh, S.A. and Chasan-Taber, L. (2001) Exercise and diabetes. *Cardiology Clinics*, **19**, 489–505.

28. Krotkiewski, M., Mandroukas, K. and Sjostrom, L. (1979) Effects of long term physical training on body fat, metabolism and blood pressure in obesity. *Metabolism: Clinical and Experimental*, **28**, 650–8.

29. Schneider, S.H., Vitug, A. and Ruderman, A.B. (1986) Atherosclerosis and physical activity. *Diabetes-Metabolism Reviews*, **1**, 445–81.

30. Hagberg, J.M., Montain, S.T., Martin, M.H. and Ehsani, A.A. (1989) Effect of exercise training in 60 to 69 year old persons with essential hypertension. *American Journal of Cardiology*, **64**, 348–53.

31. National Institutes of Health (1998) *National Heart, Lung and Blood Institute: The Practical Guide. Identification, Evaluation, and Treatment of Overweight and Obesity in Adults*, NIH, Bethesda.

32. Lee, C., Blair, S.N. and Jackson, A.S. (1999) Cardiorespiratory fitness, body composition, and all cause and cardiovascular disease mortality in men. *American Journal of Clinical Nutrition*, **69**, 373–80.

33. Ainsworth, B.E., Haskell, W.L., Whitt, M.C. *et al.* (2000) Compendium of physical activities: an update of activity codes and MET intensities. *Medicine and Science in Sports and Exercise*, **32**(9 Suppl), S498–S504.

34. Ferro-Luzzi, A. and Martino, L. (1996) Obesity and physical activity, in *The Origins and Consequences of Obesity: Ciba Foundation Symposium 201*, John Wiley & Sons, Chichester, UK.

35. Ekelund, U., Yngve, A., Brage, S. *et al.* (2004) Body movement and physical activity related energy expenditure in children and adolescents: implications for the interpretation of physical activity data. *American Journal of Clinical Nutrition*, **79**, 851–6.

36. McArdle, W.D., Katch, F.I. and Katch, V.L. (1996) *Exercise Physiology, Energy, Nutrition and Human Performance*, 4th edn, Williams & Wilkins, Baltimore.

37. Ravussin, E. and Swinburn, B.A. (1992) Pathophysiology of obesity. *Lancet*, **340**, 404–8.

38. Ravussin (1995) Energy expenditure and body weight, in *Eating Disorders and Obesity* (eds K.D. Brownell and C.G. Fairburn), Guilford Press, New York.

39. Harrison, M.H., Bruce, D.L., Brown, G.A. and Cochrane, L.A. (1980) A comparison of some indirect methods of predicting maximal oxygen uptake. *Aviation Space and Environmental Medicine*, **51**, 1128.

40. Astrand, P.O. and Ryhming, I. (1954) A nomogram for the calculation of aerobic capacity (physical fitness) from pulse rate during submaximal work. *Journal of Applied Physiology*, **7**, 218.

41. Heyward, V. (1998) *Advanced Fitness Assessment and Exercise Prescription*, 3rd edn, Human Kinetics, Champaign.

42. Cooke, C.B. (2001) Metabolic rate and energy balance, in *Kinanthropometry and Exercise Physiology Laboratory Manual: Tests procedures and data. Volume 2: Exercise Physiology*, 2nd edn (eds R. Eston and T. Reilly), Routledge, London.

43. American College of Sports Medicine (1995) *ACSM's Guidelines for Exercise Testing and Prescription*, Williams & Wilkins, Baltimore.

44. Borg, G.V. and Linderholm, H. (1967) Perceived exertion and pulse rate during graded exercise in various age groups. *Acta Medica Scandinavica*, **472**(Suppl), 194–206.

45. Birk, T.J. and Birk, C.A. (1987) Use of ratings of perceived exertion for exercise prescription. *Sports Medicine*, **4**, 1–8.

46. Dunbar, C.C., Robertson, R.J., Baun, R. *et al.* (1992) The validity of regulating exercise intensity by ratings of perceived exertion. *Medicine and Science in Sports and Exercise*, **24**, 94–9.

47. Goran, M.I. (1998) Measurement issues related to studies of childhood obesity: Assessment of body composition, body fat distribution, physical activity and food intake. *Paediatrics*, **101**, 505–19.

48. Delaney, J.P. (1998) Role of energy expenditure in the development of paediatric obesity. *American Journal of Clinical Nutrition*, **68**, 950–5.

49. Roberts, S.B. and Leibel, R.L. (1998) Excess energy intake and low energy expenditure as predictors of obesity. *International Journal of Obesity*, **22**, 385–6.

50. Gately, P.J., Cooke, C.B., Barth, J.H. and Butterly, R.J. (1997) Exercise tolerance in a sample of morbidly obese subjects. *Procedings of the European Congress on Obesity*, Trinity College, Dublin, Ireland.

51. Surgeon General's Report (1996) *Physical Activity and Health: A Report of the Surgeon General*, US Department of Health and Human Services, Washington, DC.

52. Albert, C.M., Mittleman, M.A., Chae, C.U. *et al.* (2000) Triggering of sudden death from cardiac causes by vigorous exertion. *NEJM*, **343**, 1355–61.

53. American College of Sports Medicine and American Diabetes Association joint position statement (1997) Diabetes mellitus and exercise. *Medicine and Science in Sports and Exercise*, **29** (12), i–vi.

54. Burke, E.J., Germain, M.J., Fitzgibbons, J.P. *et al.* (1987) A comparison of the physiologic effects of submaximal exercise during and off hemodialysis treatment. *Journal of Cardiopulmonary Rehabilitation*, **7**, 68–72.

55. Schulz, L.O. and Schoeller, D.A. (1994) A compilation of total daily energy expenditures and body weights in healthy adults. *American Journal of Clinical Nutrition*, **60**, 676–81.

56. Black, A.E., Coward, W.A., Cole, T.J. and Prentice, A.M. (1996) Human energy expenditure in affluent societies: an analysis of 574 doubly-labelled water measurements. *European Journal of Clinical Nutrition*, **50**, 72–92.

57. Seidell, J.C. (1998) Epidemiology: Definition and classification of obesity, in *Clinical Obesity* (eds P.G. Kopelman, and M.J. Stock), Blackwell Science, London.
58. Haapanen, N., Miilumnpalo, S., Pasanen, M. *et al.* (1997) Association between leisure time physical activity and 10 year body mass change among working aged men and women. *International Journal of Obesity*, **21**, 288–96.
59. Coakley, E.H., Rimm, E.B., Colditz, G. *et al.* (1998) Predictors of change in men: Results from the health professionals follow up study. *International Journal of Obesity*, **22**, 89–96.
60. Schmitz, K.H., Jacobs, D.R., Leon, A.S. *et al.* (2000) Physical activity and body weight associations over ten years in the CARDIA study. *International Journal of Obesity*, **24**, 1475–87.
61. Wareham, N.J., van Sluijs, E.M.F. and Ekelund, U. (2005) Physical activity and obesity prevention: a review of the current evidence. *Proceedings of the Nutrition Society*, **64**, 229–47.
62. Miller, W.C., Koceja, D.M. and Hamilton, E.J. (1997) A meta-analysis of the past 25 years weight loss research using diet, exercise or diet plus exercise intervention. *International Journal of Obesity*, **21**, 941–7.
63. Ballor, D.L. and Poehlman, E.T. (1995) A meta-analysis of the effects of exercise and/or dietary restriction on resting metabolic rate. *European Journal of Applied Physiology*, **71**, 535–42.
64. Epstein, L.H. and Myers, M.D. (1998) Treatment of pediatric obesity. *Paediatrics*, **101**, 554–71.
65. Miller, W.C. (1999) How effective are traditional dietary and exercise interventions for weight loss? *Medicine and Science in Sports and Exercise*, **31** (8), 1129–34.
66. Garner, D.M. and Wooley, S.C. (1991) Confronting the failure of behavioural and dietary treatment for obesity. *Clinical Psychology Review*, **11**, 729–80.
67. Garrow, J.S. and Summerbell, C.D. (1995) Meta-analysis: effects of exercise, with or without dieting, on the body composition of overweight subjects. *European Journal of Clinical Nutrition*, **49**, 1–10.
68. Klem, M.L., Wing, R.R., McGuire, M.T. *et al.* (1997) A descriptive study of individuals successful at long-term maintenance of substantial weight loss. *The American Journal of Clinical Nutrition*, **66**, 239–46.
69. Anderson, J.W., Konz, E.C., Frederich, R.C. and Wood, C.L. (2001) Long-term weight loss maintenance: a meta-analysis of US studies. *American Journal of Clinical Nutrition*, **74**, 579–84.
70. Dunn, A.L., Garcia, M.E., Marcus, B.H. *et al.* (1998) Six-month physical activity and fitness changes in project active, a randomised trial. *Medicine and Science in Sports and Exercise*, **30**, 1076–83.
71. Epstein, L.H. and Goldfield, G.S. (1999) Physical activity in the treatment of childhood overweight and obesity: Current evidence and research issues. *Medicine and Science in Sports and Exercise*, **31**, S553–S559.
72. Epstein, L.H., Wing, R.R., Koeske, R. and Valoski, A. (1985) A comparison of lifestyle exercise, aerobic exercise and calisthenics on weight loss in obese children. *Behavior Therapy*, **16**, 345–56.
73. Hills, A.P. and Parker, A.W. (1988) Obesity management via diet and exercise intervention. *Child: Care, Health and Development*, **14**, 409–16.
74. Gutin, B., Owens, S., Okuyama, T. *et al.* (1999) Effect of physical training and it's cessation on percent body fat and bone density of children with obesity. *Obesity Research*, **7** (2), 208–14.
75. Epstein, L.H., Valoski, A., Wing, R.R. and McCurley, J. (1994) Ten-year outcomes of behavioural family-based treatment for childhood obesity. *Health Psychology*, **13**, 373–83.

76. Epstein, L.H., Valoski, L.S., McCurley, J. *et al.* (1995) Effects of decreasing sedentary behaviour and increasing activity on weight change in obese children. *Health Psychology*, **14**, 109–15.

77. Gutin, B., Cucuzzo, N., Isalm, S. *et al.* (1995) physical training improves body composition of black obese 7- to 11-year-old girls. *Obesity Research*, **3** (4), 305–12.

78. Diabetes Prevention Program Research Group (2002) Reduction in the incidence of type 2 diabetes with lifestyle intervention or metformin. *The New England Journal of Medicine*, **346**, 393–403.

79. Tuomilehto, J., Lindstrom, J., Eriksson, J.G. *et al.* (2001) Prevention of type 2 diabetes mellitus by change in lifestyle among subjects with impaired glucose tolerance. *New England Journal of Medicine*, **344**, 1343–50.

80. Pan, X.R., Li, G.W., Hu, Y.H. *et al.* (1997) Effects of diet and exercise in preventing NIDDM in people with impaired glucose tolerance: the Da Qing IGT and Diabetes Study. *Diabetes Care*, **20**, 537–44.

81. Helmrich, S.P., Ragland, D.R., Leung, P.W. and Paffenbarger, R.S., Jr (1991) Physical activity and reduced occurrence of non-insulin dependant diabetes mellitus. *The New England Journal of Medicine*, **325**, 147–52.

82. Manson, J.E., Rimm, E.B., Stampfer, M.J. *et al.* (1991) Physical activity and incidence of non-insulin dependant diabetes mellitus in women. *Lancet*, **338**, 774–8.

83. Manson, J.E., Nathan, D.M., Krolewski, A.S. *et al.* (1992) A prospective study of exercise and incidence of diabetes among US male physicians. *Journal of the American Medical Association*, **268**, 63–7.

84. Eriksson, K.F. and Lindgarde, F. (1998) No excess 12 year mortality in men with impaired glucose tolerance who participated in the Malmo preventive trial with diet and exercise. *Diabetologia*, **41**, 1010–16.

85. Boulé, N.G., Haddad, E., Kenny, G.P. *et al.* (2001) Effects of exercise on glycemic control and body mass in type 2 diabetes mellitus: a meta-analysis of controlled clinical trials. *Journal of the American Medical Association*, **286**, 1218–27.

86. Boulé, N.G., Kenny, G.P., Haddad, E. *et al.* (2003) Meta-analysis of the effect of structured exercise training on cardiorespiratory fitness in type 2 diabetes mellitus. *Diabetologia*, **46**, 1071–81.

87. Church, T.S., Cheng, Y.J., Earnest, C.P. *et al.* (2004) Exercise capacity and body composition as predictors of mortality among men with diabetes. *Diabetes Care*, **27**, 83–8.

88. Hu, F.B., Sigal, R.J., Rich-Ewards, J.W. *et al.* (1999) Walking compared with vigorous physical activity and risk of type 2 diabetes in women. *Journal of the American Medical Association*, **282** (5), 1433–7.

89. Wei, M., Gibbons, L.W., Kampert, J.B. *et al.* (2000) Low cardiorespiratory fitness and physical inactivity as predictors of mortality in men with type 2 diabetes. *Annals of Internal Medicine*, **132**, 605–11.

90. Brown, S.A., Upchurch, S., Anding, R. *et al.* (1996) Promoting weight loss in type 2 diabetes. *Diabetes Care*, **19**, 613–24.

91. McAuley, K.A., Williams, S.M., Mann, J.I. *et al.* (2002) Intensive lifestyle changes are necessary to improve insulin sensitivity. *Diabetes Care*, **25**, 445–52.

92. Dunstan, D.W., Daly, R.M., Owen, N. *et al.* (2002) High intensity resistance training improves glycemic control in older persons with type 2 diabetes. *Diabetes Care*, **25**, 1729–35.

93. Castaneda, C., Layne, J.E., Munoz-Orians, L. *et al.* (2002) A randomized controlled trial of resistance exercise training to improve glycemic control in older adults with type 2 diabetes. *Diabetes Care*, **25**, 2335–41.

94. Wadden, T.A. and Foster, G.D. (2000) Behavioral Treatment of Obesity. *Medical Clinics of North America*, **84** (2), 441–61.

95. Dishman, R.K. (1994) *Advances in Exercise Adherence*, Human Kinetics, Champaign.

96. Sallis, J.F. and Owen, N. (1997) *Physical Activity and Behavioural Medicine*, Sage, California.

97. Rodin, J., Silberstein, L.R. and Striegel-Moore, R.H. (1985) Women and weight: a normative discontent. *Psychology and Gender*, **32**, 20–35.

98. Gortmaker, S.L., Must, A., Perrin, J.M. *et al.* (1993) Social and economic consequences of overweight in adolescent and young adulthood. *New England Journal of Medicine*, **329**, 1008–12.

99. Sullivan, M., Sullivan, M., Karlsson, J. *et al.* (1993) Swedish obese subjects (SOS) – an intervention study of obesity. Baseline evaluation of health and psychosocial functioning in the first 1743 subjects examined. *International Journal of Obesity*, **17**, 503–12.

100. Fox, K. (1988) Children's participation motives. *British Journal of Physical Education*, **19**, 79–82.

101. Gould, D. (1984) Psychosocial development and children's sport, in *Motor Development During Childhood and Adolescence* (ed. J.R. Thomas), Burgess, Minneapolis, MN.

102. Wankel, L.M. and Kreisel, P.S.J. (1985) Factors underlying enjoyment of youth sports: sport and age group comparisons. *Journal of Sport Psychology*, **7**, 51–64.

103. Parker, D.L. (1991) Juvenile obesity. The importance of exercise and getting children to do it. *Physician and Sports Medicine*, **19**, 113–25.

104. Stucky-Ropp, R.C. and Dilorenzo, T.M. (1993) Determinants of exercise in children. *Preventive Medicine*, **22**, 880–9.

105. Bar-Or, O. and Baranowski, T. (1994) Physical activity, adiposity and obesity among adolescents. *Pediatric Exercise Science*, **6**, 348–60.

106. Wadden, T.A., Sarwer, D.B. and Berkowitz, R.I. (1999) Behavioural treatment of the overweight patient. *Baillière's Clinical Endocrinology and Metabolism*, **13** (1), 93–107.

107. Faith, M.S., Fontaine, K.R., Cheskin, L.J. and Allison, D.B. (2000) Behavior approaches to the problems of obesity. *Behavior Modification*, **24** (4), 459–93.

108. Gately, P.J., Cooke, C.B., Barth, J.H. *et al.* (2005) Children's residential weight-loss programs can work: a prospective cohort study of short-term outcomes for overweight and obese children. *Paediatrics*, **116**, 73–7.

109. Gately, P.J., Cooke, C.B., Butterly, R.J. *et al.* (2000) The effects of a children's summer camp programme on weight loss, with a 10 month follow up. *International Journal of Obesity*, **24**, 1445–52.

9

Diabetes, obesity and cardiovascular disease – therapeutic implications

Jayadave Shakher and Anthony H. Barnett
Department of Medicine/Diabetes/Endocrinology, Birmingham Heartlands Hospital, Birmingham, UK

9.1   Introduction

Obesity is a worldwide problem. The prevalence of obesity is no longer confined to western populations as shown in two large international studies. (INTERHEART, IDEA) Obesity and overweight are independent risk factors for cardiovascular morbidity and mortality [1,2]. These figures were mainly based on epidemiological studies in white populations. The INTERHEART study was the first large international study to establish that obesity is a significant cardiovascular disease risk factor across world's populations. Risk of morbidity and mortality begins to rise at body mass index (BMI) $>25 \, \text{kg/m}^2$ and the risk increases sharply at BMI $>30 \, \text{kg/m}^2$. Although BMI is used as a surrogate indicator of cardiovascular risks, central or abdominal obesity is considered to be a better predictor.

The mechanism by which obesity causes increased cardiovascular morbidity and mortality is attributed to associated co-morbidities and risk factors such as hypertension, dyslipidaemia, type 2 diabetes and insulin resistance. The co-occurrence of some or all of these risk factors along with obesity is termed the cardiometabolic syndrome.

Until recently the mechanism of atherosclerosis in obesity was not well understood. The recognition of adipose tissue as a metabolically active endocrine organ, capable of synthesizing and secreting mediators like tumour necrosis factor-alpha (TNF-α), interleukin-6 (IL-6), plasminogen activator inhibitor1 (PAI-1) and angiotensin II (AII) may help explain the process of accelerated atherosclerosis. Endothelial dysfunction,

Obesity and Diabetes, Second Edition   Edited by Anthony H. Barnett and Sudhesh Kumar
© 2009 John Wiley & Sons, Ltd

which is a recognized complication of obesity and type 2 diabetes mellitus, plays an important role in thrombus formation.

Altered secretion of adipocytokines may be implicated in the pathogenesis of type 2 diabetes mellitus. Therefore by modifying lipids, decreasing blood pressure, achieving near normoglycaemia, and reducing pro-inflammatory cytokines and adhesion molecules through weight loss and pharmacotherapy, may prevent progression of atherosclerosis or occurrence of acute coronary syndrome events in obese high risk populations with type 2 diabetes.

9.2   Obesity and mortality

A number of large epidemiological studies have indicated that the greater the BMI the higher the mortality. The association between excess body weight and death is seen in The Nurses' Health Study, with mortality rising progressively in woman with BMI >29 kg/m² [3]. The increased mortality was also noted in the American Cancer Society's Cancer Prevention Study I and II [4].

A prospective study involving 527 265 US men and women, aged 50–71 years from National Institutes of Health-AARP cohort, followed up for 10 years, showed an increased risk of death for the highest and lowest categories of BMI among both sexes, in all racial or ethnic groups and at all ages. This study also addresses potential biases related to pre-existing chronic disease and smoking status, some of the factors apart from diet and exercise habits, which may explain the wide variability in the annual excess deaths attributable to obesity.

Among the individuals aged ≥50 years, who never smoked and with low prevalence of chronic disease, the risk of death increased by 20–40% in overweight persons and by two to over three fold among obese persons [5].

9.3   Obesity and cardiovascular disease

Obesity is a major contributor to the risk of cardiovascular disease. In the Framingham Heart Study, the 26 year incidence of CHD was increased by a factor of 2.4 in obese women and 2 in obese men under age of 50 years [6]. Excess weight was an independent predictor of coronary artery disease, coronary death and congestive heart failure after adjusting for other known recognized risk factors.

In the Nurses' Health Study from the United States, the risk of developing CHD increased 3.3-fold with BMI >29 kg/m² and 1.8-fold between 25 and 29 kg/m² compared to those women with BMI < 21 kg/m². (4,7) Each kilogram of weight gained from the age of 18 years was associated with 3.1% higher risk of cardiovascular disease [3,7]. Excess weight in adolescence is a predictor of these risks in adulthood [8].

This increased risk extends to overweight children and adolescents, who may be at risk of premature cardiovascular morbidity and death [9]. As an example, in an autopsy study of 3000 subjects under age 35 years (who had died of external causes), increasing

BMI was associated with fatty streaks and raised atherosclerotic lesions in the coronary arteries in young men [10].

The increased CHD risk is better correlated with abdominal or central obesity than body mass index [11]. In the Nurses' Health Study, a waist–hip ratio (WHR) of >0.88 versus WHR <0.72 was associated with an increased relative risk of CHD of 3.25 [12]. Analysis of the INTERHEART study showed a simple measure of WHR is a better predictor of obesity-associated CVD risk than BMI [13]. A second large trial, the International Day for the Evaluation of Abdominal Obesity (IDEA) study also shown that waist circumference is a stronger predictor of CVD outcomes than BMI [14].

The prevalence of subclinical CVD was also higher in overweight and obese individuals compared to those with normal BMI and correlated better in individuals with increased waist circumference than normal WC in 1938 Framingham Study participants as measured by five tests (ECG, echocardiogram, carotid ultrasound, ankle brachial pressure and urinary micro-albumin excretion) [15]. WHR appears to be better marker of subclinical atherosclerosis than BMI and waist circumference as measured by coronary artery calcium imaging [16,17].

Along with an increased risk of CHD, obese populations experience a higher recurrence of cardiac event rates after acute myocardial infarction. The relative risk of recurrent infarction or death was 1.5 with BMI 30–34.5 kg/m^2 and 1.8 with BMI >35 kg/m^2 compared to BMI 16–24 kg/m^2 as seen in a population-based study of 2541 patients [18].

There is also an important association between obesity and heart failure. In the Framingham Heart Study, increased in BMI was associated with an increased risk of heart failure with doubling of the risk in obese subjects compared with subjects with a normal BMI. After adjustment for traditional risk factors, there was an increase in the risk of heart failure of 5% for men and 7% for women for each increment of 1 in BMI [19].

The increased CHD morbidity and mortality could be related to traditional risk factors like hypertension and dyslipidaemia or due to the effect of obesity per se on the cardiovasculature. Obesity is associated with disturbances in cardiac function and structural changes in the absence of hypertension and underlying organic heart disease. There is an increase in total blood volume in proportion to body weight resulting in higher cardiac output. Volume overload of the left ventricle results in increased left ventricular stress, which stimulates eccentric hypertrophy of the ventricle with resultant diastolic dysfunction. Over time, excessive wall stress causes ventricular dilatation resulting in systolic dysfunction, termed obesity cardiomyopathy. The presence of hypertension in obesity exacerbates left ventricular wall changes which can increase progression towards heart failure [20].

Left ventricular wall abnormality is implicated in the propensity for sudden death seen in obesity. The reason for sudden death from cardiomyopathy may be due to complex ventricular arrhythmias. Prolonged Q-T interval, which predisposes to cardiac arrhythmias, occurs in up to one-third of obese subjects [21]. Other ECG changes observed in a study of 100 obese subjects compared with 100 normal subjects, without any evidence of cardiac disease included more leftward shift of P, QRS and T axes, evidence of left ventricular hypertrophy and left atrial abnormality and T-wave flattening seen in the inferior and lateral leads [22].

An analysis from Framingham and another population-based-cohort study, the Danish Diet, Cancer and Health Study, showed obese individuals (BMI ≥ 30) were at increased risk of developing either atrial fibrillation or flutter when compared to normal (BMI < 25) [23,24]. An increase in BMI was also found to be associated for sustained atrial fibrillation [25].

The structural and functional changes are also seen in the right side of the heart in obesity. Right ventricular dysfunction could be secondary to left ventricular dysfunction or due to obstructive sleep apnoea and/or obesity hypoventilation syndrome which occurs in 5% of morbidly obese individuals [26].

9.4   Obesity and hypertension

A rise in blood pressure is associated with increased body weight. Epidemiological studies indicate that obesity is a strong independent risk factor for hypertension [27,28]. In the Framingham Study, for example, the prevalence of hypertension among obese individuals was twice that of those individuals with normal weight irrespective of sex and age [6]. In the Swedish Obesity Study, hypertension was present at baseline in approximately one-half of subjects [29,30]. The INTERSALT Study involving 10 000 men and women showed that a 10 kg increase in weight was associated with 3 mmHg rise in systolic and 2.3 mmHg rise in diastolic blood pressure [31]. This level of blood pressure elevation is associated with a 12% increase risk for CHD and 24% increase for stroke. In the Nurses' Health Study, the relative risk of hypertension in those women who gained 5.0–9.9 kg and greater than 25.0 kg was 1.7 and 5.2, respectively. The risk of hypertension was even higher with abdominal obesity (WHR > 0.9 in men and >0.85 in women) [32].

The exact mechanism of the association of central obesity and hypertension is not fully defined. Insulin resistance may provide a metabolic link perhaps through hyperinsulinaemia. Hyperinsulinaemia enhances sodium reabsorption directly through its effects on distal renal tubules [33] and indirectly through the stimulation of central sympathetic nervous system [34,35]. It also augments AII-mediated aldosterone secretion [36]. The resultant hypervolaemia causes an increase in cardiac output, yet the total peripheral resistance remains near normal with failure of vasodilatation of the systemic vasculature. Vasodilatation is thought to be mediated by nitric oxide (NO) and this vasodilatory effect is blunted in obese and hypertensive subjects [37,38].

Another mechanism that may cause increased vascular tone is through alterations in cation transport. Insulin has been shown to stimulate NA/K ATPase activity with accumulation of intracellular sodium along with increase in intracellular calcium leading to vascular resistance and hypertension. [39]. This link between hyperinsulinaemia and hypertension is not seen in Pima Indians despite commonly having hyperinsulinaemia, insulin resistance and obesity [40]. These discrepancies might be explained by difference in genetic susceptibility to the development of hypertension or to the effects of insulin on blood pressure. Another explanation is that there might be 'selective insulin resistance' with impaired ability of insulin to cause glucose uptake, but preservation of some actions such as renal sodium retention, activation of the renin-angiotensin system, alteration in cation flux and stimulation of the sympathetic nervous system.

9.5 Obesity and dyslipidaemia

Obesity is associated with alteration in lipoprotein metabolism resulting in an athero-genic lipid profile with increase in total cholesterol (TC), triglycerides (TG), low density lipoprotein cholesterol (LDLc), very low density lipoprotein cholesterol (VLDL) and reduced level of high density cholesterol (HDLc) [6,41].

Dyslipidaemia associated with obesity is multi-factorial and frequently associated with different components of metabolic syndrome; the relationship is strongest particularly for visceral adipose tissue (VAT), clinically correlated with measurement of waist circumference.

The common underlying driver appears to be insulin resistance (IR). IR results in lipolysis with increased availability of free fatty acids (FFA) to liver and subsequent increased production of atherogenic lipid particles. Each of the individual components of this dyslipidaemic profile is associated with increased risk of cardiovascular disease. (see Lipid metabolism in adipose tissue.)

Epidemiological studies such as the Framingham Heart Study and the Multiple Risk Factor Intervention Trial (MRFIT) showed a significant positive correlation between plasma cholesterol levels and increased risk of death due to CHD [28].

In the PROCAM study, involving 4407 German men aged between 40 and 65 years without cardiac disease at the start of the study, the combination of high triglyceride and total cholesterol and low HDL levels for example was associated with the increased risk of coronary heart disease. In men with plasma cholesterol levels above 6.5 mmol/l with HDLc less than 0.9 mmol/l, the risk of myocardial infarction over 6 years was as high as 20–30% [42].

Indeed, epidemiological studies confirm that low plasma HDL cholesterol is a better predictor of risk of CHD. The univariate analysis of the data from PROCAM indicates a significant association between CHD and HDL ($p < 0.001$) which remained after adjustment for other risk factors [43]. The Framingham Study also shows a clear correlation between low HDLc and increased risk of CHD mortality and morbidity, regardless of LDL cholesterol levels [6]. The ratio of total/HDLc is a good index of the relative contribution of atherogenic vs. antiatherogenic lipoprotein to CHD risk.

Although there is an inverse relationship between low HDL and elevated TG levels, TG concentration as an independent risk factor of coronary heart disease remains controversial. Studies such as the PROCAM, the Stockholm Prospective Study and the Paris Prospective Study showed positive correlations between TG and CHD risks. ([42,44,45]) The meta-analyses of sixteen population-based studies showed that after adjusting for HDLc, every 1 mmol/l increase in TG was associated with relative risk increase in CHD by 14% in men and 37% in women [46].

Despite the controversy, there is a growing consensus that TG lipoprotein directly causes atherosclerotic cardiovascular disease or at least acts as a marker for CHD risk factors. The pathogenesis of atherosclerosis is believed to be related to TG-rich lipoproteins (TGRLPs) which include VLDL, chylomicrons and their remnants and IDL, all of which contain more cholesterol than LDLc [47–49].

These small TGRLPs appear to possess atherogenic potential similar to small dense LDLc, with the ability to infiltrate arterial wall and leads to atherosclerosis [50].

The role of LDLc in the pathogenesis of CHD has been well established and indeed the predominance of small, dense LDL particles is reported to be more prevalent in CHD patients than in healthy controls [51]. This was confirmed in Québec Cardiovascular Study which showed dense LDL particles are associated with increase risk of CHD over 5 years and the combination of small dense LDLc and elevated apolipoprotein B (ApoB) concentration resulted in a sixfold increase in risk of CHD. Further analyses of LDL subclasses indicate absolute levels of small LDL are a more significant predictor of CHD risk than reduced peak LDL size alone [52,53].

Though ApoB and LDLc are considered good predictors of CHD, the use of ApoB in clinical practice is limited by lack of standardization and calculation of LDLc using the Friedewald equation

$$LDLc = (TC - HDLc\text{-}TG)/2.17 \text{ in mmol/l} \quad \text{or} \quad TG/5 \text{ in mg/dl}$$

is less accurate with increasing TG levels and inapplicable at TG > 4.52 mmol/l [54].

Recently, non-HDLc was considered to be a better predictor of CHD risk as it encompasses all cholesterol present in atherogenic lipoprotein particles (VLDL, IDL, LDL, lipoprotein A) and there appears to be a correlation between non-HDLc and ApoB. The measurement of non-HDLc (TC minus HDLc) required only TC and HDLc which can be measured in non-fasting sample [55].

9.6　Metabolic syndrome, obesity, type 2 diabetes and insulin resistance

Insulin resistance is a common feature of obesity and its incidence rises with increasing BMI. Visceral obesity is an even better predictor than BMI of hyperinsulinaemia, insulin resistance and type 2 diabetes [56,57]. The clustering of cardiovascular risk factors with insulin resistance was first described as syndrome X by Reaven in 1988 and included central obesity, hypertension, glucose intolerance and dyslipidaemia ('deadly quartet') [58–60]. Other features of the syndrome have since been added to include a procoagulant state and accelerated atherosclerosis, appropriately called the 'cardio-metabolic syndrome'.

The National Cholesterol Education Programme (Adult Treatment Panel III, ATP III) suggests that clinical criteria for definition of insulin resistance or metabolic syndrome should be based upon any three of the following [61] (Table 9.1).

The WHO definition requires insulin resistance as the baseline criteria. The International Diabetes Federation's definition focuses on abdominal obesity rather than insulin resistance with different waist circumference thresholds set for different race/ethnicity groups (Table 9.2) (Figure 9.1).

Table 9.1 ATP III Metabolic syndrome

Waist circumference	>102 cm/40 in (in men)
	>88 cm/35 in (in women)
TG level	>150 mg/dl (1.7 mmol/l)
HDL cholesterol	<40 mg/dl (<1 mmol in men)
	<50 mg/dl (<1.3 mmol in women)
Blood pressure	>130/85 mmHg
Fasting glucose	>110 mg/dl (>6.1 mmol/l)

Based on these criteria, the Third National Health and Nutrition Examinations Survey (NHANES), found an overall prevalence of metabolic syndrome at 22% and the prevalence increasing steadily with age. African/American women have approximately 57% higher prevalence and Hispanic women have approximately 26% high prevalence than their male counterparts. Ford and colleagues found that in men and women with metabolic syndrome from NHANES, approximately 50% showed evidence of insulin resistance suggesting that the link between obesity and IGT or type 2 diabetes may be through this mechanism [62].

The Third National Health and Nutrition Survey (NHANES III) data showed that there is an increased prevalence of CHD among adults with metabolic syndrome [63]. An epidemiological study ($N = 4483$) showed patients with metabolic syndrome had

Table 9.2 Metabolic syndrome

Components	WHO (Modified)	NCEP (ATP III)	IDF
IR	Presence		
IFG (FPG) (mmol/l)	≥6.1	≥6.1	≥5.6
IGT (2 hour PG) mmol/l	≥7.8		
WHR	>0.9 (>0.85)		
Waist circumference (cm)		>102 (>88)	>94 (>80)+
BMI (kg/m²)	>30		
BP (mmHg)	≥140/90	≥130/85	≥130/85
Triglycerides (mmol/l)	≥1.7	≥1.7	≥1.7
HDL cholesterol (mmol/l)	<0.9 (1/0)	<1.04 (<1.29)	≥0.9 (<1.1)
Number of components for diagnosis	IR or IFG or IGT plus ≥2 other components: central obesity (using WHR and/or BMI), ↑BP, dyslipidaemia (↑TG and/or ↓HDL cholesterol)	≥3 of the components above	Central obesity (waist circumference) plus two other components. Waist circumference defined ethnic groups

FPG, fasting plasma glucose; IFG, impaired fasting glycaemia; IR, insulin resistance; WHR, waist–hip ratio; BP, blood pressure.

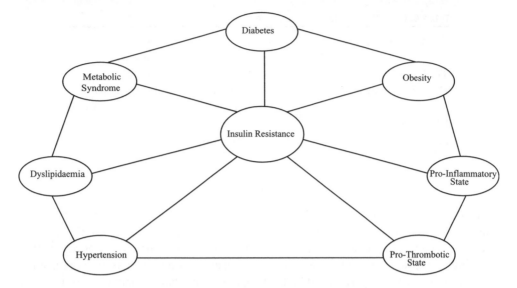

Figure 9.1   Insulin resistance syndrome

significant morbidity and mortality compared with normal patients with a relative risk of 2.96 for CHD, 2.63 for myocardial infarction (MI), 2.27 for stroke and 1.81 for death (median follow-up of 6.9 years) (Botnia study; [64]). The increased cardiovascular mortality was also seen in the Kuopio ischaemic heart study, involving 1209 Finnish men without CVD or diabetes at baseline. (Hazard ratio 3.55) [65]. In the San Antonia Heart Study, the hazard ratio for CVD mortality in people with metabolic syndrome is 2.1 in women and 2.0 in men. The risk increased to 8.19 in women and 3.09 in men, who have both metabolic syndrome and diabetes [66]. A recent meta-analysis drawn from a large number of longitudinal studies that included 172 573 people, indicates a significantly increased risks of cardiovascular events and death in people with metabolic syndrome [67].

There are a variety of factors that contribute to insulin resistance, including the distribution of body fat, the role of FFA, adipocytokines, pro-inflammatory mediators and genetic factors.

In obese individuals there is increased release of FFA from the visceral fat, which is more resistant to the metabolic effect of insulin and more sensitive to lipolytic hormones. An increased delivery of FFA to the liver may reduce insulin binding to hepatocytes, and impair insulin action with increased hepatic glucose production. Along with increased production of FFA, there is decreased utilization with defects in uptake and oxidation of FFA by the skeletal muscle in obesity and type 2 diabetes [68,69]. Regular exercise induces an increase in type 1 (aerobic, red) muscle fibres with enhanced insulin sensitivity by utilizing FFA, whereas type 2 (anaerobic, white) fibres predominate in sedentary subjects contributing to insulin resistance [70].

Fat cells produce adiponectin, which may play a role in development of insulin resistance and type 2 diabetes. A low concentration of adiponectin is related to insulin resistance and hyperinsulinaemia and with increased risk of type 2 diabetes in human subjects. The administration of thiazolidinediones in insulin-resistant subjects increases serum adiponectin levels [71,72].

TNF-α, an inflammatory cytokine, also secreted by adipocytes, is elevated in animal models of obesity and insulin resistance and neutralization of TNF-α ameliorates insulin resistance in obese rats. TNF-α mRNA expression is increased in obesity and levels of TNF-α correlate with serum insulin and body mass index.

TNF-α is implicated in causing insulin resistance by different mechanisms. It increases hormone sensitive lipase activity with resultant FFAs release from adipose tissue stores to the liver. At the post receptor level, TNFα interferes with insulin signalling and IRS proteins formation. This impairs insulin mediated glucose uptake by adipocytes through down regulation of the GLUT4, insulin responsive glucose transporters. It also down regulates peroxisome proliferator activator receptor expression [73,74].

9.7   Obesity and type 2 diabetes

Obesity is a powerful risk factor for the development of type 2 diabetes and more than two thirds of patients with type 2 diabetes are obese. The risk of type 2 diabetes correlates positively with increasing obesity [75,76]. In the Nurses' Health Study, the risk of developing diabetes increased fivefold in women with BMI 25 kg/m^2 compared with those with BMI 22 kg/m^2. The risk becomes higher reaching 28-fold with BMI 30 kg/m^2 and 93-fold with BMI >35 kg/m^2 [77]. In the same study, those who gained 5.0–7.9 kg had a relative risk of 1.9; this risk is increased to 2.7 for women who gained 8.0–10.9 kg.

The risk of obesity and type 2 diabetes was better defined by a high waist-to-hip circumference ratio and waist circumference [78]. Additionally, the duration of obesity was directly related to the risk of diabetes [79]. The risk of type 2 diabetes from obesity is more prevalent across certain ethnic groups such as South Asians and Afro-Caribbeans [80].

The increasing prevalence of type 2 diabetes is paralleled by the rise in the level of obesity in the general population. This process occurred over too short a period to implicate genetic factors per se. It is most likely that environmental factors interact with genetic susceptibility in the pathogenesis of type 2 diabetes. The 'thrifty genotype hypothesis' has been proposed as an explanation for the increased prevalence of type 2 diabetes. This suggests that during times of famine alternating with times of plenty, the ability to store fat efficiently leads to a survival advantage. In Western Style society, when there is permanent 'plenty', this genetic 'advantage' has become a liability with increased risk of development of obesity and diabetes [81].

9.8   Insulin resistance and cardiovascular disease

Various studies have shown that hyperinsulinaemia is a predictor of cardiovascular disease. The Québec Study showed that fasting insulin concentrations are independent predictors CHD. Plasma insulin levels were found to be 18% higher in men who develop CHD compared to men who remain healthy and fasting plasma insulin concentration was found to be an independent CHD risk factor after taking into account lipid and lipoprotein concentration [82].

Haffner and colleagues found that people who developed diabetes had higher fasting glucose and insulin concentrations along with elevated BP, lower HDLc and higher TG than in those whose glucose metabolism remained normal. Thus, for the macrovascular complications of type 2 diabetes like stroke or MI, the period of increased risk begins or 'the clock starts ticking' even before the onset of hyperglycaemia [83].

Evidence is emerging that inflammation and endothelial dysfunction are likely to be the important contributors to the accelerated atherosclerosis seen in people with IR, obesity and type 2 diabetes. Atherosclerosis precedes the development of type 2 diabetes and inflammation may be involved in the underlying process [84].

Yudkin [85] showed that inflammatory markers like C-reactive protein (CRP), pro-inflammatory cytokines, IL-6 and TNF-α correlate with obesity and IR. In a prospective study, Pradhan [86] followed 27 628 women free of diagnosis of diabetes and cardio-vascular disease for 4 years and found that baseline elevated markers of systemic inflammation like CRP and IL-6 powerfully predict the development of type 2 diabetes. Ridker *et al.* found that elevated level of CRP in the previously healthy women predicted the development of type 2 diabetes as well as likelihood of developing MI [87].

Increased levels of circulating inflammatory markers are also found in groups at risk of developing type 2 diabetes such as obese children, women with polycystic ovarian syndrome, women with a family history of type 2 diabetes and people of South Asian origin and Pima Indians, independently of BMI ([88–90]) These studies showed that inflammatory markers which are related to atherosclerosis also predicted the onset of cardiovascular disease and type 2 diabetes ('Common soil hypothesis') [87,91].

Loss of normal endothelial cell (EC) function is thought to be an early marker of development of atherosclerosis. In type 2 diabetes, there is early endothelial injury probably as a result of hyperglycaemia, hypertension and dyslipidaemia and insulin resistance. Impaired EC dysfunction is also seen in the early stages of diabetes, IGT and in first degree relatives of type 2 diabetes (Figures 9.2 and 9.3).

Endothelial cells serve as a metabolically active barrier between the lumen and the vessel wall and play a pivotal role in vascular homeostasis. Normal endothelial function includes regulation of vasomotor tone, homeostasis, leucocyte trafficking and vascular smooth muscle cell proliferation and migration. Endothelial cells elaborate NO, which mediates vasodilatation, antagonises thrombosis, and has anti-inflammatory properties and inhibits growth of vascular smooth muscle cells (VSMC) [92,93]. In dysfunctional states, apart from loss of NO secretion, ECs release substances such as AII and endothelin. They mediate vasoconstriction, aggravate thrombosis and activate plate-lets. These substances are proinflammatory and in the absence of NO, promote growth of VSMC and stimulate adhesion molecules like ICAM and VCAM (intracellular and vascular cell adhesion molecules [94] (Figure 9.3).

The mechanisms of EC dysfunction are secondary to hyperglycaemia and resistance to insulin. Hyperglycaemia contributes to EC dysfunction in several ways (glucose

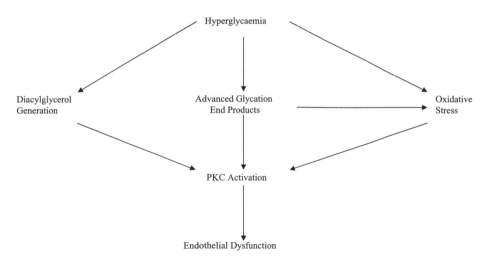

Figure 9.2 Mechanisms of hyperglycaemia-induced endothelial dysfunction. PKC, protein kinase C

hypothesis). Exposure to a high glucose level results in intracellular hyperglycaemia which damages the cells by multiple mechanisms. These include increased activity of the aldose reductase/sorbitol pathway, increased formation of advanced glycation end products (AGE), increased synthesis of diacylglycerol and increased oxidative stress with generation of protein kinase C (PKC). The adverse effect of oxidative stress on the cardiovascular system can be implicated into effects on NO availability, inflammatory response and lipid and lipoprotein modifications. Oxidative stress is increased during

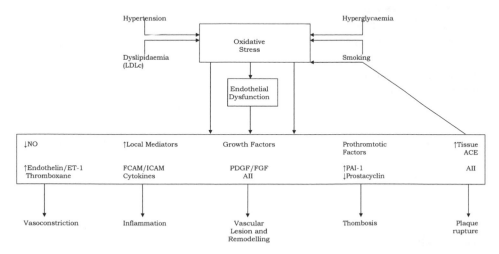

Figure 9.3 Endothelial dysfunction and mediators of vascular injury. NO, nitric oxide; VCAM, vascular cell adhesion molecule, ICAM intracellular adhesion molecule; PDGF, platelet-derived growth factor; FGF, fibroblast growth factor; AII, angiotensin II; PAI-1, plasminogen activator inhibitor-1

acute hyperglycaemia including postprandial hyperglycaemia. This results in overpro-duction of reactive oxygen species (ROS), in particular superoxide anion by the mitochondrial electron transport chain. Generation of excess superoxide anion reduces the availability of NO by reacting with NO to form the strong oxidant peroxynitrite which is directly toxic to endothelial cells (despite paradoxical increase in NO due to stimulation of NO synthase by the superoxide anion). ROS activate nuclear factor-κB with resultant expression of inflammatory cytokines like TNF-α, IL-1, -6, -8 and -18. ROS may be involved in initiation of lipid peroxidation which results in formation of advanced lipoxidation end products, which like AGEs contribute towards the athero-genic process [95–99] (Figures 9.2 and 9.3).

IR has shown to be associated with EC dysfunction even in the absence of hyperglycaemia (insulin hypothesis). IR is implicated in the development of cardio-vascular disease. A post receptor pathway involving phosphoinositol-3 (PI-3) kinase activity is implicated in IR. Insulin normally binds to its receptors and phosphorylates insulin receptor substrate 1 (IRS-1), which in turn activates the PI-3 kinase. PI-3 kinase plays a major role in both insulin mediated glucose disposal in adipose tissue and also in NO production by the EC.

The insulin stimulation of PI-3 kinase is reduced in obese subjects and almost absent in type 2 diabetes, [100] whereas, insulin action on the mitogen-activated protein kinase (MAPK) is unaffected. This 'selective insulin resistance' results in enhancement of the mitogenic pathway with increased VSMC growth and migration and increase in PAI-1 and endothelin. This pathway is present in vessels, heart and kidneys [101].

Adipocytes also contribute towards endothelial dysfunction. Adipocytes release IL-6 and TNF-α. IL-6 is one of the key promoters of hepatic CRP synthesis. CRP in turn has been shown to downregulate endothelial nitric oxide synthase *in vitro* and also regulates PAI-1 synthesis and secretion. TNF-α may have a direct effect on EC [102].

Endothelial dysfunction predisposes to atherosclerosis in the presence of increased prothrombotic factors like coagulation abnormalities, increased platelet activation, inflammatory mediators and presence of oxidized lipoproteins.

Visceral obesity and insulin resistance are associated with an increased level of PAI-1, increased plasma level of fibrinogen, factor VII, and factor VIII C coagulant activities. High levels of PAI-1 predisposes to CHD. Hyperinsulinaemia, hypergly-caemia and AII are all important simulators of PAI-1 gene expression and PAI-1 production [70,103]. Elevated PAI-1 levels have been found in non-diabetic first degree relatives of type 2 diabetic probands and in patients with established cardiovascular disease. Hyperfibrinogenaenimia is a strong independent risk factor for CHD and act synergistically with dyslipidaemia and hypertension to promote atherosclerosis [104].

9.9 Type 2 diabetes and dyslipidaemia

Dyslipidaemia is common in type 2 diabetes and contributes significantly to the increased risk of CHD. The characteristic dyslipidaemia consists of elevated triglycerides and low HDLc [105,106]. The Framingham Heart Study reported no difference with regards to total and LDL cholesterol levels between diabetic men and women compared with their non diabetic counterparts. People with diabetes, however, have an increased proportion of small dense atherogenic LDL particles and twice the prevalence of low HDLc with high TG compared with non diabetics [107,108]. A 'normal' LDL level can be misleading in a patient with diabetes as there are many more small dense particles than large buoyant particles will comprise the reported LDL value. Small dense LDL gets oxidized more readily and able to penetrate the vascular wall easily to initiate the formation of atheromatous plaque.

Low HDL levels are independent predictors of CHD and have a strong inverse relationship with TG levels. The risk weakens as the HDLc concentration rises above 1 mmol/l. In the UKPDS, there was a significant association between the risk of CHD and elevated levels of LDLc and TG and decreased concentration of HDLc. For each 1 mmol/l increase in LDL concentration, there was 1.57-fold increase in the risk of CHD and for each increase in 0.1 mmol/l of HDL cholesterol the risk was decreased by 0.15-fold [109].

Some studies have reported that TG are better predictor of CHD risks than LDLc. The Diabetes Intervention Study and the PARIS prospective study demonstrated that TG levels were significantly higher in people who died from CHD than who survived [110,111]. The mechanism by which raised triglycerides cause atherosclerosis is attributed to the presence of TGRLP, as described above.

There are also changes to apolipoprotein composition in diabetic patients with increased susceptibility of apolipoproteins A1 and B to glycation which results in decreased affinity for HDL receptors and increased susceptibility to oxidative modification [112].

9.10   Type 2 diabetes and hypertension

The prevalence of hypertension in the diabetic population is 1.5–3 times higher than that of the non-diabetic age-matched population [113]. In type 2 diabetes, hypertension may be present at the time of the diagnosis or precedes the development of hyperglycaemia [114] and is implicated in development of both micro- and macrovascular complications.

Epidemiological studies indicate that diabetic individuals with hypertension have greatly increased risks of cardiovascular disease, renal inefficiency and retinopathy. In UKPDS, every 10 mmHg rise in systolic blood pressure was associated with a 15% increase in risk of coronary artery disease [115].

A recent study from Finland evaluated the joint effects of different stages of hypertension and type 2 diabetes at baseline and at follow-up on the risk of CHD incidence and mortality in nearly 50 000 Finnish adults from 24 to 75 years old. There was increased CHD of 22% in men and 26% in women for each 20 mmHg increment in systolic blood pressure and by 18% for men and 23% in women for each 10-mm Hg increment in diastolic pressure, in a group which had no history of CHD or stroke [116].

The pathophysiology of hypertension in diabetes is postulated to be related to hyperinsulinaemia. (for mechanisms, see obesity and hypertension). Apart from the functional changes, diabetes can cause arterial wall structural changes. This may be due to non-enzymatic glycation of proteins including collagen and other matrix proteins to form AGEs [97].

9.11   Type 2 diabetes and CHD

Type 2 diabetes predisposes to macrovascular complications such as MI, peripheral vascular disease and stroke. Epidemiological studies have shown that the risk of CHD is increased two- to sixfold in patients with type 2 diabetes compared with non-diabetic subjects [28,117]. Indeed, in the non diabetic subjects, there has been a substantial decline in mortality from coronary heart disease in many parts of the world in recent years. The effect was considerably less in adults with diabetes with perhaps even an increase in women with diabetes [118].

There is also a high prevalence of subclinical CHD in the diabetic population [119] Conversely, among people with established CHD, there is a high prevalence of diabetes. In fact, one quarter of patients who had myocardial infarction in the PROCAM Study have diabetes [120].

CHD is responsible for more than three quarters of deaths in type 2 diabetic patients and mortality from CHD is approximately three times higher in diabetic patients than in the general population [121,122]. In the PROCAM study, there were 419 diabetic patients among the cohort of 4849 men and overall mortality was twice as high in diabetic group compared with non-diabetic subjects. The excess mortality was largely explained by cardiovascular mortality [120].

The cardioprotective effect in females is lost in diabetes and the proportionate increase in CHD mortality is significantly greater in women than in men [123].

There is also an ethnic variation in the prevalence CHD, with lower rate of prevalence in the Japanese population in both diabetic and non diabetic persons [124]. This is in contrast to the high risk of CHD among South Asian migrants to the UK and elsewhere [80]. This population has increased susceptibility to insulin resistance and type 2 diabetes with a tendency to abdominal fat deposition and abnormal lipid profile. Pima Indians who are obese with a high prevalence of diabetes, however, have a lower risk of dying from CHD compared with the non diabetic population in the Framingham study [125]. This may be due to genetic susceptibility and/or a better lipid profile with low concentration of LDLc and TC.

CHD is also more severe in patients with diabetes and tends to occur at a younger age, with higher rates of diffuse multi-vessel disease, low ejection fraction, and increased tendency to develop congestive cardiac failure. They have a poorer outcome following myocardial infarction with higher rates of cardiac failure and death in the early post infarction period [123,126,127]. In the Bypass Angioplasty Revascularisation Investigation (BARI), the diabetic subgroup awaiting revascularization, showed a higher incidence of triple vessel disease, greater left ventricular dysfunction and a lower

5 year survival rate. The BARI Study also showed that 5 year survival was significantly higher in diabetic patients undergoing coronary artery bypass grafting (CABG) compared to percutaneous coronary angioplasty (PTCA), and CABG may therefore be the preferred procedure in diabetic patients with diffuse atherosclerosis [120].

The increased risk of CHD in type 2 diabetes is not entirely explained by traditional risk factors, though the diabetic population tends to have lower HDLc, higher total cholesterol/HDLc ratio and more hypertension. In the MRFIT, increasing the number of traditional risk factors like hypercholesterolaemia, smoking or hypertension increased the cardiovascular mortality, but the diabetic patients had approximately three times the risk compared with non-diabetic subjects for the same given number of risk factors [28]. The CHD mortality of diabetic patients without a history of myocardial infarction has been found to be similar to that of patients without diabetes who have had a previous MI [129].

Several mechanisms may be involved which explain this increased risk of CHD in type 2 diabetes. These include: increased inflammatory and prothrombotic mediators; endothelial dysfunction; increased oxidative stress; AGEs; platelet hyperactivity; reduce fibrinolytic capacity; as well autonomic neuropathy predisposing patients to ventricular arrhythmia.

Hyperglycaemia is a well-established risk factor for small vessel disease in diabetes and improving glycaemic control reduces the risk of severe microvascular complications [130]. The link between hyperglycaemia and the risk of CHD is unclear in type 2 diabetes. In the UKPDS study, a reduction 0.9% in glycated haemoglobin did not demonstrated significant benefit with regards to macrovascular disease, although a reduction of 16% in myocardial infarction in the intensive treated group was almost significant ($p = 0.052$)[109] The group of patients treated intensively with Metformin, however, had a 39% reduction in incidence of myocardial infarction compared with the conventional group and those in the intensively treated group who received insulin or sulfonylurea. From an 'epidemiological updated HbA1c model', the rate of MI doubled comparing HbA1c 5.5% with 11%, but there was a 10-fold increase in microvascular events.

The reasons for the relatively poor correlation between glycaemia and CHD have been debated. It has been suggested that post-prandial hyperglycaemia measured by 2 hour glucose concentration after an oral glucose tolerance test may be more strongly related to CHD morbidity and mortality than fasting blood glucose concentration or HbA1c [131]. It is also believed that the risk factor for cardiovascular disease appear even before diabetes becomes recognisable ('ticking clock hypothesis').

Apart from chronic hyperglycaemia, acute hyperglycaemia influences CHD outcome in people with MI as seen in the DIGAMI Study. In this trial, people who were intensively treated with insulin therapy (insulin glucose infusion for 24 hours followed by intensive subcutaneous insulin treatment), compared with a controlled group managed by conventional therapy, showed a reduction in mortality to 33% compared with 44% in the conventional group. The exact mechanism may not be related to improvement in hyperglycaemia and could be through indirect effects on improving platelet function, lipoprotein abnormalities and prothrombotic factors [132]. However, in DIGAMI-2 trial, there was no difference in mortality rates among three glucose management strategies. This could be partly explained by similar glucose control in the intensive outpatient subcutaneous insulin therapy group and the other two groups of standard treatment and care according to local practice [133].

9.12 Benefits of weight loss

Weight loss programmes need to involve lifestyle modification with changes in dietary intake, physical activity and behaviour therapy; these measures, as well as the role of anti-obesity drugs are discussed in detail elsewhere.

9.13 Management of hypertension

Weight reduction has been shown to be an effective non-pharmacological approach to improve blood pressure in several studies [134,135]). Loss of 1 kg body weight is associated with a mean decrease in blood pressure of 1 mmHg [136]. Weight reduction can also reduce the number of antihypertensive medications prescribed [137].

The role of sodium restriction is controversial. The INTERSALT Study showed that dietary sodium restriction can independently lower blood pressure and is additive with weight loss [137]. Studies have shown that moderate sodium restriction to 100 mmol (2300 mg) per day can reduce systolic pressure by 5 mmHg and diastolic pressure by 2–3 mmHg [138]. In addition, the response to antihypertensive therapy appears to be more effective in salt restricted subjects.

A number of randomized controlled trials involving large numbers of hypertensive diabetic patients have shown important benefits in CHD outcomes from lowering blood pressure ([115,139]; Losartan Intervention For Endpoint Reduction in Hypertension study, [140]; Antihypertensive and Lipid-Lowering Treatment to Prevent Heart Attack Trial, [141]). The UKPDS showed that tight blood pressure group was associated with significant reduction in macrovascular complications compared to the less intensive treated group (10/5 mmHg difference between the groups). In the HOPE study, there was a 22% relative risk reduction (RRR) in the primary composite endpoint defined as a combination of cardiovascular death, non-fatal MI and non-fatal stroke. The diabetic subgroup (MICRO-HOPE) had better cardiovascular outcome events (cardiovascular deaths RRR of 37% vs. 26%). Similar benefits were seen in the diabetic subgroup of the Captopril Prevention Project (CAPPP) Trial (Table 9.2).

Two other large placebo-controlled trials, EUROPA and PEACE, looked at the benefit of angiotensin-converting enzyme (ACE)-I in reducing cardiovaslcular events in high-risk populations.

The EUROPA trial was similar in design to HOPE with stable CHD patients but at lesser risk. (hypertension 27% vs. 47%, diabetes 12% vs. 38%) There was a significant reduction in the primary endpoint (20% RRR) and the diabetic population also had a significant reduction in major cardiovascular events [142].

However, the PEACE trial which involved over 8000 patients with stable CHD of whom 46% were hypertensive and 17% had diabetes, showed lack of benefit on the primary endpoint. The lack of benefit of trandalopril may be due in part to a lower average baseline BP than in HOPE and EUROPA, more patients on lipid lowering therapy and 72% had prior revascularization [143].

Further studies involving ACE inhibitors, the FACET (Fosinopril vs. Amlodipine Cardiovascular Randomized Events Trial) and the ABCD trial (Appropriate Blood Pressure Control in Diabetes) appeared to suggest that calcium channel blockers might be inferior to ACE-I in the context of cardiovascular disease and/or the beneficial outcome observed is a reflection of the cardio-protective effect of an ACE inhibitor. These studies should be interpreted with caution as the trials were not designed and powered to assess a difference between two treatment groups with regard to cardio-vascular events [144,145].

The reported difference with calcium antagonist therapy with regard to adverse cardiovascular events were not replicated in the Systolic Hypertension Europe (SYS-Eur) Trial and the Hypertension Optimal Treatment Study (HOT) (Table 9.2) [146,147].

The HOT Study also looked at the optimal diastolic target blood pressure. Felodipine was used as an initial treatment with other agents introduced in a five step regime to achieve the diastolic target value <90 mmHg, <85 mmHg or <80 mmHg. Among the diabetic group, aggressive diastolic blood pressure lowering in the less than 80 mmHg group was associated with a 51% reduction in risk of major cardiovascular events and 43% reduction in risk of cardiovascular mortality [148].

Similarly, much has been debated about the adverse effects of diuretic therapy especially in diabetic subjects. The beneficial effect of Chlorthalidone as an antihypertensive agent was seen in the Systolic Hypertension in the Elderly Program (SHEP), which demonstrated reduction in major cardiovascular events in older type 2 diabetic patients and non-diabetics who had isolated systolic hypertension (ISH) (Table 9.2) [149].

The data from the largest hypertensive trial, ALLHAT, (33 357 subjects) compared the effect on cardiovascular endpoints of three newer agents (amlodipine, lisinopril or doxazosin) with a diuretic (chlorthalidone). After a mean follow up of 4.9 years, there was no difference in the relative risk of the primary outcome (combined fatal CHD or nonfatal myocardial infarction) or all cause mortality between Amlodipine, Lisinopril and Chlorthalidone (Table 9.2) [141].

The results of a number of trials suggest that, at the same level of blood pressure control, most antihypertensive drugs provide same degree of cardiovascular protection. The trials include STOP-Hypertension-2, NORDIL, INSIGHT and INVEST found similar outcome between older agents like diuretics and beta blockers and newer drugs like ACE inhibitors and calcium channel blockers [148,150].

The ASCOT trial was stopped prematurely due to worse cardiovascular outcomes in atenolol-treated group. This difference may be partially due to a slightly lower BP in the Amlodipine group who also had slightly lower mean BMI, TG, serum creatinine and glucose and fractionally higher HDLc (Table 9.2). The lipid arm of ASCOT indicated that active treatment with atorvastatin resulted in significant reductions in the primary endpoint (non-fatal MI and fatal CHD) of 36%, and in secondary endpoints of all coronary events (29%), fatal and non-fatal stroke (27%), and all cardiovascular events and procedures (21%) [151,152].

A recent large international trial, GEMINI AALA evaluated the efficacy of combination Amlodipine/Atorvastatin in achieving recommended guidelines (JNC 7, NCEP ATP III) in over 1600 hypertensive patients with elevated LDLc. Fifty-five percent of patients achieved BP and LDLc goals leading to approximately 50% reduction in the 10 year risk for a cardiovascular event. The mean BP was reduced by 20.2/11.4 mm Hg from baseline of 146.5/88.3 mm Hg and LDLc reduction by 28.6% by 1.1 mmol/l from baseline value of 3.4 mmol/l [153].

The recently published ADVANCE trial is a major placebo-controlled randomized trial which evaluates the benefit of antihypertensive therapy in patients with diabetes. It compares fixed dose combination of perindopril and indapamide to placebo in over 11 000 type 2 diabetic patients. After 4.3 years, the relative risk of death from cardiovascular disease was reduced by 18% and all cause mortality by 14% in the active treatment arm, with significant reduction also seen in total coronary events (14%) and total renal events (21%). (average BP 134.7/74.8 in active arm vs. 140.3/77.0 mm Hg in placebo) (Action in Diabetes and Vascular Disease; [154]).

ACCOMPLISH, (Avoiding Cardiovascular Events in Combination Therapy in Patients Living with Systolic Hypertension) a major morbidity and mortality trial was stopped early as ACE-I benazepril plus calcium channel blocker, amlodipine was found to be more effective than treatment with the ACE-I plus diuretic (20% risk reduction in cardiovascular morbidity and mortality; March 2008, American College of Cardiology Session).

The understanding of the role of AII in the pathogenesis of atherosclerosis and its' effect on myocardial tissues might suggest that AII type 1 receptor blockers (ARB) show genuine drug class differences in relation to cardiovascular outcomes.

Indeed, the LIFE (Losartan Intervention for Endpoint reduction) Study looked at the effect of Losartan or Atenolol on 9193 hypertensive patients with left ventricular hypertrophy. Losartan not only reduced the cardiovascular outcomes, but there was approximately a twofold greater ECG-left ventricular hypertrophy regression compared with the Atenolol group. More impressive results were seen in sub-set of 1195 patients with diabetes, with 39% risk reduction in all cause mortality compared with the Atenolol group. These benefits were above and beyond those attributable to BP reduction alone (Table 9.2) [140]. However, the VALUE trial comparing Valsartan with Amlodipine in 15 000 high-risk hypertensive patients showed the rates of the primary composite endpoints, cardiac morbidity and mortality were the same in both arms. (Valsartan Antihypertensive Long-term Use Evaluation, [155]) (Table 9.3).

Micro-albuminuria is considered as a harbinger of CHD and a predictor of renal decline in patients with type 2 diabetes. The IRMA 2 showed treatment with irbesartan significantly reduced the rate of progression from micro-albuminuria to diabetic nephropathy compared to placebo. Two other ARB studies (IDNT and RENAAL) showed reduction in doubling of creatinine and development of end-stage renal disease,

Table 9.3   Major hypertension trials in subjects with diabetes

Study	No. randomized	No. diabetes	Follow up (years)	Main comparison	End point reduction (diabetes)
UKPD	1148	1148	9	Captopril vs. atenolol	Diabetes-related death – 32%, stroke 44%
SHEP	4736	583	5	Chlorthalidone vs. placebo	All cardiovascular events (46–66%)
CAPP	10 985	572	6	Captopril vs. β blocker or thiazide	Captopril Group fatal/non-fatal 34%
SYST-EURO	4695	492	2	Nitrendipine vs. placebo	All major cardiovascular events (41–70%)
HOT	18 790	1501	4	Felodipine	All cause mortality 39%
MICRO-HOPE		3577	4.5	Ramipril vs. placebo	Total mortality – 29% CV deaths – 37% MI – 22%
ALLHAT	24 335	8633	4.9	Amlodipine, doxazosin lisinopril chlorthalidone	Total mortality – 39%
LIFE	9193	1195	4.8	Losartan vs. atenolol	Losartan group all cause mortality 39%
ABCD	470	470	5	Nisoldipine Vs. enalapril	
ADVANCE		11 140	4.3	Fixed dose perindopril/ indapamide	All cause mortality 14% CV death 18%

but neither affected cardiovascular death, though this was not the primary endpoint [156–158] (Table 9.6).

The DETAIL study is the first study to compare the effects of ACE-I vs. ARBs on renal function in type 2 diabetes and did not demonstrate any difference in renal parameters between the two groups. Though this was a small study with high drop-out rates, it demonstrated that use of ARBs is safe and not inferior to ACE-I in these patients (Diabetics Exposed to Telmisartan and Enalapril Study; [159]).

Recently published large trial, ONTARGET, (The Ongoing Telmisartan Alone and in Combination With Ramipril Global Endpoint Trial) enrolled 25 620 with CHD or diabetes with additional risk factors and patients were randomized to receive ramipril 10 mg, telmisartan 80 mg or the combination of the two. The combination therapy group had better mean blood pressure reduction (2.4/1.3 mmHg) than the Telmisartan and the Ramipril group. However, this resulted in higher rates of hypotensive symptoms, syncope, renal dysfunction, and hyperkalaemia, with a trend toward an increased renal dysfunction requiring dialysis in the combination therapy group. The primary composite end point (cardiovascular death, MI, stroke, or heart failure hospitalization) had occurred in a similar number of patients in all three groups. This study shows that Telmisartan is equally effective to Ramipril in patients with vascular disease or diabetes without heart failure and could be considered as alternate agent in ACE-I intolerant subjects [160].

The message from ONTARGET study was similar to that found in VALIANT, Valsartan had a similar effect in reducing mortality as captopril alone, but the combination had no extra benefit, but did have additional side effects. The benefit of combination therapy which was seen in two heart failure trials (Val-HeFT, valsartan and CHARM, candesartan) did not use full dose of ACE-I and the subjects had HF rather than stable CHD, which may explain the different results [161,162].

9.14   Management of dyslipidaemia

Weight loss and exercise can reduce TG, increase HDLc and in some persons lower LDLc levels [163,164]. Regular physical activity should be a standard part of any lipid management programme. NCEP and ADA recommend drug therapy only after lifestyle interventions has been tried except for those patients with clinical evidence of CHD or with very high LDLc levels or in people with diabetes.

Several studies have shown that aggressive dietary therapy alone or in combination with exercise has beneficial effects on lipid levels and CHD.

The St. Thomas' Atherosclerosis Regression Study (STARS) randomized men with CHD and total cholesterol level above 6.0 mmol/l to conventional care or a low fat diet. Weight reduction measures and exercise programmes were provided for overweight subjects. After 3 years, the progression rate of coronary atherosclerosis slowed in the diet treated group [165]. The clinical trials involving omega 3 fatty acid also showed significant benefit on cardiovascular end points. In the Diet and Reinfarction Trial (DART), men recovering from MI, who were randomized to dietary advice consisting of increased fatty fish consumption had a 29% reduction on all cause mortality at 2 year follow up [166].

In the GISSI Prevention Trial, post MI patients randomized to receive omega 3 fatty acid supplementation (1 g/day) had a significant 10–15% reduction in combined primary endpoints of death, and fatal/non-fatal stroke [167]. In the Lyon Diet Heart Study, patients randomized to receive a Mediterranean-type diet instead of a Western-type diet had a risk reduction in the combined primary end point of death from cardiovascular causes or non fatal acute MI of 73%, cardiovascular mortality of 76% and all cause mortality of 70%. These benefits persisted at extended follow-up (mean of 46 months). The study consisted of a sample of 605 patients less than 70 years old who had an MI within the prior 6 months (302 experimental and 303 control subjects). Limitations of the study are the methodology and the small sample size (American Heart Association Science Advisory) [168–170].

Table 9.4 CHD prevention trials with statins in patients with diabetes – subgroups analysis

Study	Drug	N	Baseline LDLc (mmol/)	LDLc lowering %	CHD risk reduction (%)	
					Overall	Diabetes
Primary prevention						
AF CAPS/ TexCAPS	Lovastatin	155	3.9	25	37	43 (NS)
HPS	Simvastatin	2982	3.4	29	24	22
Secondary prevention						
CARE	Pravastatin	586	3.6	27	23	25
4S	Simvastatin	202	4.8	36	32	55
LIPID	Pravastatin	782	3.9	25	24	19 (NS)
HPS	Simvastatin	1978	3.3	30	24	18
4S-Extended	Simvastatin	483			32	42

NS, not significant.

Several large-scale, controlled, randomized clinical trials have established that intervention with statins reduces CHD risk. This is seen in both the primary and secondary prevention settings and it is mediated mainly by reduction in LDL cholesterol (Table 9.4).

The landmark Scandinavian Simvastatin Survival Study (4S) convincingly demonstrated that coronary events and total mortality were decreased by 30% with LDLc reduction of 36%. The Cholesterol and Recurrent Events (CARE) and Long Term Intervention with Pravastatin in Ischemic Disease (LIPID) demonstrated similar benefits in patients with relatively average total cholesterol and LDLc [171,172].

The link between increasing LDL and CHD is well established in statin trials with a roughly linear relationship between CHD events rates and LDLc levels. Those at the highest CHD risk experience the greatest benefit from the decrease in LDLc and tend to plateau at lower LDLc levels. The lowest event rate is in the CARE Pravastatin group, who achieved a mean LDLc of less than 2.6 mmol/l, which is in accordance with the NCEP guideline of LDLc target <2.6 mmol/l. The baseline LDLc level in 4S was 4.88 mmol/l, in CARE 3.6 mmol/l and 3.88 mmol/l in LIPID. In all these trials, statins approximately reduced LDLc level by about one third. In the recent Heart Protection Study, (HPS) 33% of the total 20 536 subjects had baseline LDLc <3 mmol/l, 25% between 3 and 3.5 mmol/l and 42% had levels 3.5 mmol/l. The simvastatin (40 mg) group when compared to placebo had significant reduction in all cause mortality, CHD deaths and major cardiovascular events. The benefit in reduction of events was similar in all the three tertiles of baseline LDL cholesterol [173].

This raises the point 'the lower the LDLc, the better?' and the issue as to whether there is a threshold LDLc below which no benefit occurs. Two studies, TNT and IDEAL, address whether intensive statin therapy is beneficial in subjects with stable CHD. TNT compared a standard 10 mg atorvastatin to 80 mg in over 10 000 patients with clinically evident CHD and LDLc level less than 3.4 mmol/l, with median follow up 4.9 years. The mean LDLc level was 2.0 mmol/l with 80 mg and 2.6 mmol/l with 10 mg and the high dose atorvastatin group had relative risk reduction of 22% in primary composite endpoints of major cardiovascular events but no difference in overall mortality. Importantly, among 5584 patients with metabolic syndrome, the risk of major cardiovascular events was high but attenuated by intensive therapy with an absolute 5 year reduction of 3.5% (Treating to New Targets, [174]). IDEAL compared Atorvastatin 80 mg to simvastatin 20/40 mg in 8888 patients with stable CHD and achieved mean LDLc of 2.69 mmol/l in the simvastatin arm and 2.12 mmol/L in the atorvastatin group. The primary end point for major coronary events (CHD death, non-fatal MI, or cardiac arrest) tended to occur less frequently with intensive therapy (RRR 11% non significant). Major cardiovascular events and any coronary events were significantly reduced by 13% ($p = 0.02$) and 16% ($p < 0.001$) respectively in atorvastatin 80 mg group (Incremental Decrease in End Points Through Aggressive Lipid Lowering, [175]).

Intensive statin therapy was also found to be beneficial in acute coronary syndrome. The Myocardial Ischaemia Reduction with Aggressive Cholesterol Lowering (MIRACL) study involved 3086 patients with unstable angina or non-Q wave MI receiving either atorvastatin 80 mg/day or placebo within 4 days of hospital admission. The primary endpoint (recurring infarction, cardiac arrest with resuscitation, worsening angina requiring hospitalization) was less frequent with atorvastatin at 16 weeks compared to placebo with a relative risk reduction of 16%, but the benefit was primarily due to a 26% reduction in hospitalization for worsening angina [176].

Two other studies comparing high and standard dose statin in acute coronary syndrome show beneficial effects in the intensive statin arm. PROVE IT (Pravastatin 40 mg and atorvastatin 80 mg) and A to Z (simvastatin 20 mg vs. 40/80 mg) achieved mean LDLc of 1.60 mmol/L and in 1.63 mmol/L in intensive arm respectively compared to 2.46 mmol/L and 1.99 mmol/L in standard dose [177,178].

The benefit of aggressive lipid lowering is also extended to the Regression Growth Evaluation Statin Study (REGRESS) where Pravastatin delayed the progression of atherosclerosis on angiography and reduction in clinical events at 24 months in the 885 men who took part. These benefits occurred at all lipid levels, including those in the lowest quintile with LDLc concentration between 2.2 and 3.8 mmol/l [179]. The Atorvastatin Versus Revascularisation Treatment Study (AVERT) compared the outcome of aggressive lipid lowering with atorvastatin (80 mg/day) to that of angioplasty in 341 stable CHD patients with coronary vessel disease.

The Atorvastatin group ($n = 164$) achieved a greater reduction of LDLc to 2.0 mmol/l as opposed to 3.0 mmol/l in angioplasty group followed by usual care. The incidence of ischaemic events was 36% lower in the atorvastatin group over 18 months. Although not statistically significant, there was lower rate of CABG and PTCA as well as hospitalization for worsening angina [180].

REVERSAL and ASTEROID are two imaging studies using intravascular ultrasound (IVUS) showed regression of atheroma volume in people treated with intensive statin therapy. (40 mg of pravastatin vs. 80 mg of atorvastatin in REVERSAL and 40 mg Rosuvastatin in ASTEROID) [181,182]. The study, known as the Justification for the Use of Statins in Primary Prevention: an Intervention Trial Evaluating Rosuvastatin (JUPITER), a large, multinational, long-term, double-blind, placebo-controlled, randomized clinical trial designed to assess directly whether statin therapy (Rosuvastatin 20 mg/day vs placebo) should be given to apparently healthy individuals with normal LDL levels but elevated CRP levels. The trial was stopped after a median follow-up of 1.9 years as Rosuvastatin significantly reduced the incidence of major cardiovascular events [191].

It has been postulated that the cardiovascular benefits of lowering LDLc may be due, at least in part, to improvement in endothelial dysfunction and the anti-inflammatory properties of statins rather than lipid lowering. In the sub study of CARE, it was shown that Pravastatin was associated with improved endothelium dependent vasodilatation and reduction of CRP.

Studies in 4S and WOSCOP demonstrated benefit within 6 months of randomization, too soon for the benefit to be explained by regression of atherosclerosis. Acute coronary syndromes arise as a result of rupture of unstable plaque which poses a greater threat than the plaque size or severity of stenosis. The vulnerability of the atherogenic plaque is related to the size of the lipid rich core, foam cells, inflammatory cells and the thickness of the fibrous cap which is contributed by the vascular smooth muscle cells. Statins reduce the lipid rich core and inflammatory cells especially macrophages and T lymphocytes and directly inhibits metalloproteinase secretion by macrophages which digests collagen in the plaque [179,183].

The beneficial effect of statins was not seen in the lipid arm of ALLHAT study. One possible explanation is that a relatively large proportion of patients taking Pravastatin (22.6%) stopped the medication and around 26% of people in the 'usual care' group had been started on a statin [141].

The role of statins in diabetic dyslipidaemia is based on subgroup analyses from a number of landmark clinical trials which established statins as effective therapy in primary and secondary prevention of CHD. Patients with diabetes benefit as much or more than non diabetics from statin treatment, but some studies did not reach statistical significance due to the small number of diabetic patients compared to non diabetic subjects (Tables 9.4 and 9.5). In the HPS study, statin therapy was associated with a significant 22% reduction in the risk of first vascular event in diabetic patients. In the CARDS study involving 2800 type 2 diabetic men and women, 10 mg of Atorvastatin vs. placebo was terminated early as the statin group showed a 37% reduction in major coronary events and 48% reduction in stroke (Collaborative AtoRvastatin Diabetes Study, [184]).

In fact, statins reduce CHD events by only approximately 30% with a residual risk of 70% which may be related to suboptimal LDLc lowering or due to the presence of other untreated lipid abnormalities. In a retrospective analysis, low baseline HDLc was found to be a strong inverse risk factor for both placebo and Pravastatin groups in the CARE and LIPID trials.

Table 9.5 CHD prevention trials with fibrates in patient with diabetes

Study	Drug	Number	CHD risk reduction (%)
Helsinki Heart Study *Secondary Prevention*	Gemfibrozil	135	68 (NS)
VA-HIT	Gemfibrozil	309	24 ($p = 0.05$)
DIAS	Fenofibrate	207	23 (NS)

NS, not significant.

In post hoc analysis of the TNT trial, HDLc was a significant predictor of major cardiovascular events and even in patients with lowest level of LDLc (<70 mg/l), the risk of CV events was reduced in those with higher rather than lower HDLc quintiles. The conclusion was that low HDLc is a powerful negative risk factor for coronary events despite treatment with statin and the risks associated with a low HDLc may not be altered by statin therapy [185].

There is evidence that fibrates which increase HDLc may be effective for secondary prevention of CHD as observed in the Veterans Affairs HDL Intervention Trial (VA-HIT) (Table 9.5) ([186]. The DIAS [187] demonstrated that the progression of focal, localized atherosclerosis was reduced by 40% on two measurements in the fenofibrate group compared with the control group. There was a non-significant trend towards reduction in combined coronary events, fewer deaths, MI and coronary intervention in the treatment arm (M) (Table 9.5) [187]. The FIELD trial which evaluated the long term effect of fenofibrate vs. placebo in subjects with type 2 diabetes, did not reach statistical significance on the primary outcome (CHD death or non-fatal MI) but significant benefit with regards to non-fatal MI, coronary revascularization and less progression to albuminuria and less retinopathy requiring laser treatment. The observed effect of fenofibrate may have been attenuated by unequal excess use of statin therapy in the placebo group [188].

Table 9.6 Ibesartan in diabetic nephropathy

	Progression of renal insufficiency IDNT ($n = 1715$)		Progression of micro-albuminuria IRMA II ($n = 590$)	
	Irbesartan 150–300 mg vs. placebo	Irbesartan 150–300 mg vs. amlodipine*	Irbesartan 150 mg vs. placebo	Irbesartan 300 mg vs. placebo
Average duration	2.6 years	2.6 years	2 years	2 years
	Primary endpoint: composite of doubling of serum creatinine, end stage renal disease or death		Primary outcome: development of clinical proteinuria	
	↓ 20% ($p = 0.02$)	↓ 23% ($p = 0.006$)	↓ 39% ($p = 0.080$)	↓ 70% (<0.001)

9.15 Conclusions

Obesity and type 2 diabetes are major risk factors for cardiovascular disease. There are a number of evidence-based treatments available to reduce cardiovascular complications in obesity. Clinicians should adopt multi-factorial therapeutic approaches to address cardio-vascular risk factors by achieving good glycaemic control, reducing lipid levels, lowering blood pressure and improving prothrombotic milieu. The benefit of multifactorial intensive vs. conventional therapy on macrovascular events in type 2 diabetes is shown in the Steno 2 study where there was a greater than 50% reduction in hard primary end points of death by cardiovascular events, MI, stroke, revascularization or amputation [189,190]. As obesity is the underlying problem in these patients, treatment of obesity itself would be a logical addition to the above therapies and can lead to significant reduction in risk factors.

References

1. Sjostrom, L.V. (1992) Mortality of severely obese subjects. *American Journal of Clinical Nutrition*, **55**, 516.
2. Allison, B.D. (1999) Annual deaths attributable to obesity in the United States. *Journal of the American Medical Association*, **282**, 1530–8.
3. Manson, J.E. (1995) Body weight and mortality among women. *New England Journal of Medicine*, **333**, 677.
4. Calle, E.E. (1999) Body mass index and mortality in a prospective cohort of U.S. adults. *New England Journal of Medicine*, **341**, 1097.
5. Adams, K.F. (2006) Overweight, obesity, and mortality in a large prospective cohort of persons 50 to 70 years old. *New England Journal of Medicine*, **355** (8), 763–8.
6. Hubert, H.B. (1983) Obesity as an independent risk factor for cardiovascular disease: a 26 year follow-up of participants in the Framingham Heart Study. *Circulation*, **67**, 968–77.
7. Manson, J.E. (1990) A prospective study of obesity and risk of coronary heart disease in women. *New England Journal of Medicine*, **322**, 882.
8. Gunnell, D.J. (1998) Childhood obesity and adult cardiovascular mortality. *American Journal of Clinical Nutrition*, **67**, 1111–18.
9. Must, A. (1992) Heart Protection Study of cholesterol lowering with Simvastatin in 20536 high-risk individuals. Long term morbidity and mortality of overweight children. *New England Journal of Medicine*, **327** (19), 1350–5.
10. McGill, H.C., Jr (2002) Obesity accelerates the progression of atherosclerosis in young men. *Circulation*, **105** (23), 2712–8.
11. Rich-Edward. (1995) The primary prevention of coronary heart disease in women. *New England Journal of Medicine*, **332**, 1758.
12. Rexrode, K.M. (1998) Abdominal obesity and coronary heart disease in women. *Journal of the American Medical Association*, **280**, 1843.
13. Yusuf, S., Hawken, S., Ounpuu, S., *et al.*; INTERHEART Study Investigators (2004) Effect of potentially modifiable risk factors associated with myocardial infarction in 52 countries (the INTERHEART Study): a case–control study. *Lancet*, **364**, 937–952.
14. Haffner, S.M. (2006) Waist circumference and BMI are both independently associated with cardiovascular disease. The International Day for the Evaluation of Abdominal Obesity (IDEA) survey. *Journal of the American College of Cardiology*. **47** (4 suppl (A)), 358.

15. Ingleson, E. (2007) Burden and prognostic importance of subclinical cardiovascular disease in overweight and obese individuals. *Circulation*, **116**, 375–84.

16. Victor, R.G., Haley, R.W., Willett, D.L. *et al.*; Dallas Heart Study Investigators (2004) The Dallas Heart Study: a population-based probability sample for the multidisciplinary study of ethnic differences in cardiovascular health. *American Journal of Cardiology*, **93** (12), 1473–80.

17. See, R. (2007) The association of differing measures of overweight and obesity with prevalent atherosclerosis. *Journal of the American College of Cardiology*, **50**(8), 752–9.

18. Rea, T.D. (2001) Body mass index and the risk of recurrent coronary events following acute myocardial infarction. *American Journal of Cardiology*, **88**, 467.

19. Kenchaiah, S. (2002) Obesity and risk of heart failure. *New England Journal of Medicine*, **347** (5), 305–13.

20. Alpert, M.A. (1993) Obesity and heart. *American Journal of the Medical Sciences*, **306**, 117.

21. Frank, S. (1986) The electrocardiogram in obesity. *Journal of the American College of Cardiology*, **7**, 295–9.

22. Alpert, M.A. (2000) The electrocardiogram in morbid obesity. *American Journal of Cardiology*, **85**, 908.

23. Wang, T.J. (2004) Obesity and the risk of atrial fibrillation. *Journal of the American Medical Association*, **292** (20), 2471–7.

24. Frost, L. (2005) Overweight and obesity as the risk of atrial fibrillation or flutter, the Danish Diet, Cancer, and Health Study. *American Journal of Medicine*, **118** (5), 489–95.

25. Dublin, S. (2006) Risk of new onset atrial fibrillation in relation to BMI. *Archives of Internal Medicine*, **166** (21), 2322–8.

26. Alpert, M.A., and Hashini, M.W. (1993) Obesity and heart. *American Journal of Medical Science* **306**, 117.

27. Modan, M., Halkin, H., Almog, S. *et al.* (1985) Hyperinsulinaemia. A link between hypertension obesity and glucose, intolerance. *Journal of Clinical Investigation*, **75**, 809–17.

28. Stalmer, J. (1993) Diabetes, other risk factors and 12 yr cardiovascular mortality for men- the Multiple Risk Factor Intervention Trial. *Diabetes Care*, **16**, 434–44.

29. Sjostrom, C.D., Lissner, L., Wedel, H., and Sjostrom, L. (1999) Reduction in incidence of diabetes, hypertension and lipid disturbances after intentional weight loss induced by bariatric surgery: the SOS Intervention Study. *Obesity Research*, **7**, 477–84.

30. Sjöström, L., Lindroos, A.-K., Peltonen, M. *et al.* (2004) Lifestyle, diabetes, and cardiovascular risk factors 10 years after bariatric surgery. *New England Journal of Medicine*, 2683–93.

31. Dyer, A.R. (1989) The INTERSALT Study: relations of body mass index to blood pressure. *Journal of Human Hypertension*, **3**, 299–308.

32. Blair, D. (1984) Evidence for increased risk for hypertension with centrally located body fat and the effect of race and sex. *American Journal of Epidemiology*, **119**, 526–40.

33. De Fronzo, R.A. (1975) The effect of insulin on renal handling of sodium, potassium, calcium, and phosphate in man. *Journal of Clinical Investigation*, **55**, 845–55.

34. Moan, A. (1995) Insulin sensitivity, sympathetic activity and cardiovascular reactivity in young men. *American Journal of Hypertension*, **8**, 268.

35. Reaven, G.M. (1996) The role of insulin resistance and the sympathoadrenal system. *New England Journal of Medicine*, **334**, 374.

36. Landsberg, L. (1992) Hyperinsulinaemia: a possible role in obesity-induced hypertension. *Hypertension*, **19** (suppl 1), 161–5.

37. Baron, A.D. (1995) Insulin mediated skeletal muscle vasodilation contributes to both insulin sensitivity and responsiveness in lean humans. *Journal of Clinical Investigation*, **96**, 786.

38. Steinberg, H.O. (1996) Obesity/insulin resistance-endothelial dysfunction. *Journal of Clinical Investigation*, **97**, 2601.

39. Sowers, J.R. (1998) Insulin, cation metabolism and insulin resistance. *Journal of Basic and Clinical Physiology and Pharmacology*, **9**, 223–33.
40. Saad, M.F. (1991) Racial differences in the relation between blood pressure and insulin resistance. *New England Journal of Medicine*, **324**, 733.
41. Grundy, S.M. (1990) Metabolic and health complications of obesity. *Disease-a-Month*, **36**, 641.
42. Assman, G. (1998) The emergence of triglycerides as a significant independent risk factor in coronary artery disease. *European Heart Journal*, **19** (suppl M), 8.
43. Assman, G. (1992) Relation of high density lipoprotein cholesterol and triglycerides to incidence of atherosclerotic coronary artery disease (The PROCAM Experience). *American Journal of Cardiology*, **70**, 733–7.
44. Carlson, L.A. (1979) Risk factors for myocardial infarction in the Stockholm prospective study (role of plasma TG and TC). *Acta Medica Scandinavica*, **206**, 351–60.
45. Cambien, F., Jacqueson, A., Richard, J.L., *et al.* (1986) Is the level of serum triglyceride a significant predictor of coronary death in 'normocholesterolemic' subjects? The Paris Prospective Study. *American Journal of Epidemiology*, **124**, 624–32.
46. Austin, M.A. (1998) Hypertriglyceridemia as a cardiovascular risk factor. *American Journal of Cardiology*, **81** (suppl 4A), 7B–12B.
47. NIH Consensus Development Panel on Triglyceride (1993) High density lipoprotein and coronary heart disease. *Journal of the American Medical Association*, **269**, 505–10.
48. Krauss, R.M. (1998) Atherogenicity of triglyceride-rich lipoproteins. *American Journal of Cardiology*, **81**, 13B–17.
49. Hodis, H.N. (1999) TGRLP remnant particles and risk of atherorosclerosis. *Circulation*, **99**, 2852–4.
50. Ross, R. (1999) Atherosclerosis – an inflammatory disease. *New England Journal of Medicine*, **340**, 115–26.
51. Fisher, W.R. (1983) Heterogeneity of plasma low density lipoprotein. *Metabolism*, **32**, 283–91.
52. Lamarche, B. (1996) Apo A1 and B levels and the risk of ischemic heart disease – five year follow-up of men in Quebec Cardiovascular Study. *Circulation*, **94**, 273–8.
53. Lamarche, B. (1997) Small dense LDLc as a predictor of ischaemic heart disease in men – Quebec Cardiovascular Study. *Circulation*, **95**, 69–75.
54. Friedewald, W.T. (1972) Estimation of the concentration of LDLc in plasma, without the use of the preparative ultracentrifuge. *Clinical Chemistry*, **18**, 499–552.
55. Frost, P.H. (1998) Rationale for use of non HDLc rather than LDLc as a tool for lipoprotein cholesterol screening and assessment of risk and therapy. *American Journal of Cardiology*, **81** (4A), 26B–31.
56. Despres, J.P. (1998) The insulin resistance syndrome of visceral obesity: effect on patients' risk. *Obesity Research*, **6** (suppl 1), 8S–17S.
57. Ferrannini, E. (1998) Relationship between IGT, NIDDM and obesity. *European Journal of Clinical Investigation*, **28**(suppl 2), 3–6, discussion 6-7.
58. De Fronzo, R.A. (1991) Insulin resistance syndrome. *Diabetes Care*, **14**, 173.
59. Reaven, G.M. (1993) Role of insulin resistance in human disease (syndrome X). *Annual Review of Medicine*, **44**, 121.
60. Williams, B. (1994) Insulin resistance: The shape of things to come. *Lancet*, **344**, 521.
61. Expert Panel on Detection, Evaluation, and Treatment of High Blood Cholesterol in Adults (2002) Executive Summary of the Third Report of National Cholesterol Education Programme. *Journal of the American Medical Association*, **285**, 2486.
62. Ford, E.S. (2002) Prevalance of the metabolic syndrome among US adults: findings from the Third National Health and Nutrition Examination Survey. *Journal of the American Medical Association*, **287**, 356.

63. Alexander, C.M. (2003) NCEP defined metabolic syndrome, diabetes and prevalence of coronary heart disease among NHANES III participants age 50 years and older. *Diabetes*, **52**, 1210–14.

64. Isomaa, B. (2001) Cardiovascular morbidity and mortality associated with the metabolic syndrome. *Diabetes Care*, **24**, 683–9.

65. Lakka, H.M. (2002) The Kuopio ischemic heart disease risk factor study. *Journal of the American Medical Association*, **288**, 2709–16.

66. Hunt, K. (2004) National Cholesterol Education Programme vs. WHO metabolic syndrome in relation to all cause mortality. *Circulation*, **110**, 1245–51.

67. Gami, A.S. (2007) Metabolic syndrome and risk of incident cardiovascular events and death. *Journal of the American College of Cardiology*, **49** (5), 403–14.

68. Jensen, M.D. (1989) Influence of body fat distribution on free fatty acid metabolism in obesity. *Journal of Clinical Investigation*, **83**, 1168–73.

69. Wiesenthal, S.R. (1999) Free fatty acids impair hepatic insulin extraction *in vivo*. *Diabetes*, **48**, 766–74.

70. McFarlane, S.I. (2001) Insulin resistance and cardiovascular disease. *Journal of Clinical Endocrinology and Metabolism*, **86** (2), 713–18.

71. Weyer, C. (2001) Hypoadiponectinemia in obesity and type 2 diabetes: close association with insulin resistance and hyperinsulinemia. *Journal of Clinical Endocrinology and Metabolism*, **86**, 1930.

72. Lindsay, R.S. (2002) Adiponectin and development of type 2 diabetes in the Pima Indian population. *Lancet*, **360**, 57.

73. Hauner, H. (1995) Effects of TNF-α on glucose transport and lipid metabolism of newly-differentiated human fat cells in cell culture. *Diabetologia*, **38**, 764–71.

74. Kern, P.A. (1995) The expression of tumour necrosis factor in human adipose tissue. Regulation by obesity, weight loss, and relationship to lipoprotein lipase. *Journal of Clinical Investigation*, **95**, 2111–19.

75. Larsson, B. (1981) The health consequences of obesity. *International Journal of Obesity*, **5**, 97–116.

76. Harris, M.I. (1989) Impaired glucose tolerance in the US population. *Diabetes Care*, **12**, 464.

77. Colditz, G.A., Willett, W.C., Stampfer, M.J. *et al.* (1990) Weight as a risk factor for clinical diabetes in women. *American Journal of Epidemiology*, **132**, 501–13.

78. Larsson, B. (1984) Abdominal obesity and risk of cardiovascular disease and death. *British Medical Journal (Clinical Research Ed.)*, **288**, 1401–4.

79. Everhart, J.E. (1992) Duration of obesity increases the incidence of NIDDM. *Diabetes*, **41**, 235–40.

80. Bhopal, R. (2002) Epidemic of cardiovascular disease in South Asians. *British Medical Journal (Clinical Research Ed.)*, **324**, 625–6.

81. Neel, J.V. (1962) Diabetes mellitus: a thrifty genotype rendered detrimental by process. *American Journal of Human Genetics*, **14**, 353–62.

82. Despres, J.P. (1996) Hyperinsulinaemia as an independent risk factor for ischemic heart disease. *New England Journal of Medicine*, **334**, 952–7.

83. Haffner, S.M. (1990) Cardiovascular risk factors in prediabetic individuals. *Journal of the American Medical Association*, **263**, 2893–8.

84. Pradhan, A.d. and Ridker, P.M. (2002) Do atherosclerosis and type 2 diabetes share a common inflammatory basis? *European Heart Journal*, **23**, 831–4.

85. Yudkin, J.S. (1999) CRP in healthy subjects: association with obesity, insulin resistance and endothelial dysfunction. *Arteriosclerosis, Thrombosis, and Vascular Biology*, **19**, 972–8.

86. Pradhan, A.D. (2001) CRP, IL-6 and risk of developing type diabetes. *Journal of the American Medical Association*, **286**, 327–34.

87. Forouhi, N.G. (2001) Relation of CRP to cardiovascular risks in European and South Asians. *International Journal of Obesity*, **25**, 1327–31.

88. Cook, D.G., Mendall, M.A., Whincup, P.H. *et al.* (2000) CRP concentration in children. Relationship to adiposity and other cardiovascular risk factors. *Atherosclerosis*, 2000, **149**, 139–50.

89. Kelly, C.C.J. (2001) Chronic inflammation in women with PCOS. *Journal of Clinical Endocrinology and Metabolism*, **86**, 2453–5.

90. Pannacciulli, N. (2002) A family history of type 2 diabetes and increased level of CRP, *Diabetic Medicine*, **19**, 689–92.

91. Stern, M.P. (1995) Diabetes and cardiovascular disease 'the common soil hypothesis'. *Diabetes*, **44**, 369–74.

92. McVeigh, G.E. (1992) Impaired endothelium dependent/independent vasodilation in patients with NIDDM. *Diabetologia*, **35**, 771–6.

93. Williams, S.B. (1996) Impaired nitric oxide-mediated vasodilation in patients with NIDDM. *Journal of the American College of Cardiology*, **27**, 567–74.

94. Lim, S.C. (1999) A soluble intracellular and vascular adhesion molecule in type 2 diabetes. *Diabetes Care*, **22**, 1865–70.

95. Wright, E., Jr (2006) Oxidative stress in type 2 diabetes; the role of fasting and postprandial glycaemia. *International Journal of Clinical Practice*, **60** (3), 308–14.

96. Hawthorne, G.C. (1989) The effect of high glucose on polyol pathway activity in cultured human endothelial cells. *Diabetologia*, **32**, 196–9.

97. Bucula, R. (1991) Advanced glycosylation endproducts – nitric oxide, in experimental diabetes. *Journal of Clinical Investigation*, **87**, 432–8.

98. Wolf, B.A. (1991) Diacylglycerol accumulation and microvascular abnormalities induced by elevated glucose levels. *Journal of Clinical Investigation*, **87**, 31–8.

99. Tesfamariam, B. (1993) Aldose reductase inhibition restores endothelial cell function in diabetic rabbit aorta. *Journal of Cardiovascular Pharmacology*, **21**, 205–11.

100. Nolan, J.J. (1997) Mechanisms of the kinetic defect in insulin action in obesity and NIDDM. *Diabetes*, **46**, 494–500.

101. Begum, N. (1998) Regulation of mitogen activated protein kinase induction by insulin in vascular smooth muscle cells. *Journal of Biological Chemistry*, **273**, 25164–70.

102. Hotamisligil, G.S. (1993) Adipose expression of TNF-α: direct role in obesity linked insulin resistance. *Science*, **259**, 87–91.

103. Meigs, J.B. (1997) Risk variable clustering in insulin resistance syndrome. The Framingham Offspring Study. *Diabetes*, **46**, 1594–1600.

104. Thompson, S.G., Kienast, J., Pyke S.D. *et al.* (1995) Hemostatic factors and the risk of myocardial infarction or sudden death in patients with angina pectoris. *New England Journal of Medicine*, 1995, **332**, 635–41.

105. Syvanne, M. (1997) Lipids and lipoproteins as coronary risk factors in NIDDM. *Lancet*, **350**(Suppl I), 20–3.

106. Haffner, S.M. (1998) Mortality from coronary heart disease in subjects with type 2 diabetes and in nondiabetic subjects with and without prior myocardial infarction. *New England Journal of Medicine*, **339**(4), 229–34.

107. Tchernof, A. (1996) The dense LDL phenotype: association with plasma lipoprotein levels, visceral obesity, and hyperinsulinemia in men. *Diabetes Care*, **19**, 629–37.

108. Laakso, M. (1997) Dyslipidemia, morbidity, and mortality in non-insulin-dependent diabetes mellitus. Lipoproteins and coronary heart disease in non-insulin-dependent diabetes mellitus. *Journal of Diabetes and its Complications*, **11** (2), 137–41.

109. Turner, R.C. (1998) Risk factors for coronary artery disease in NIDDM. UKPDS-23. *British Medical Journal (Clinical Research Ed)*, **316**, 823–8.

110. Fontbonne, A. (1989) Hypertriglycerideamia as a risk factor for CHD, 11 yr follow up. *Paris Prospective Study. Diabetologia*, **32**, 300–4.

111. Hanefeld, M. (1996) The Diabetes Intervention Study, 11 yr follow up. *Diabetologia*, **39**, 1577–83.

112. Hedrick, C.C. (2000) Glycation impairs HDLc function. *Diabetologia*, **43**, 312–20.

113. Wingard, D.L. (1995) Heart disease and diabetes, in Diabetes in America, US Govt. Printing Office, Washington, DC, pp. 429–48. (NIH publ. no. 95-1468).

114. Hypertension in Diabetic Study (HDS). (1993) prevalence of hypertension in newly presenting type 2 diabetic patients and the association with risk factors for cardiovascular and diabetic complications. *Journal of Hypertension*, **11**, 309–17.

115. UK Prospective Diabetes Study Group (1998) Tight blood pressure control and risk of macrovascular and microvascular complications in type 2 diabetes: UKPDS 38. *British Medical Journal (Clinical Research Ed)*, **317**, 703–13

116. Hu, G., Jousilahti, P. and Tuomilehto, J. (2007) Joint effects of history of hypertension at baseline and type 2 diabetes at baseline and during follow-up on the risk of coronary heart disease. *European Heart Journal*, **28**, 3059–66.

117. Pyörälä, K. (1987) Diabetes and atherosclerosis: an epidemiologic view. *Diabetes-Metabolism Reviews*, **3** (2), 463–524.

118. Gu, K. (1999) Diabetes and decline in heart disease mortality in US adults. *Journal of the American Medical Association*, **282**, 1291–97.

119. Kuller, L.H. (2000) Diabetes mellitus: subclinical cardiovascular disease. *Arteriosclerosis, Thrombosis, and Vascular Biology*, **20**, 823–29.

120. Assmann, G., Schulte, H., and Cullen, P. (1997) New and classical risk factors – the Munster heart study (PROCAM). *European Journal of Medical Research*, **2**, 237–42.

121. Kannel, W.B. (1979) Diabetes and cardiovascular risk factors: the Framingham study. *Circulation*, **59**, 8–13.

122. Jarrett, R.J. (1985) Mortality and associated risk factors in diabetes. *Acta Endocrinologica (Suppl)*, **272**, 21–6.

123. Smith, J.W. (1984) Prognosis of patients with diabetes mellitus after myocardial infarction. *American Journal of Cardiology*, **54**, 718–21.

124. Sasaki, A. (1989) Mortality in type 2 diabetic patients. A long term follow up study in Osaka District, Japan. *Diabetes Research and Clinical Practice*, **7**, 33–40.

125. Nelson, R.G. (1990) Low incidence of fatal coronary heart disease in Pima Indians. *Circulation*, **81**, 987–95.

126. Singer, D.E. (1989) Diabetic myocardial infarction. Interaction of diabetes with other pre-infarction risk factors. *Diabetes*, **38**, 350–57.

127. Aronson, D. (1997) Mechanisms of determining course and outcome of diabetic patients who have had acute myocardial infarction. *Annals of Internal Medicine*, **126**, 296–306.

128. Bypass Angioplasty Revascularization Investigation Investigators (2000) Seven-year outcome (BARI). *Journal of the American College of Cardiology*, **35**, 1122–9.

129. Haffner, S.M. (1998) Management of dyslipidemia in adults with diabetes. *Diabetes Care*, **21** (1), 160–78.

130. The Diabetes Control and Complications Trial Research Group (1993) The effect of intensive treatment of diabetes on the development and progression of long-term complications in insulin-dependent diabetes mellitus. *New England Journal of Medicine*, **329**, 977–86.

131. Barzilay, J.I. (1999) Cardiovascular disease in older adults with glucose disorders: comparison of ADA criteria for diabetes mellitus with WHO criteria. *Lancet*, **354**, 622–5.

132. Malmberg, K. (1997) Diabetes Mellitus, Insulin-Glucose Infusion in Acute Myocardial Infarction (DIGAMI). *British Medical Journal*, **314**, 1512–5.

133. Malmberg, K. (2005) DIGAMI 2. *European Heart Journal*, **26**, 650.

134. Schotte D.E. and Stunkard A.J. (1990) The effects of weight reduction on blood pressure in 301 obese patients. *Archives of Internal Medicine*, **150**, 1701–4.

135. Krezesinki, J.M. (1993) Importance of weight loss and sodium restriction in the treatment of mild and moderate essential hypertension. *Acta Clinica Belgica*, **48**, 234–45.

136. Staessen, J. (1989) Body weight, sodium intake and blood pressure. *Journal of Hypertension*, **7** (Suppl 1), S19–S23

137. Faberberg B. (1984) Blood pressure control during weight reduction in obese hypertensive men. *British Medical Journal*, **119**, 11–4.

138. Cutler, J.A. (1997) Randomized trials of sodium reduction: an overview. *American Journal of Clinical Nutrition*, **65** (Suppl. 2), 643S–651S.

139. Heart Outcomes Prevention Evaluation Study Investigators (2000) Effects of ramipril on cardiovascular and microvascular outcomes in people with diabetes mellitus: results of the HOPE study and MICRO-HOPE substudy. *Lancet*, **355**, 253–9.

140. Dahlof, B., Devereux, R.B., Kjeldsen, S.E., *et al.* (2002) Cardiovascular morbidity and mortality in the Losartan Intervention For Endpoint reduction in hypertension study (LIFE): a randomised trial against atenolol. *Lancet*, **359** (9311), 995–1003.

141. ALLHAT Collaborative Group (2002) Major outcomes in high risk hypertensive patients randomized to ACE inhibitor or calcium channel blocker vs diuretic. *Journal of the American Medical Association*, **287**, 2981–97.

142. Fox, K.M. (2003) Efficacy of perindopril in reduction of cardiovascular events among patients with stable coronary artery disease: randomised, double-blind, placebo-controlled, multicentre trial (the EUROPA study). *Lancet*, **6, 362** (9386), 782–8.

143. Braunwald, E. (2004) Angiotensin-converting-enzyme inhibition in stable coronary artery disease. *New England Journal of Medicine*, **351** (20), 2058–68.

144. Tatti, P. (1998) Outcome results of fosinopril versus amlodipine cardiovascular events randomised trial (FACET) in patients with hypertension and NIDDM. *Diabetes Care*, **21**, 597–603.

145. Estacio R. (2000) Effect of blood pressure control on diabetic microvascular complications in patients with hypertension and type 2 diabetes. *Diabetes Care*, **23** (Suppl. 2), B54–B64.

146. Hansson, L. (1998) Effects of intensive blood-pressure lowering and low-dose aspirin on patients with hypertension: principal results of the Hypertension Optimal Treatment (HOT) randomised trial. *Lancet*, **351**, 1755–62 [Medline].

147. Tuomilehto, J. (1999) Effects of calcium channel blockade in older patients with diabetes and systolic hypertension. *New England Journal of Medicine*, **340**, 677–84.

148. Hansson, L. (1999) STOP 2. Randomised trial of old and new antihypertensive drugs in elderly patients: cardiovascular mortality and morbidity the Swedish Trial in Old Patients with Hypertension-2 study. *Lancet*, **354** (9192), 1751–6.

149. Curb, J.D., (1996) Effect of diuretic-based antihypertensive treatment on cardiovascular disease risk in older diabetic patients with isolated systolic hypertension: Systolic Hypertension in the Elderly Program Cooperative Research Group. *Journal of the American Medical Association*, **276**, 1886–92.

150. Hansson, L. (2000) Randomised trial of effects of calcium antagonists compared with diuretics and beta-blockers on cardiovascular morbidity and mortality in hypertension: the Nordic Diltiazem (NORDIL) study. *Lancet*, **29**, (9227) 359–65.

151. Dahlof, B. (2005) Anglo-Scandinavian Cardiac Outcomes Trial-Blood Pressure Lowering Arm (ASCOT-BPLA): a multicentre randomised controlled trial. *Lancet*, **366** (9498), 895–906, 10–16.

152. Sever, P.S., Dahlof, B., Poulter, N.R., Wedel, H., *et al.,* ASCOT investigators. (2003) Prevention of coronary and stroke events with atorvastatin in hypertensive patients who have average or

lower-than-average cholesterol concentrations, in the Anglo-Scandinavian Cardiac Outcomes Trial - Lipid Lowering Arm (ASCOT-LLA): a multicentre randomised controlled trial. *Lancet*, **361**, 1149–58.

153. Erdine, S., The GEMINI-AALA Investigators (2007) Multiple-risk intervention with single-pill amlodipine besylate/atorvastatin calcium therapy helps patients with diverse ethnicity attain recommended therapeutic goals for blood pressure and lipids. *Journal of Hypertension*, **25** (suppl 2), S277, Abstract 7C.6.

154. Patel A., ADVANCE Collaborative Group, MacMahon S., *et al.* (2007) Effects of a fixed combination of perindopril and indapamide on macrovascular and microvascular outcomes in patients with type 2 diabetes mellitus (the ADVANCE trial): a randomised controlled trial. *Lancet*, **370**, 829–840.

155. Julius, S. (2004) Outcomes in hypertensive patients at high cardiovascular risk treated with regimens based on valsartan or amlodipine: the VALUE randomised trial. *Lancet*, **19**, **363** (9426), 2022–31.

156. Brenner, B.M. (2001) Effects of losartan on renal and cardiovascular outcomes in patients with type 2 diabetes and nephropathy. *New England Journal of Medicine*, **345**, 861–9.

157. Lewis, E.J. (2001) Renoprotective effect of the angiotensin-receptor antagonist irbesartan in patients with nephropathy due to type 2 diabetes. *New England Journal of Medicine*, **345**, 851–60.

158. Parving, H.H. (2001) The effect of irbesartan on the development of diabetic nephropathy in patients with type 2 diabetes. *New England Journal of Medicine*, **345**, 870–8.

159. Barnett, A. *et al.* (2004) Comparison of angiotensin-II receptor blocker and angiotensin-converting enzyme inhibition in subjects with type 2 diabetes and nephropathy. *New England Journal of Medicine*, **351**, 1952–61.

160. Yusuf, S., Teo, K.K., Pogue, J. *et al.* for the ONTARGET Investigators (2008) Telmisartan, ramipril, or both in patients at high risk for vascular events. *New England Journal of Medicine*, **358**, 1547–59.

161. Pfeffer, M.A. (2003) Valsartan in Acute Myocardial Infarction Trial Investigators. Valsartan, captopril, or both in myocardial infarction complicated by heart failure, left ventricular dysfunction, or both. *New England Journal of Medicine*, **349**, 1893–1906.

162. Young, J.B. (2004) Mortality and morbidity reduction with Candesartan in patients with chronic heart failure and left ventricular systolic dysfunction: results of the CHARM trial. *Circulation*, **26, 110** (17), 2618–26.

163. Wood, P.D. (1988) Changes in plasma lipids and lipoproteins in overweight men during weight loss through dieting as compared with exercise. *New England Journal of Medicine*, **319**, 1173–9.

164. Goldstein, D.J., (1992) Beneficial health effects of a modest weight loss. *International Journal of Obesity*, **16**, 397–415.

165. Watts, G.F. (1992) Effects on coronary artery disease of lipid-lowering diet or diet plus cholestyramine in the St. Thomas' Atherosclerosis Regression Study (STARS). *Lancet*, **339**, 563.

166. Burr, M.L. (1989) Effects of changes in fat, fish and fibre intakes on death and myocardial infarction: Diet and Reinfarction Trial (DART). *Lancet*, **2**, 757–61.

167. GISSI Prevenzione Investigators (1999) Dietary supplementation with n-3 polyunsaturated fatty acids and vitamin E after myocardial infarction. *Lancet*, **354**, 447–55.

168. De Lorgeril, M. (1996) Effect of a Mediterranean type of diet on the rate of cardiovascular complications in patients with coronary heart disease. Insights into the cardioprotective effect of certain nutriments. *Journal of the American College of Cardiologists*, **28**, 1103.

169. Kris-Etherton, P., Eckel, R.H., Howard, B.V., St. Jeor, S., Bazzarre, T.L.; Nutrition Committee Population Science Committee and Clinical Science Committee of the American Heart

Association. (2001) AHA Science Advisory: Lyon Diet Heart Study. Benefits of a Mediterranean-style, National Cholesterol Education Program/American Heart Association Step I Dietary Pattern on Cardiovascular Disease. *Circulation*, **103**, 1823–5.

170. De Lorgeril, M. (1999) Mediterranean diets, traditional risk factors, and the rate of cardiovascular complications after myocardial infarction. Final report of the Lyon Diet Heart Study. *Circulation*, **99**, 779.

171. Sacks, F.M. (1996) The effect of pravastatin on coronary events after myocardial infarction in patients with average cholesterol levels. Cholesterol and Recurrent Events Trial investigators. *New England Journal of Medicine*, **335**, 1001.

172. The Long-Term Intervention with Pravastatin in Ischaemic Disease (LIPID) Study Group (1998) Prevention of cardiovascular events death with pravastatin in patients with coronary heart disease a broad range of initial cholesterol levels. *New England Journal of Medicine*, **339**, 1349.

173. MRC/BHF (2002) Heart protection Study of cholesterol lowering with Simvastatin in 20 536 high-risk individuals: a randomised placebo-controlled trial. *Lancet*, **360**, 7.

174. LaRosa, J.C. (2005) Intensive lipid lowering with atorvastatin in patients with stable coronary disease. *New England Journal of Medicine*, **7, 352** (14), 1425–35.

175. Pedersen, T.R. (2005) High-dose atorvastatin vs usual-dose simvastatin for secondary prevention after myocardial infarction: the IDEAL study: a randomized controlled trial. *Journal of the American Medical Association*, **16, 294** (19), 2437–45.

176. Schwartz, G.G. (2001) Effects of atorvastatin on early recurrent ischaemic events in acute coronary syndromes. The MIRACL Study: A randomized controlled trial. *Journal of the American Medical Association*, **285**, 1711.

177. Cannon, C.P. (2004) Intensive versus moderate lipid lowering with statins after acute coronary syndromes. *New England Journal of Medicine*, **8350** (15), 1495–504.

178. deLemos, J.A. (2004) Early intensive vs a delayed conservative simvastatin strategy in patients with acute coronary syndromes: phase Z of the A to Z trial. *Journal of the American Medical Association*, **15, 292** (11), 1307.

179. Jukema, J.W. (1995) Effects of lipid lowering by pravastatin on progression and regression of coronary artery disease in men with normal to moderately elevated serum cholesterol levels: The Regression Growth Evaluation Statin Study (REGRESS). *Circulation*, **91**, 2528.

180. Pitt, B. (1999) Atorvastatin Versus Revascularization Treatment Investigators. Aggressive lipid-lowering therapy compared with angioplasty in stable coronary artery disease. *New England Journal of Medicine*, **341**, 70.

181. Nissen, S.E. (2004) Effect of intensive compared with moderate lipid-lowering therapy on progression of coronary atherosclerosis: a randomized controlled trial. *Journal of the American Medical Association*, **3, 291** (9), 1071–80.

182. Nissen, S.E. (2006) Effect of very high-intensity statin therapy on regression of coronary atherosclerosis: the ASTEROID trial. *Journal of the American Medical Association*, **5, 295** (13), 1556–65.

183. Corti R. (2001) Effects of lipid-lowering by simvastatin on human atherosclerotic lesions: a longitudinal study by high-resolution, noninvasive magnetic resonance imaging. *Circulation*, **104**, 249.

184. Colhoun, H.M. (2004) Primary prevention of cardiovascular disease with atorvastatin in type 2 diabetes in the Collaborative Atorvastatin Diabetes Study (CARDS): multicentre randomised placebo-controlled trial. *Lancet*, **364** (9435), 685–96.

185. Barter, P. (2007) HDLc, very low levels of LDLc and cardiovascular events. *New England Journal of Medicine*, **357**, 1301–10.

186. Rubins, H.B. for the Veterans Affairs High-Density Lipoprotein Cholesterol Intervention Trial Study Group (1999) Gemfibrozil for the secondary prevention of coronary heart disease in men

with low levels of high-density lipoprotein cholesterol. *New England Journal of Medicine*, **341**, 410.

187. Diabetes Atherosclerosis Intervention Study Investigators (2001) Effect of fenofibrate on progression of coronary-artery disease in type 2 diabetes: the Diabetes Atherosclerosis Intervention Study, a randomised study. *Lancet*, **357**, 905–10.
188. Keech, A. (2005) Effects of long-term fenofibrate therapy on cardiovascular events in 9795 people with type 2 diabetes mellitus (the FIELD study): randomised controlled trial. *Lancet*, **26**, **366** (9500), 1849–61.
189. Gæde, P. (2003) Multifactorial intervention and cardiovascular disease in patients with type 2 diabetes. *New England Journal of Medicine*, **348**, 383–93.
190. Gæde, P. and Pedersen, O. (2004) Target intervention against multiple risk markers to reduce cardiovascular disease in patients with type 2 diabetes. *Annals of Medicine*, **36**, 355–66.
191. Ridker, P. (2008) Rosuvastatin to prevent vascular events in men and women with elevated CRP, *New England Journal of Medicine*, **359**, 2195–2207.

10

Drug therapy for the obese diabetic patient

John P.H. Wilding

Clinical Sciences Centre, University Hospital Aintree, Liverpool, UK

10.1   Introduction

Type 2 diabetes is strongly associated with obesity and overweight, such that the majority of patients (at least 80% in Caucasian populations) will have a body mass index of at least 25 kg/m², and well over 50% will be clinically obese [1]. Hence any discussion of drug therapy in patients with type 2 diabetes must give serious consideration to the special problems encountered when treating obese subjects. This is particularly important as polypharmacy is now the norm for patients with type 2 diabetes, given the evidence that an aggressive, multifactorial approach to risk factor reduction is of benefit when attempting to reduce the risk of micro- and macrovascular complications [2,3]. More specifically, there is good evidence that weight loss can be an effective treatment for type 2 diabetes, resulting in improved control and reducing risk from cardiovascular disease [4–6] (Figure 10.1). In this Chapter 1 will discuss those aspects of pharmacotherapy in patients with type 2 diabetes that are relevant to obesity; namely the effects of drugs used to treat hyperglycaemia on body weight, the choice of drugs used to treat other risk factors such as hypertension, drugs used to treat complications and consider the role of specific therapy for weight reduction and weight maintenance in the treatment and prevention of type 2 diabetes.

10.2   Drugs for hyperglycaemia

Treatment of hyperglycaemia is arguably the most difficult task when treating obese patients with type 2 diabetes. For example in the United Kingdom Prospective Diabetes

Obesity and Diabetes, Second Edition   Edited by Anthony H. Barnett and Sudhesh Kumar
© 2009 John Wiley & Sons, Ltd

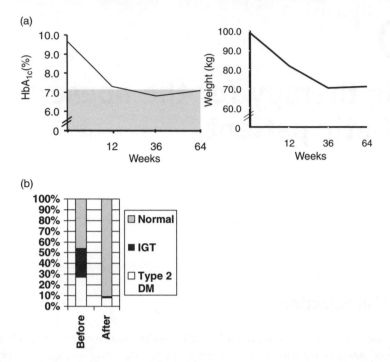

Figure 10.1   Benefits of weight loss in type 2 diabetes. (a) Changes in weight and HbA1c in subjects who succeeded in losing at least 13.6 kg during a behavioural weight loss programme (redrawn using data from Wing *et al.* 1987 [4]). (b) Change in glucose tolerance status after gastric bypass surgery (data from Pories *et al.* 1995 [5])

Study (UKPDS), the progressive worsening of glycaemic control over time, despite regular stepwise increases in therapy in an attempt to maintain predetermined levels of fasting glycaemia [7] was particularly apparent in obese patients [8]. Furthermore, many drugs used to treat hyperglycaemia often lead to further weight gain in patients with diabetes, which will tend to increase insulin resistance, sometimes creating a vicious cycle of increasing weight and drug dose, and adversely affecting risk factors such as blood pressure and low density lipoprotein (LDL)-cholesterol [9]. Newer strategies, either combining drugs such as metformin with glucagon-like peptide-1 (GLP-1) analogues or dipeptidylpeptidase IV (DPP-IV) inhibitors minimize weight gain, or treating obesity itself with drugs may be more appropriate strategies than those used in the UKPDS study.

Metformin

There is now good evidence that whenever possible, metformin should be used as first-line therapy in overweight and obese patients with type 2 diabetes, when hypergly-caemia cannot be adequately controlled by lifestyle changes alone. In the UKPDS, early treatment of obese patients with metformin, both improved hyperglycaemia, resulting in average HbA1c values 0.6% lower compared to patients predominantly treated with diet alone, and prevented most of the weight gain that occurred in subjects treated with insulin or sulfonylureas [8,10]. Overweight or obese subjects randomized to metformin had a 32% reduction in the composite endpoints for both micro- and macrovascular complications, including retinopathy, nephropathy, peripheral neuro- pathy, myocardial infarction, and stroke, compared to lifestyle change alone [10]. This is in contrast to other treatments, which only significantly reduced microvascular complications. It is tempting to speculate that the apparent additional protective effect of metformin on the incidence of macrovascular disease was due to its effects on body weight, although it is not possible to determine this from the UKPDS data. Some studies have suggested that metformin causes modest weight loss [11], and this may be the case in some patients; however its potency as a weight loss agent is not sufficient for it to be classed as such. The mechanism whereby metformin influences body weight is not known; many patients report nausea and gastrointestinal disturbance as a side effect, and this leads to withdrawal of the drug in about 5% of patients. This suggests that metformin may act predominantly by reducing energy intake, and there is evidence that this is the case [12]. Recent reports have also proposed that metformin may be a weak DPP-IV inhibitor, and that some of its beneficial effects may occur by enhancement of incretin action [13] or by prolonging post-meal suppression of the appetite stimulating hormone, ghrelin [14]. There has been some concern about lactic acidosis as a side effect of metformin therapy, which precludes its use in many patients due to contra- indications that include renal impairment, cardiac and hepatic failure, that are common in the obese diabetic population. Despite this, there is evidence that it is widely used in patients with contraindications, without much evidence of adverse effects (lactic acidosis remains very rare) and there have been recent calls for these to be reviewed in the light of this experience [15]. Metformin also has a potential role in the prevention of diabetes, with a 30% reduction seen over 4 years in the US diabetes prevention program, although this was less than with an intensive diet and exercise programme (that reduced diabetes incidence by 58%), it may be a suitable choice for people unable or unwilling to undertake such an approach, particularly in younger patients [16].

Sulfonylureas

Weight gain, in the range of 3–4 kg over the first 6–12 months of therapy is usual with drugs such as glibenclamide and chlorpropramide, as was seen in the UKPDS and in the ADOPT study [11]. Similar effects are usually seen with newer agents, such as glipizide and gliclazide, although some studies report no weight gain with glipizide, this may be because these studies were of short duration [17,18]. Such drugs should therefore be considered as second-line agents in obese patients with type 2 diabetes, usually as add- on therapy to metformin, and only used as monotherapy only if metformin is contra- indicated or poorly tolerated. The mechanisms whereby sulfonylureas cause weight gain are not fully understood, and have not been studied in detail. Improved metabolic control, with reduction of glycosuria has been suggested as one possible mechanism, but weight gain also occurs in patients without glycosuria. Studies of energy intake and metabolic rate in diabetic patients on sulfonylureas versus metformin show little difference in energy expenditure, but this is slightly lower in those on sulfonylureas after adjusting for fat free mass [19]. Hyperglycaemia itself is correlated with basal metabolic rate, perhaps due to the energy costs of increased gluconeogenesis and futile glucose cycling; so part of the weight gain could be due to a reduction in metabolic rate related to improvements in hyperglycaemia during therapy [20,21]. Hyperinsulinaemia, leading to increased deposition of lipid in adipose tissue might also increase metabolic efficiency. Hypoglycaemia increases hunger and food intake [22], and is a known side-effect of sulponylureas, but hypoglycaemia is uncommon in poorly-controlled obese patients with type 2 diabetes. A recent report suggesting that the sulfonylurea receptor is expressed in adipocytes and increases expression of lipogenic enzymes such as fatty acid synthase could be of relevance, but the clinical significance of this *in vitro* observation remains uncertain [23]. Receptors for sulfonylureas are also present in the hypothalamus and other appetite-regulating areas of the central nervous system, but the possibility of direct effects on appetite and/or central nervous system (CNS) modulation of energy expenditure by sulfonylureas and related compounds has not been systematically investigated [24].

Non-sulfonylurea insulin secretagogues

Newer insulin secretagogues, acting on the K-ATP channel, glitinides, such as nateglinide and repaglinide are very short acting, and are therefore given prior to meals to control post-prandial hyperglycaemia. They appear to be equivalent to sulfonylureas in terms of their effects on overall glycaemic control as measured by HbA1c. There have been some claims that these newer agents cause less weight gain than sulfonylureas, but these have been in relatively short-term studies, or from observational data and there are no definitive data from comparative long-term randomized trials to substantiate claims of superiority in this respect [25]. It is also of interest that nateglinide has also been shown to inhibit DPP-IV activity [26].

Acarbose

Acarbose is an α-glucosidase inhibitor that inhibits the breakdown of some complex sugars to glucose within the intestinal lumen, thus reducing the rise in glucose seen after a carbohydrate meal. This undigested carbohydrate is eventually broken down by bacterial fermentation in the large bowel, and most of the sugars are therefore eventually absorbed. Acarbose therefore does not usually cause weight loss, although this has been reported in some studies [27], but it does reduce HbA1c by about 0.6% on average, without weight gain [28]. It can therefore be helpful in obese patients with type 2 diabetes, but its use is frequently limited by gastrointestinal side-effects.

Thiazolidinediones

Thiazolidinediones are agonists at the peroxisome proliferator activated receptor-γ (PPARγ), a nuclear receptor found predominantly in adipose tissue, the function of which is thought to be regulation of aspects of adipocyte differentiation and adipocyte function [29]. These drugs act to sensitize tissues such as adipose tissue and muscle to insulin, via a range of effects that include a reduction in circulating non-esterified fatty acids, and alterations in expression of adipocytokines such as tumour necrosis factor-α (TNF-α), leptin and adiponectin that may influence insulin sensitivity [24,25,30]. Weight gain and redistribution of body fat appear to be closely linked to the therapeutic effects of this class of drugs. In animal models weight gain is dose dependent, and occurs in all animal models of obesity studied to date, including the fatty Zucker rat, that lacks functional leptin receptors (thus dispelling the notion that weight gain is secondary to the reduction in leptin synthesis seen with thiazolidinedione treatment) [31]. The effect is also dependent on diet, with greater effects seen when rats are provided with a highly palatable diet [32]. Part of the weight gain may be due to increased energetic efficiency as weight gain still occurs when animals are pair-fed to controls [33]. Thiazolidinediones also cause fluid retention, possibly via an aldosterone-dependent mechanism [34] but the majority of weight gain is due to an increase in adipose tissue rather than body water. In humans, the average weight gain over 12 months of treatment is in the range of 3–4 kg, which is similar to that observed with sulfonylureas [35]; however longer-term studies, such as the ADOPT study, indicate that the effect may be progressive, reaching 6 kg after 4 years, in contrast to the plateau reached with SUs (Figure 10.2) [11]. The changes in fat distribution are of

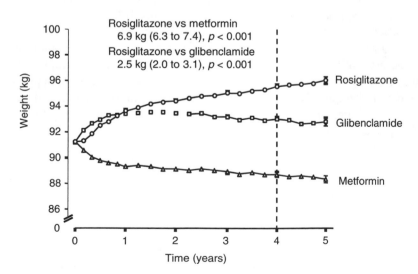

Figure 10.2   Effect of different oral hypoglycaemic agents on body weight (data from Kahn *et al.* 2006 [11])

some interest, and been claimed to be beneficial, as investigation using magnetic resonance imaging or computerized tomography has shown decreases in visceral adipose tissue whilst subcutaneous adipose tissue mass increases [36]. Animal and human studies have also demonstrated the synergistic effect of drug treatment plus lifestyle changes – thus avoidance of weight gain enhances the therapeutic effect [33, 37]. Thiazolidenediones have recently been the subject of some controversy with respect to cardiovascular safety, with the consensus view now emerging that whilst there is some supportive data for pioglitazone (mainly from the ProActive study) [38–40], the effects of rosiglitazone at best neutral, and may possibly increase the risk of myocardial infarction [40, 41]. Both drugs in this class are now contra-indicated in the presence of heart failure.

Incretin mimetics and DPP-IV inhibitors

The most recent therapeutic advances in the treatment of type 2 diabetes have been the development of drugs that act on the incretin system. Incretins are hormones, released from the gastrointestinal tract after food ingestion. They potentiate the insulin secretory response to oral glucose, and suppress glucagon release. The main incretin hormones in humans are glucagon-like peptide 1 (GLP-1) (7–36) amide, produced by the L-cells in the jejunum and ileum, and glucose-dependent insulinotropic polypeptide (GIP), produced from K-cells in the duodenum and jejunum. GLP-1 is the more potent of the two, and although its secretion is impaired in patients with type 2 diabetes, the pancreatic response to GLP-1 is preserved. In contrast, although GIP secretion is normal in diabetes, the insulin secretory response to exogenous GIP is lost [42]. Furthermore, GLP-1 has been shown to be a physiological satiety signal in rodents [43], and effects on appetite have also been shown with GLP-1 at supraphysiological concentrations, and with potent GLP-1 analogues in humans [44]. The naturally produced hormones have a short half-life, due mainly to rapid degradation by serum proteases, predominantly DPP-IV, so are not suitable for use as therapy in humans, although early studies using sc injections and infusions were successful in proving that GLP-1-based therapies had potential for the treatment of type 2 diabetes. Two approaches have been used to target GLP-1 for diabetes treatment; the first is to use modified peptides, given by sc injection that are resistant to DPP-IV degradation and thus long acting, these include exenatide (Byetta) [45], and liraglutide [46]. The main side effect with these drugs is nausea, which may lead to discontinuation in some subjects. The alternative approach has been to develop orally-active drugs that prevent breakdown of GLP-1, DPP-IV inhibitors such as sitagliptin (Januvia), and vildagliptin (Galvus) [47,48]. In general the peptide analogues have been found to result in modest weight loss (2–3 kg), whereas DPP-IV inhibitors are generally weight neutral. Both groups of drugs are efficacious in the management of diabetes, with significant improvements in glycaemic control, with falls in glycated haemoglobin of between 0.7 and 1.1% depending on the particular study. GLP-1 analogues have been proposed as an alternative to insulin in obese patients with type 2 diabetes, and the trial data

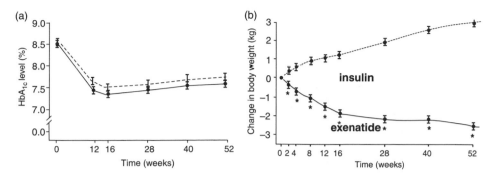

Figure 10.3 Comparison of effects of premixed insulin and exenatide on glycaemic control and body weight (data from Nauck *et al.* 2007 [51])

suggests that the differential in weight may be significant (up to 5.4 kg), with similar effects on glycaemic control [49–51] (Figure 10.3). Longer acting preparations, including a once weekly version of exenatide are undergoing clinical trials [52].

Insulin

The natural history of type 2 diabetes is that of declining β-cell function, such that insulin therapy is often required, either as a substitute or as add-on therapy to oral agents. In the UKPDS 53% of sulfonylurea-treated patients required insulin during the course of the study. Insulin treatment is frequently, but not invariably associated with significant weight gain; in the UKPDS the average weight gain in subjects randomized to insulin was 7.5 kg over 10 years (compared to 2.5 kg in those randomized to diet alone) [7]. In one study in the US of intensive insulin therapy in type 2 diabetes, good control (average glucose fell from 17.5 to 7.7 mmol/l) was only achieved at the expense of weight gain of nearly 9 kg in just 6 months. Weight gain with insulin treatment can be attenuated by up to 80% with the addition or continuation of metformin, and where possible this should be considered standard treatment of obese patients with type 2 diabetes when insulin therapy is required. However more intensive regimens are often required which can result in greater and sometimes progressive weight gain [53].

10.3 The role of anti-obesity drugs in diabetic management

Given the overwhelming evidence that obesity is of fundamental importance in the aetiology of type 2 diabetes, as well as many of its comorbid conditions such as hypertension, dyslipidaemia and other aspects of the metabolic syndrome, it is surprising how little attention has been given to weight management, compared to the extensive studies that have been conducted with drugs to control hyperglycaemia, hypertension and dyslipidaemia. There is little doubt that reduction of excess body

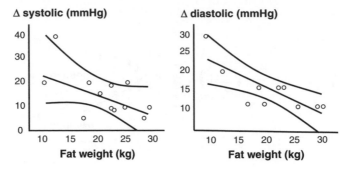

Figure 10.4 Obese patients respond less well to nifedipine as antihypertensive treatment. Data redrawn from reference [51]

weight can be very effective treatment. Dietary intervention studies suggest that a weight loss of approximately 10% is required to significantly improve HbA1c in subjects with established type 2 diabetes, although some subjects may respond dramatically to lesser degrees of weight loss [4]. Modest weight loss early in the course of the disease, combined with other changes to diet and lifestyle can also be extremely effective, as was shown during the first three months of dietary treatment in the UKPDS [54], and the first year of the ongoing Look Ahead study [55]. Prevention studies, conducted in obese and overweight subjects with impaired glucose tolerance, have shown that weight loss of only 3 or 4 kg can have dramatic effects to prevent or delay the onset of type 2 diabetes [16,56] (Figure 10.4). Thus there is heterogeneity of response to weight loss in type 2 diabetes that may be in part related to the duration of the disease with weight loss becoming less effective as β-cell dysfunction develops. Nevertheless, even in insulin-requiring patients, weight loss can be beneficial, and on occasion can result in normalization of blood glucose, especially after surgical intervention, such as gastric bypass [5].

What then, is the role of anti-obesity drugs? The fenfluramines have now been withdrawn on grounds of safety, following reports of development of carcinoid-like valvular heart lesions in some patients in the United States. Phentermine and diethyl-propion remain available for short-term use (up to 3 months), despite of lack of long-term trial data of sufficient quality to support their continued use. Two newer agents, orlistat and sibutramine are now in widespread use, and data is available regarding their role in the management of patients with type 2 diabetes. A third agent, rimonabant, is available in Europe and a number of other countries, but not in the United States.

Orlistat

Orlistat is an inhibitor of pancreatic and intestinal lipases, and therefore prevents the breakdown of dietary fat into fatty acids and glycerol within the gut lumen, resulting in approximately 30% malabsorption of dietary fat. For individuals on a Western diet, this typically results in a daily caloric deficit of about 200–300 kcal; without dietary restraint, this should result in a weight loss of about 0.2–0.3 kg per week, or 5–7.5 kg over 6 months. This will of course be somewhat attenuated by the fall in metabolic rate that occurs with weight loss, so weight loss tends to gradually reach a plateau after 6–9 months of treatment. Clinical trials with orlistat have usually included dietary advice to help weight loss, and recommendations about increasing physical activity; hence the average weight loss achieved in non-diabetic subjects is on average about 10 kg (compared to 6 kg with diet and exercise alone). There is some evidence that the early response to treatment is a good predictor of future weight loss [57]. Once weight loss has stopped, the role of continued drug use is to promote weight maintenance, as weight is soon regained if the drug is stopped. Side-effects of orlistat are confined to the gastrointestinal tract, as the drug is not systemically absorbed and include loose fatty stools, oily spotting and, rarely, faecal incontinence. These side-effects tend to reduce with time, as patients learn to avoid foods that are high in fat. Circulating concentrations of fat-soluble vitamins and beta-carotene fall by about 10%, but clinical vitamin deficiency is very rare, and can be prevented by use of a multivitamin supplement.

Several studies have been conducted using orlistat in diabetic patients, either treated with diet or with a variety of oral agents and insulin. Typically, subjects with type 2 diabetes find it more difficult to lose weight than those without diabetes [58], and in general the weight loss observed is less; for example in sulfonylurea-treated patients with type 2 diabetes, weight loss over 12 months was 6 kg with orlistat compared to 3 kg with placebo, so that twice as many patients achieved 5 and 10% weight loss with orlistat. This modest weight loss did however result in improvements in glycaemic control that were proportional to weight loss, and moreover, there were also favourable changes in the lipid profile [59]. Similar results have been shown in metformin and insulin-treated patients, but these trials have yet to be reported in full [60,61]. The Xendos trial, a trial of diabetes prevention with orlistat has also recently reported, and supports the use of orlistat as an adjunct to diet and exercise in subjects at high risk of developing type 2 diabetes, as well as demonstrating efficacy at weight maintenance for up to 4 years [62].

Sibutramine

Sibutramine is a centrally-acting drug that is an inhibitor of serotonin and noradrenaline reuptake. As a reuptake inhibitor, it is in some ways pharmacologically similar to reuptake inhibitors used as antidepressants, but sibutramine does not have antidepressant or euphoric properties. It is pharmacologically distinct from serotonin releasing agents, such as dexfenfluramine, that have been reported to cause cardiac valvular lesions similar to those seen in carcinoid syndrome [63–65]. Sibutramine is thought to act by both increasing post-prandial satiety (the feeling of fullness after a meal), and by increasing thermogenesis, particularly by attenuating the usual fall in energy expenditure that occurs with weight loss [66,67]. CNS-mediated side-effects include dry mouth, insomnia and constipation; there is also a modest increase in sympathetic nervous system activity, which is responsible for the change in thermogenesis, but also can result in increases in heart rate and blood pressure in some patients, although the average changes seen in clinical trials are of 2–4 bpm in heart rate, and 1–2 mmHg of systolic and diastolic blood pressure, although no significant changes are seen in obese hypertensive patients whose blood pressure is well controlled [68]. The efficacy of sibutramine for both weight loss and weight maintenance has been tested in clinical trials of up to two years duration. For example in the Sibutramine Trial Of weight Reduction and Maintenance (STORM) study, conducted in non-diabetic patients, mean weight loss of 12% occurred over the first 6 months of the study; this was largely maintained for a further 18 months in those subjects in whom the active drug was continued, whereas significant weight regain occurred in subjects switched to placebo, despite continuing dietary and lifestyle advice. Nearly 50% of patients maintained weight loss of at least 10% for the duration of the study. As well as inducing weight loss, there were significant improvements in the lipid profile with weight loss in this study, with reduction in LDL, very low density lipoprotein cholesterol, triglycerides and an increase in high density lipoprotein (HDL) cholesterol, such that the cholesterol HDL ratio fell by 13.3% [69]. These beneficial effects may have been offset to some extent by increases in blood pressure, although a metanalysis of such changes suggests an overall decrease in cardiovascular risk, as assessed using the Framingham risk equation [70]. Sibutramine has also been evaluated in diabetic patients treated with diet, metformin and sulfonylureas [71]. As with orlistat, weight loss proved more elusive in trials in diabetic patients, but, for example, in metformin-treated patients, an average weight loss of about 5% was achieved and maintained for 12 months, compared to virtually no weight loss in placebo-treated subjects, despite intensified dietary advice. This was associated with improvements in HbA1c, lipid profile and little change in blood pressure in subjects who lost weight, although there was an increase in heart rate, and more sibutramine-treated patients experienced a rise in blood pressure [49]. These encouraging results, together with legitimate concerns regarding the cardiovascular effects of sibutramine, has led to the design of the Sibutramine Cardiovascular Outcomes Trial (SCOUT), that is investigating the effects of weight loss with sibutramine on cardiovascular end-points in high risk patients, including many with type 2 diabetes. Data from the 6 week single blind lead-in from the SCOUT study has recently been published, and sibutramine appeared well tolerated in this group, with a mean fall in blood pressure of 3/1 mmHg, and with less than 5% of participants having a rise in blood pressure of more than 10 mmHg [72].

Rimonabant

Rimonabant is the most recently available drug for weight loss; it is an inverse agonist which blocks the action of endogenous endocannabinoids such as anandamide and 2-anhydroglycerol at the cannabinoid-1 (CB-1) receptor. The endocannabinoid neuro-modulatory system has been implicated in a wide range of metabolic processes, including appetite and body weight regulation and lipid metabolism. There is some evidence from rodent and human studies that this system has higher levels of activity in obesity, providing some support for this as a logical approach. In clinical trials rimonabant has been found to be effective at producing weight loss, and studies have been conducted in non-diabetic and diabetic patients with obesity. Efficacy is similar to that seen with sibutramine, with weight loss of 8–9% from randomization after 1 year in non-diabetic patients, and slightly less (6%) in those with diabetes [73–75]. The effects largely persist if the drug is continued for 2 years (7.9% weight loss), but as expected, weight is likely to return to baseline levels if the drug is stopped [74]. As might be expected lipid profile and diabetes improve with weight loss, but there is some evidence that rimonabant may have independent effects to improve these parameters, although most of the evidence supporting this is indirect. Cannabinoid receptors are present in fat tissue and the liver, and preclinical studies suggest a role in regulation of fat metabolism; analysis of data from clinical trials suggests that improvements in lipid profile, particularly increases in HDL cholesterol and lowering of HbA1c in diabetes are greater than would be expected with weight loss alone; thus it is estimated that about half of the 0.6% reduction in HbA1c seen in the RIO diabetes study was due to weight loss, and the remainder to other effects of the drug.

Adverse effects of rimonabant have been a cause for concern; in clinical trials overall withdrawal rates for adverse events were 13.8 % for rimonabant vs. 7.2% for placebo. The events of most concern relate to mood disorders (particularly anxiety and depression), and associated feelings of suicidality. Anxiety and depressed mood occurred about twice as often in patients treated with rimonabant 20 mg (3.2% vs. 1.6% for depression, and 5.6% vs. 2.4% for anxiety). A similar odds ratio for suicidality was found in an independent analysis carried out for an FDA advisory committee, but the numbers of events was very small. It is of interest that the rates of adverse events compared to placebo were similar in the second year of treatment, suggesting that patients either stop treatment, or that such effects diminish over time with continued therapy. Other adverse effects include gastrointestinal disorders, dizziness and insomnia – most of these are mild in severity. These concerns initially led to a strengthening of the warnings in Europe (where rimonabant was licensed) to include a contraindication in depression and a recommendations for monitoring for mood disorders, and to the FDA advisory panel to vote against recommending approval for rimonabant in July 2007, pending availability of further data. However ongoing concerns and reports of suicide and suicidality in clinical trials led to the withdrawal of the marketing authorisation for rimonabant in the European Union in October 2008, and the suspension of ongoing clinical trials. It now seems unlikely that the overall potential for rimonabant and other CB1 antagonists for treatment and prevention of vascular disease will ever be fully evaluated.

In summary, there is now good evidence that use of drugs for weight loss can be a useful adjunct to improve glycaemic, lipid and possibly blood pressure control in patients with type 2 diabetes, however at present, careful selection of motivated patients is important, as with any weight loss programme, and definitive trials examining hard endpoints are yet to be conducted.

Drugs in development

Given the high level of recent interest in developing drugs for weight loss, it seems likely that newer, perhaps more effective agents will eventually become available. Agents currently under evaluation include new lipase inhibitors, mitochondrial transfer protein inhibitors, combinations of existing agents such as phentermine with anticonvulsants such as topiramate and new serotonin agonists. The role of newer drug treatments, such as incretin enhancers and agonists that promote weight loss or are weight neutral is likely to increase. Diabetes management would be transformed if a safe, highly effective weight loss agent became available, but this seems unlikely in the near future.

10.4　Antihypertensive treatment

Although many intervention trials have been conducted using different antihypertensive agents in diabetic and non-diabetic subjects, few studies have been conducted exclusively in obese subjects, and some studies have specifically excluded very obese patients. The average BMI in the UKPDS study was approximately $29 \, \text{kg/m}^2$, but no sub-group analysis based on BMI has been reported. There is clear evidence from the literature that obese hypertensive patients have higher circulating catecholamine concentrations and greater activity of the renin-angiotensin system than non-obese patients, but it is unknown whether this is also the case in diabetic patients. It is therefore difficult to draw firm conclusions about the optimal antihypertensive strategy for obese patients with type 2 diabetes. Angiotensin-converting enzyme (ACE) inhibitors are certainly effective, and may have other advantages in subjects with cardiovascular disease, nephropathy and retinopathy; they have been shown to reduce complication rates in the UKPDS study [76]; angiotensin 2 receptor blockers have similar effects, and can be used if patients are intolerant of ACE inhibitors, combination with ACE inhibitors may be indicated in patients with microalbuminuria. Low dose thiazide diuretics are safe, but slightly less efficacious than ACE inhibitors – they are useful add-on agents as second- or third-line therapy. β-Blockers are certainly effective antihypertensive drugs, but they can cause weight gain, and were less well tolerated than ACE inhibitors in the UKPDS, so should perhaps be considered as second-line agents, although they may be specifically indicated in patients with angina, some dysrhythmias, and in heart failure. Calcium channel blockers seem to be less effective in patients with obesity-related hypertension [77], but are useful as add-on therapy [78] (Figure 10.5). Other drugs such as α-blockers, methyldopa and clonidine and may have a role as adjunctive therapy where blood pressure is difficult to control.

Lipid-lowering treatment

Although weight loss may have beneficial effects on lipids, particularly on HDL cholesterol and triglycerides, the evidence for use of lipid-lowering agents in subjects at

Table 10.1   Drugs causing weight gain

Class	Examples	Mechanism of effect
Anticonvulsants	Sodium valproate Phenytoin Gabapentin	Unknown
Antidepressants	Citalopram Mirtazepine	Serotonin
Antipsychotics	Chlorpromazine Risperidone Olanzepine	? Dopamine agonism
Beta-blockers	Atenolol	? inhibition of thermogenesis
Corticosteroids	Prednisolone Dexamethasone	Promote fat deposition Increase appetite
Insulin	All formulations	
Sex steroids	Medroxyprogesterone acetate Progesterone Combined oral contraceptives	Increase appetite
Insulin secretagogues	Glibenclamide Gliclazide Repaglinide	Changes in metabolic rate, and increased appetite implicated
Thiazolidinediones	Rosiglitazone Pioglitazone	Changes in metabolic rate, and increased appetite implicated
Drugs for migraine	Pizotifen	Serotonin antagonist
Protease inhibitors	Indinavir Ritonavir	Promotes site-specific fat deposition

high risk of cardiovascular disease is now very strong, and it would therefore be difficult to justify withholding such treatment on the grounds of expected effects of weight loss. Clearly, if substantial weight loss is achieved, then the continuing need for lipid-lowering drugs should be reviewed (Table 10.1).

10.5   Use of other drugs that may cause weight gain

There is a long list of drugs, mainly centrally-acting, that can cause weight gain, and these are often prescribed to patients with diabetes. Of particular note are tricyclic antidepressants and anticonvulsants such as carbemazepine and gabapentin used for symptom control in painful neuropathy. Other drugs include antipsychotic drugs, notably the newer atypical antipsychotic agents, such as clozapine and olanzapine, that can cause substantial weight gain, and have been suggested to independently worsen insulin resistance and perhaps increase diabetes risk in non-diabetic subjects [79]. Pizotifen, a serotonin antagonist used in the management of migraine, may cause increased appetite and therefore weight gain [80]. Corticosteroids and some progesterone preparations, such as medroxyprogesterone acetate may also cause substantial weight gain, and in the case of corticosteroids, worsen insulin resistance and impair β-cell function. Finally, antiretroviral therapy, used in the management of human immunodeficiency virus infection, may cause lipodystrophy with increased central adiposity and thus either predispose to diabetes, or exacerbate exisiting glucose intolerance [81]. Whilst it may not be possible to avoid the use of many of these drugs, it is important to be aware of their potential effects on body weight, keep doses to the minimum, and give appropriate advice to patients, with regard to dietary restraint when they are taking drugs that may result in weight gain.

References

1. Daousi, C., Casson, I.F., Gill, G.V. *et al.* (2006) Prevalence of obesity in type 2 diabetes in secondary care: association with cardiovascular risk factors. *Postgraduate Medical Journal*, **82** (966), 280–4.
2. Gaede, P., Vedel, P., Larsen, N. *et al.* (2003 January 30) Multifactorial intervention and cardiovascular disease in patients with type 2 diabetes. *New England Journal of Medicine*, **348** (5), 383–93.
3. Gaede, P., Lund-Andersen, H., Parving, H.H. and Pedersen, O. (2008) Effect of a multifactorial intervention on mortality in type 2 diabetes. *New England Journal of Medicine*, **358** (6), 580–91.
4. Wing, R.R., Koeske, R., Epstein, L.H. *et al.* (1987) Long-term effects of modest weight-loss in type-ii diabetic patients. *Archives of Internal Medicine*, **147**, 1749–53.
5. Pories, W.J., Swanson, M.S., MacDonald, K.G. *et al.* (1995) Who would have thought it – an operation proves to be the most effective therapy for adult-onset diabetes-mellitus. *Annals of Surgery*, **222**, 339–52.
6. Lean, M.E., Powrie, J.K., Anderson, A.S. and Garthwaite, P.H. (1990) Obesity, weight loss and prognosis in type 2 diabetes. *Diabetic Medicine*, **7** (3), 228–33.
7. Turner, R.C. (1999) Intensive blood-glucose control with sulphonylureas or insulin compared with conventional treatment and risk of complications in patients with type 2 diabetes (UKPDS 33) (vol 352, pg 837, 1998). *Lancet*, **354**, 602.
8. Turner, R.C., Cull, C.A., Frighi, V. and Holman, R.R. (1999) Glycemic control with diet, sulfonylurea, metformin, or insulin in patients with type 2 diabetes mellitus – progressive requirement for multiple therapies (UKPDS 49). *Journal of the American Medical Association*, **281**, 2005–12.
9. Yki-Jarvinen, H., Ryysy, L., Kauppila, M. *et al.* (1997) Effect of obesity on the response to insulin therapy in noninsulin-dependent diabetes mellitus. *Journal of Clinical Endocrinology and Metabolism*, **82** (12), 4037–43.
10. Turner, R.C., Holman, R.R., Stratton, I.M. *et al.* (1998) Effect of intensive blood-glucose control with metformin on complications in overweight patients with type 2 diabetes (UKPDS 34). *Lancet*, **352**, 854–65.
11. Kahn, S.E., Haffner, S.M., Heise, M.A. *et al.* (2006) Glycemic durability of rosiglitazone, metformin, or glyburide monotherapy. *New England Journal of Medicine*, **355** (23), 2427–43.

12. Makimattila, S., Nikkila, K. and Yki-Jarvinen, H. (1999) Causes of weight gain during insulin therapy with and without metformin in patients with type II diabetes mellitus. *Diabetologia*, **42** (4), 406–12.

13. Lindsay, J.R., Duffy, N.A., McKillop, A.M. *et al.* (2005) Inhibition of dipeptidyl peptidase IV activity by oral metformin in type 2 diabetes. *Diabetic Medicine*, **22** (5), 654–7.

14. English, P.J., Ashcroft, A., Patterson, M. *et al.* (2007) Metformin prolongs the postprandial fall in plasma ghrelin concentrations in type 2 diabetes. *Diabetes-Metabolism Research and Reviews*, **23** (4), 299–303.

15. Jones, G.C.A.W.M. and Macklin, J.P. (2003) Contraindications to the use of metformin. *British Medical Journal*, **326**, 4–5.

16. Diabetes Prevention Program Research Group (2002) Reduction in the incidence of type 2 diabetes with lifestyle intervention or metformin. *New England Journal of Medicine*, **346**, 393–403.

17. Simonson, D.C., Kourides, I.A., Feinglos, M. *et al.* (1997) Efficacy, safety, and dose-response characteristics of glipizide gastrointestinal therapeutic system on glycemic control and insulin secretion in NIDDM – results of two multicenter, randomized, placebo-controlled clinical trials. *Diabetes Care*, **20** (4), 597–606.

18. Cefalu, W.T., Bell-Farrow, A., Wang, Z.Q. *et al.* (1998) Effect of glipizide GITS on insulin sensitivity, glycemic indices, and abdominal fat composition in NIDDM. *Drug Development Research*, **44** (1), 1–7.

19. Chong, P.K.K., Jung, R.T., Rennie, M.J. and Scrimgeour, C.M. (1995) Energy-expenditure in type-2 diabetic-patients on metformin and sulfonylurea therapy. *Diabetic Medicine*, **12** (5), 401–8.

20. Efendic, S., Wajngot, A. and Vranic, M. (1985) Increased activity of the glucose cycle in the liver – early characteristic of type-2 diabetes. *Proceedings of the National Academy of Sciences of the United, States of America*, **82** (9), 2965–9

21. Franssilakallunki, A. and Groop, L. (1992) Factors associated with basal metabolic-rate in patients with type-2 (non-insulin-dependent) diabetes-mellitus. *Diabetologia*, **35** (10), 962–6.

22. Dewan, S., Gillett, A., Mugarza, J.A. *et al.* (2004) Effects of insulin-induced hypoglycaemia on energy intake and food choice at a subsequent test meat. *Diabetes-Metabolism Research and Reviews*, **20** (5), 405–10.

23. Shi, H., Moustaid-Moussa, N., Wilkison, W.O. and Zemel, M.B. (1999) Role of the sulfonylurea receptor in regulating human adipocyte metabolism. *FASEB Journal*, **13** (13), 1833–8.

24. Treherne, J.M. and Ashford, M.L. (1991) The regional distribution of sulphonylurea binding sites in rat brain. *Neuroscience*, **40**, 523–31.

25. Landgraf, R., Frank, M., Bauer, C. and Dieken, M.L. (2000) Prandial glucose regulation with repaglinide: its clinical and lifestyle impact in a large cohort of patients with Type 2 diabetes. *International Journal of Obesity*, **24**, S38–S44.

26. Duffy, N.A., Green, B.D., Irwin, N. *et al.* (2007) Effects of antidiabetic drugs on dipeptidyl peptidase IV activity: nateglinide is an inhibitor of DPP IV and augments the antidiabetic activity of glucagon-like peptide-1. *European Journal of Pharmacology*, **568** (1–3), 278–86.

27. Wolever, T.M.S., Chiasson, J.L., Josse, R.G. *et al.* (1997) Small weight loss on long-term acarbose therapy with no change in dietary pattern or nutrient intake of individuals with non-insulin-dependent diabetes. *International Journal of Obesity*, **21** (9), 756–63.

28. Holman, R.R., Cull, C.A. and Turner, R.C. (1999) A randomized double-blind trial of acarbose in type 2 diabetes shows improved glycemic control over 3 years (UK Prospective Diabetes Study 44). *Diabetes Care*, **22**, 960–64.

29. Spiegelman, B.M. (1998) PPAR-gamma: adipogenic regulator and thiazolidinedione receptor. *Diabetes*, **47**, 507–14.

30. Sewter, C.P., Digby, J.E., Blows, F. *et al.* (1999) Regulation of tumour necrosis factor-alpha release from human adipose tissue in vitro. *Journal of Endocrinology*, **163**, 33–8.

31. Wang, Q., Dryden, S., Frankish, H.M. *et al.* (1997) Increased feeding in fatty Zucker rats by the thiazolidinedione BRL 49653 (rosiglitazone) and the possible involvement of leptin and hypothalamic neuropeptide Y. *British Journal of Pharmacology*, **122**, 1405–10.

32. Pickavance, L.C., Tadayyon, M., Widdowson, P.S. *et al.* (1999) Therapeutic index for rosiglitazone in dietary obese rats: separation of efficacy and haemodilution. *British Journal of Pharmacology*, **128**, 1570–6.

33. Pickavance, L.C., Buckingham, R.E. and Wilding, J.P.H. (2001) Insulin-sensitizing action of rosiglitazone is enhanced by preventing hyperphagia. *Diabetes Obesity & Metabolism*, **3** (3), 171–80.

34. Guan, Y.F., Hao, C.M., Cha, D.R. *et al.* (2005) Thiazolidinediones expand body fluid volume through PPAR gamma stimulation of ENaC-mediated renal salt absorption. *Nature Medicine*, **11** (8), 861–6.

35. Raskin, P., Rendell, M., Riddle, M.C. *et al.* (2001) A randomized trial of rosiglitazone therapy in patients with inadequately controlled insulin-treated type 2 diabetes. *Diabetes Care*, **24** (7), 1226–32.

36. Kelly, I.E., Han, T.S., Walsh, K. and Lean, M.E.J. (1999) Effects of a thiazolidinedione compound on body fat and fat distribution of patients with type 2 diabetes. *Diabetes Care*, **22**, 288–93.

37. Reynolds, L.R., Konz, E.C., Frederich, R.C. and Anderson, J.W. (2002) Rosiglitazone amplifies the benefits of lifestyle intervention measures in long-standing type 2 diabetes mellitus. *Diabetes Obesity & Metabolism*, **4** (4), 270–5.

38. Dormandy, J.A., Charbonnel, B., Eckland, D.J.A. *et al.* (2005) Secondary prevention of macrovascular events in patients with type 2 diabetes in the PROactive Study (PROspective pioglitAzone Clinical Trial In macroVascular Events): a randomised controlled trial. *Lancet*, **366** (9493), 1279–89.

39. Lincoff, A.M., Wolski, K., Nicholls, S.J. and Nissen, S.E. (2007) Pioglitazone and risk of cardiovascular events in patients with type 2 diabetes mellitus – A meta-analysis of randomized trials. *Journal of the American Medical Association*, **298** (10), 1180–8.

40. Singh, S., Loke, Y.K. and Furberg, C.D. (2007) Long-term risk of cardiovascular events with rosiglitazone – a meta-analysis. *Journal of the American Medical Association*, **298** (10), 1189–95.

41. Nissen, S.E. and Wolski, K. (2007) Effect of rosiglitazone on the risk of myocardial infarction and death from cardiovascular causes. *New England Journal of Medicine*, **356** (24), 2457–71.

42. Drucker, D.J. (2006) The biology of incretin hormones. *Cell Metabolism*, **3** (3), 153–65.

43. Turton, M.D., Oshea, D., Gunn, I. *et al.* (1996) A role for glucagon-like peptide-1 in the central regulation of feeding. *Nature*, **379** (6560), 69–72.

44. Edwards, C.M.B., Stanley, S.A., Davis, R. *et al.* (2001) Exendin-4 reduces fasting and postprandial glucose and decreases energy intake in healthy volunteers. *American Journal of Physiology-Endocrinology and Metabolism*, **281** (1), E155–E161.

45. Kendall, D.M., Riddle, M.C., Rosenstock, J. *et al.* (2005) Effects of exenatide (exendin-4) on glycemic control over 30 weeks in patients with type 2 diabetes treated with metformin and a sulfonylurea. *Diabetes Care*, **28** (5), 1083–91.

46. Harder, H., Nielsen, L., Thi, T.D.T. and Astrup, A. (2004) The effect of liraglutide, a long-acting glucagon-like peptide 1 derivative, on glycemic control, body composition, and 24-h energy expenditure in patients with type 2 diabetes. *Diabetes Care*, **27** (8), 1915–21.

47. Hermansen, K., Kipnes, M., Luo, E. *et al.* (2007) Efficacy and safety of the dipeptidyl peptidase-4 inhibitor, sitagliptin, in patients with type 2 diabetes mellitus inadequately controlled on

glimepiride alone or on glimepiride and metformin. *Diabetes Obesity & Metabolism*, **9** (5), 733–45.

48. Ahren, B., Pacini, G., Foley, J.E. and Schweizer, A. (2005) Improved meal-related beta-cell function and insulin sensitivity by the dipeptidyl peptidase-IV inhibitor vildagliptin in metformin-treated patients with type 2 diabetes over 1 year. *Diabetes Care*, **28** (8), 1936–40.

49. Heine, R.J., Van Gaal, L.F., Johns, D. *et al.* (2005) Exenatide versus insulin glargine in patients with suboptimally controlled type 2 diabetes – a randomized trial. *Annals of Internal Medicine*, **143** (8), 559–69.

50. Davis, S.N., Johns, D., Maggs, D. *et al.* (2007) Exploring the substitution of exenatide for insulin in patients with type 2 diabetes treated with insulin in combination with oral antidiabetes agents. *Diabetes Care*, **30** (11), 2767–72.

51. Nauck, M.A., Duran, S., Kim, D. *et al.* (2007) A comparison of twice-daily exenatide and biphasic insulin aspart in patients with type 2 diabetes who were suboptimally controlled with sulfonylurea and metformin: a non-inferiority study. *Diabetologia*, **50** (2), 259–67.

52. Kim, D., MacConell, L., Zhuang, D.L. *et al.* (2007) Effects of once-weekly dosing of a long-acting release formulation of exenatide on glucose control and body weight in subjects with type 2 diabetes. *Diabetes Care*, **30** (6), 1487–93.

53. Holman, R.R., Thorne, K.I., Farmer, A.J. *et al.* (2007) Addition of biphasic, prandial, or basal insulin to oral therapy in type 2 diabetes. *New England Journal of Medicine*, **357**, 1716–30.

54. Manley, S.E., Stratton, I.M., Cull, C.A. *et al.* (2000) Effects of three months' diet after diagnosis of yype 2 diabetes on plasma lipids and lipoproteins (UKPDS 45). UK Prospective Diabetes Study Group. *Diabetic Medicine*, **17** (7), 518–23.

55. Look AHEAD Research Group, Pi-Sunyer, X., Blackburn, G., Brancati, F.L. *et al.* (2007) Reduction in weight and cardiovascular disease risk factors in individuals with type 2 diabetes: one-year results of the look AHEAD trial. *Diabetes Care*, **30** (6), 1374–83.

56. Tuomilheto, J., Lindstrom, J., Erickson, J.G. *et al.* (2001) Prevention of type 2 diabetes mellitus by changes in lifestyle amongst subjects with impaired glucose tolerance. *New England Journal of Medicine*, **344**, 1343–50.

57. Sjostrom, L., Rissanen, A., Andersen, T. *et al.* (1998) Weight loss and prevention of weight regain in obese patients: a 2-year, European, randomised trial of orlistat. *Lancet*, **352**, 167–72.

58. Wing, R.R., Marcus, M.D., Epstein, L.H. and Salata, R. (1987) Type-ii diabetic subjects lose less weight than their overweight nondiabetic spouses. *Diabetes Care*, **10**, 563–6.

59. Hollander, P.A., Elbein, S.C., Hirsch, I.B. *et al.* (1998) Role of orlistat in the treatment of obese patients with type 2 diabetes – a 1-year randomized double-blind study. *Diabetes Care*, **21**, 1288–94.

60. Miles, J., Aronne, L., Hollander, P. and Klein, S. (2001) Effect of orlistat in overweight and obese type 2 diabetes patients treated with metformin. *Diabetologia*, **44**, 890.

61. Bray, G.A., Pi-Sunyer, F.X., Hollander, P. and Kelley, D.E. (2001) Effect of orlistat in overweight patients with type 2 diabetes receiving insulin therapy. *Diabetes*, **50**, A107.

62. Anon (2002) Xendos study: orlistat plus diet prevents, delays diabetes onset in obese patients. *Formulary*, **37** (10), 504.

63. Gundlah, C., Martin, K.F., Heal, D.J. and Auerbach, S.B. (1997) *In vivo* criteria to differentiate monoamine reuptake inhibitors from releasing agents: Sibutramine is a reuptake inhibitor. *Journal of Pharmacology and Experimental Therapeutics*, **283**, 581–91.

64. Connolly, H.M., Crary, J.L., McGoon, M.D. *et al.* (1997) Valvular heart disease associated with fenfluramine-phentermine. *New England Journal of Medicine*, **337** (9), 581–8.

65. Bach, D.S., Rissanen, A.M., Mendel, C.M. *et al.* (1999) Absence of cardiac valve dysfunction in obese patients treated with sibutramine. *Obesity Research*, **7**, 363–9.

66. Halford, J.C.G., Heal, D.J. and Blundell, J.E. (1994) Investigation of a new potential antiobesity drug, sibutramine, using the behavioral satiety sequence. *Appetite*, **23**, 306–7.

67. Hansen, D.L., Toubro, S., Stock, M.J. *et al.* (1998) Thermogenic effects of sibutramine in humans. *American Journal of Clinical Nutrition*, **68**, 1180–6.

68. Hazenberg, B.P. (2000) Randomized, double-blind, placebo-controlled, multicenter study of sibutramine in obese hypertensive patients. *Cardiology*, **94** (3), 152–8.

69. James, W.P.T., Astrup, A., Finer, N. *et al.* (2000) Effect of sibutramine on weight maintenance after weight loss: a randomised trial. *Lancet*, **356** (9248), 2119–25.

70. Lauterbach, K. (2000) Framingham analysis: Coronary heart disease risk reduction with weight loss in obesity on sibutramine treatment. *Obesity Research*, **8**, B83.

71. Serrano-Rios, M., Meichionda, N. and Moreno-Carretero, E. (2002) Role of sibutramine in the treatment of obese type 2 diabetic patients receiving sulphonylurea therapy. *Diabetic Medicine*, **19** (2), 119–24.

72. Torp-Pedersen, C., Caterson, I., Coutinho, W. *et al.* (2007) Cardiovascular responses to weight management and sibutramine in high risk subjects: an analysis from the SCOUT trial. *European Heart Journal*, **28**(23), 2830–1. doi:10.1093/eurheartj/ehm217.

73. Van Gaal, L.F., Rissanen, A.M., Scheen, A.J. *et al.* (2005) Effects of the cannabinoid-1 receptor blocker rimonabant on weight reduction and cardiovascular risk factors in overweight patients: 1-year experience from the RIO-Europe study. *Lancet*, **365** (9468), 1389–97.

74. Pi-Sunyer, F., Aronne, L.J., Heshmati, H.M. *et al.* (2006) Effect of rimonabant, a cannabinoid-1 receptor blocker, on weight and cardiometabolic risk factors in overweight or obese patients – RIO-North America: a randomized controlled trial. *Journal of the American Medical Association*, **295** (7), 761–75.

75. Scheen, A.J., Finer, N., Hollander, P. *et al.* (2006) Efficacy and tolerability of rimonabant in overweight or obese patients with type 2 diabetes: a randomised controlled study (vol 368, pg 1660, 2006). *Lancet*, **368** (9548), 1650.

76. Stearne, M.R., Palmer, S.L., Hammersley, M.S. *et al.* (1998) Tight blood pressure control and risk of macrovascular and microvascular complications in type 2 diabetes: UKPDS 38. *British Medical Journal*, **317**, 703–13.

77. Stoabirketvedt, G., Thom, E., Aarbakke, J. and Florholmen, J. (1995) Body-fat as a predictor of the antihypertensive effect of nifedipine. *Journal of Internal Medicine*, **237** (2), 169–73.

78. Sharma, A.M., Pischon, T., Engeli, S. and Scholze, J. (2001) Choice of drug treatment for obesity-related hypertension: where is the evidence? *Journal of Hypertension*, **19** (4), 667–74.

79. Hedenmalm, K., Hagg, S., Stahl, M. *et al.* (2002) Glucose intolerance with atypical antipsychotics. *Drug Safety*, **25** (15), 1107–16.

80. Galanopoulou, P., Giannacopoulos, G., Theophanopoulos, C. *et al.* (1990) Behavioural changes on diet selection and serotonin (5-HT) turnover in rats under pizotifen treatment. *Pharmacology, Biochemistry, and Behavior*, **37**, 461–4.

81. Carr, A., Samaras, K., Chisholm, D.J. and Cooper, D.A. (1998) Pathogenesis of HIV-1-protease inhibitor-associated peripheral lipodystrophy, hyperlipidaemia, and insulin resistance. *Lancet*, **351**, 1881–3.

11

The role of metabolic surgery in the management of type 2 diabetes

David Kerrigan[1] and Jon Pinkney[1,2]
[1]Gravitas, Murrayfield Hospital, Wirral, UK
[2]Royal Cornwall Hospital, Truro, UK

11.1 Introduction

The epidemic of obesity afflicting much of the developed world has gone hand in hand with an explosion in the incidence of type 2 diabetes. Bariatric surgery (Greek *baros* weight, *iatrikos* the art of healing) is a rapidly evolving branch of surgical science, which aims to bring about substantial weight loss in those whose obesity places them at risk of developing serious health problems. Surgery can produce dramatic weight loss, but also induces startling improvements in many of the metabolic sequelae of obesity. This has led to a recent re-branding of bariatric surgery as the 'new' sub-specialty of *metabolic surgery*, shifting the emphasis of treatment away from 'cosmetic' weight loss to amelioration of seemingly intractable medical complications as diverse as hypertension, sleep apnoea, and of course, diabetes.

For many individuals, the risk of metabolic complications does not become acute until they are more than 50% overweight (corresponding to a body mass index (BMI) of 40 kg/m^2) [1], a condition known as *morbid* obesity. In an attempt to balance the risks of surgery against the benefits of weight loss, bariatric operations have traditionally been restricted to the morbidly obese, or those with a BMI >35 kg/m^2 who have already developed co morbidity [2]. However, there is currently an intense debate on the advisability of lowering the threshold for surgical intervention to 30 kg/m^2 in type 2 diabetes, given the advent of less invasive laparoscopic techniques and the increasing body of evidence that surgical bypass of the foregut induces profound improvements in glycaemic control.

Obesity and Diabetes, Second Edition   Edited by Anthony H. Barnett and Sudhesh Kumar
© 2009 John Wiley & Sons, Ltd

11.2   Obesity and type 2 diabetes

Obesity is the most significant risk factor for type 2 diabetes, which is three times more common in overweight individuals (BMI > 25 kg/m²) than in those of normal body weight [3–5]. In the morbidly obese, the relative risk of type 2 diabetes is at least 5% for men and 8–20% in women [6–8]. Approximately 30% of those considered for weight reduction surgery have type 2 diabetes [9–13], and a further 5–27% have impaired glucose tolerance [9,10,12].

Even allowing for a degree of selection bias in these surgical reports, obesity is clearly a major problem for a significant proportion of type 2 diabetics, particularly as treatment of the diabetes with oral hypoglycaemics can often exacerbate further weight gain.

It has been suggested that modest weight loss in type 2 diabetics may prolong survival [14] and reduces the incidence of new diabetes by 58% within 4 years in overweight populations with impaired glucose tolerance [15,16]. Several short-term studies of diet and exercise programmes in obese type 2 diabetics have also shown significant improvements in glycaemic control with weight loss [17–25]. However, in clinical practice, it is far more difficult to reproduce these encouraging results in an unselected group of diabetics. Even those who do lose weight usually relapse because maintenance of weight loss using low-calorie diets and lifestyle changes is beyond most patients [26].

Although diabetic patients may struggle to maintain a beneficial degree of weight loss with non-surgical treatment, there is an increasing body of evidence to suggest that surgically induced weight loss can ameliorate many of the pathophysiological abnormalities found in type 2 diabetes, or even offer the prospect of a 'surgical cure' for the condition. This chapter explores the evidence behind these claims.

11.3   Surgical techniques

Broadly speaking, weight reduction operations fall into one of two groups, *restrictive* procedures, and those that combine restriction of gastric size with a degree of *malabsorption*. In experienced hands, these are all safe procedures with an operative mortality of 0.05–0.5%, and an acceptably low risk of serious long-term complications.

Restrictive procedures

Purely restrictive procedures limit the patients' capacity for food intake by creating a very small pouch from the proximal stomach, just beneath the gastro-oesophageal junction (Figures 11.1 and 11.2). The pouch is constructed in such a way that it must drain via a narrow opening, which effects a degree of resistance to the emptying of solid food (although liquids empty normally). The aim is to produce enough resistance to retain food in the gastric pouch so that the patient feels full after a relatively small meal. Ingested food drains through into the more distal stomach, but this happens gradually,

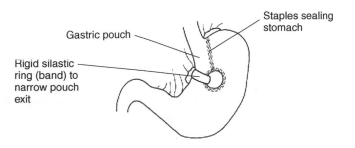

Gastric pouch

Staples sealing stomach

Rigid silastic ring (band) to narrow pouch exit

Figure 11.1   Vertical banded gastroplasty (VBG)

and so the sensation of satiety lasts for longer than usual. In this way, calorie intake is dramatically reduced.

The most widely practised restrictive operation in the 1980s and early 1990s was the vertical banded gastroplasty (VBG) (Figure 11.1). Although VBG is an effective means of inducing sustained weight loss, it is associated with a fairly high risk (4–48%) of disruption of the stapled gastric partition and weight regain [27–32]. Consequently, the VBG has largely been superseded by laparoscopic adjustable gastric banding as the restrictive operation of choice.

Laparoscopic banding (Figure 11.2) is a 'keyhole' technique in which the upper stomach is encircled by an inflatable silicone cuff, or 'band'. Postoperatively, the band is progressively inflated with small volumes of fluid (injected into an access port hidden beneath the patient's skin) until the desired degree of compression of the stomach is obtained and an adequate rate of weight loss commences.

Both VBG and laparoscopic banding produce a similar degree of weight loss, with a typical patient losing 50–60% of their excess body weight over the first 2 years post-op [33–40].

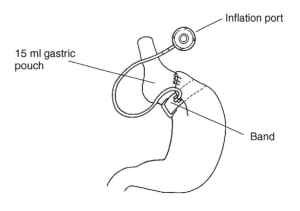

Inflation port

15 ml gastric pouch

Band

Figure 11.2   Laparoscopic gastric band

Restrictive/malabsorptive procedures

There are two types of operation that utilize a combination of restricted gastric size and a variable degree of small intestinal bypass to achieve superior weight loss.

The Roux-en-Y gastric bypass (Figure 11.3) is the most widely performed operation for weight reduction in the United States. Creating a 15 ml gastric pouch beneath the gastro-oesophageal junction induces a similar degree of gastric restriction to the VBG and laparoscopic band. However, after gastric bypass, food is separated from digestive juices by surgically diverting it away from the duodenum and proximal jejunum. The amount of bowel bypassed is varied according to the patient's BMI, but in general the total length of small bowel available for calorie absorption is reduced by about 150–300 cm. Nevertheless, malabsorptive symptoms are rare after gastric bypass, which is thought to work largely by affecting satiety signals to the brain and through reduced stomach capacity.

Biliopancreatic diversion (BPD) involves a much more extensive intestinal bypass, with diverted food rejoining bile and pancreatic secretions in the terminal ileum, just 50–100 cm from the ileocaecal valve (Figure 11.4). This situation leads to a greater degree of malabsorption, which, after compensatory bowel hypertrophy, means only 60% of ingested calories are absorbed [41]. Unlike the obsolete jejunoileal bypass operations performed in the 1970s, BPD is not associated with excessive diarrhoea and malnutrition, as it does not create a 'blind loop' of unused, excluded small bowel prone to toxic bacterial overgrowth (although a milder degree over bacterial overgrowth still occurs). BPD patients malabsorb proportionately more fat and starch, with relative sparing of protein absorption. However, protein loss from the gut is still increased by five times the normal rate [42] (approximately 30 g/day), and so it essential that patients quickly resume a fairly normal eating pattern if they are to achieve the target protein intake of 70–100 g daily. For this reason, a much larger 200–400 ml stomach remnant is

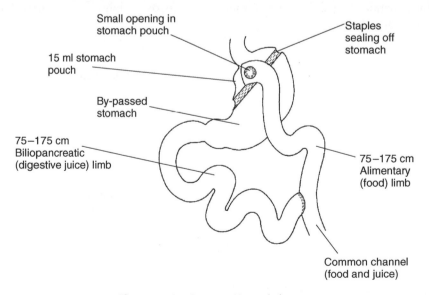

Figure 11.3   Roux-en-Y gastric bypass

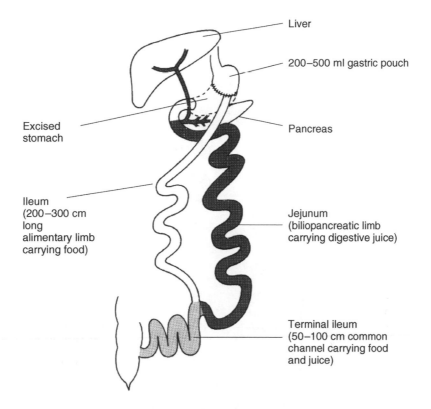

Liver

200–500 ml gastric pouch

Excised
stomach

Pancreas

Ileum
(200–300 cm
long
alimentary limb
carrying food)

Jejunum
(biliopancreatic limb
carrying digestive juice)

Terminal ileum
(50–100 cm common
channel carrying food
and juice)

Figure 11.4   Biliopancreatic diversion

retained, although some gastric restriction is still required to initiate weight loss and reduce the risk of peptic ulceration.

The duodenal switch (DS) procedure (Figure 11.5) is a modification of the BPD in which the vagus nerves, antrum, pylorus and proximal duodenum are preserved [43], thereby reducing the incidence of post-operative diarrhoea and dumping syndrome to less than 10% [44]. Stomach size is reduced by excising the greater curvature and fundus of the stomach, creating a long, thin gastric tube. This part of the operation, known as a sleeve gastrectomy, has recently been advocated as a primary bariatric procedure in its own right [45].

Sleeve gastrectomy does not produce any calorie malabsorption and results in similar weight loss to other restrictive operations, but it differs from banding and VBG in that it involves removal of the gastric fundus, the area which produces the appetite-stimulating hormone ghrelin [46–48]. Ghrelin levels have been shown to fall markedly after sleeve gastrectomy, gastric bypass and DS [49,50] and the resulting anorectic effect may be a contributory factor in the mechanism by which these operations produce weight loss.

All malabsorptive operations bypass the duodenum and proximal jejunum and thus carry a risk of trace element deficiency (particularly calcium, iron and zinc). Reduction in gastric size can also result in poor vitamin B12 absorption in up to a third of patients.

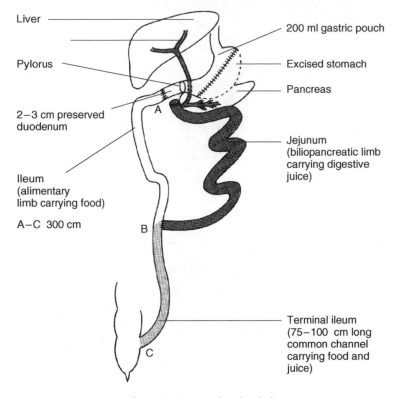

Figure 11.5   Duodenal switch

Most vitamin and mineral deficiencies are equally prevalent after gastric bypass and BPD, but generally tend to be minor as long as a daily multivitamin supplements are taken [51]. An exception is the malabsorption of fat soluble vitamins seen after BPD and DS. High dose vitamin D and calcium replacement is mandatory after these procedures, with regular monitoring of parathormone, vitamin D and vitamin A.

Although they were developed as open surgical procedures, BPD/DS, sleeve gastrectomy [52–55] and Roux-en-Y gastric bypass [12,56–60] are now routinely performed using laparoscopic minimally invasive techniques. Over 2 years, one would expect to see excess body weight reduced by 70%, although there is some evidence that sleeve gastrectomy alone may be somewhat less effective (60% excess weight loss) [45] and that BPD/DS produces better and more sustained weight loss, particularly in those with a BMI > 50 [9,41,61–65].

11.4   Resolution of diabetes after bariatric surgery

The best known report of diabetes remission after weight reduction surgery came from Walter Pories and his team in Greenville, in the United States, not least because of its provocative title 'Who would have thought it? An operation proves to be the most effective therapy for adult-onset diabetes mellitus' [9]. In an uncontrolled observational series, Pories studied 165 patients with type 2 diabetes (and a further 165 with impaired glucose tolerance) after gastric bypass surgery. A remarkable 83% of the diabetic patients (and 99% of those with impaired glucose tolerance) were rendered eugly-caemic. Furthermore, 10 of the 27 patients who remained diabetic were found to have technical failures due to disruption of the gastric staple line, leaving just 17 true non-responders. Analysis of this subgroup showed them to be older than euglycaemic patients (by about 7 years) and to have been diagnosed with diabetes for significantly longer. Retrospectively, Pories also noted that 9-year mortality in a group of diabetics who had not undergone surgery (because of personal preference or their insurance company's refusal to pay) was 28% compared to 9% in the surgical group (including perioperative deaths). The percentage of control subjects treated with oral hypogly-caemics or insulin increased from 56 to 87% during the period of review, but fell from 32 to 9% after gastric bypass [66]. These two groups were not particularly well-matched, but the results are intriguing.

The second major study with important data on this issue is the Swedish Obese Subjects (SOS) study. This is a well-designed prospective, but non-randomized com-parison of patients who had undergone a variety of bariatric operations and those who had been treated with best medical therapy (which at the time did not include orlistat or sibutramine). Within the study group were 156 patients with type 2 diabetes. After 2 years of follow-up, the requirement for on-going drug treatment to control hyperglycaemia in the surgical arm was half that in the non-surgical group [7]. Furthermore, in a matched population of non-diabetic patients observed for 8 years, surgically treated patients with (by surgical standards) a reasonably poor degree of maintained weight loss (16%) showed a dramatic reduction in the incidence of newly diagnosed diabetes. No weight loss was observed in the non-surgical control group over the 8 years of study [67].

The surgical literature is littered with other enthusiastic, personal and largely uncontrolled series which appear to confirm the widely held view that most diabetics can be 'cured' by surgically-induced weight loss [10,60,63,68–82]. A problem that is frequently overlooked when assessing these reports is that none of these studies were specifically designed to test the efficacy of bariatric surgery as a treatment for diabetes. The recruitment of diabetics into these studies was haphazard and unintentional. Furthermore, many patients were only diagnosed with diabetes at baseline screening, and may not therefore represent a typical type 2 diabetic clinic population with emerging macrovascular disease. It is essential that any diabetes study looks at the progression of microvascular complications: unfortunately, we have no data on how bariatric surgery affects this important end-point.

11.5   How could surgery 'cure' diabetes?

The simplistic explanation for observed improvements in glycaemic control after bariatric surgery is the rapid weight loss induced by decreased food intake and post-operative malabsorption. However, although our understanding is far from complete, there is increasing evidence that weight loss is simply a surrogate marker for improved diabetes control and not the direct cause of any observed benefit.

Modification of dietary intake

Bariatric surgery results in a substantial reduction in nutrient intake, which may account for the normalization of plasma glucose reported. In a recent study, a sham operated individual who followed the same strict post-operative diet recommended to Roux-en-Y gastric bypass patients showed similar improvements in insulin and glucose levels. This suggests that calorific restriction is a major factor in promoting glycaemic control after weight loss surgery [9]. Furthermore, there are some indications that gastric bypass may alter the type of food patients ingest. Induction of the 'dumping syndrome' or postoperative changes in taste and food preference result in a preferential reduction in carbohydrate ingestion [83]. This may enhance diabetic control because it is known that obese individuals with a high carbohydrate intake (especially simple sugars), have increased insulin secretion. Hyperinsulinaemia favours anabolic metabolism [84, 85] and stimulates hyperphagia with carbohydrate craving, producing yet further increases in insulin secretion. Consequently, insulin receptor down-regulation occurs, followed by insulin resistance, and a vicious cycle of increasing carbohydrate consumption and weight gain. Successful weight loss is almost impossible by conventional means under these circumstances, but bariatric surgery may allow the cycle to be broken.

Although this evidence provides a cogent argument for the role of reduced calorie intake mediating improved diabetes control, other observations indicate that this cannot be the sole explanation. Whilst energy intake is drastically reduced immediately after surgery, over the ensuing months it progressively increases without adversely affecting glucose and insulin levels. This is particularly true in the case of patients undergoing BPD/DS, who achieve excellent long-term glycaemic control, even though their eating capacity is usually fully restored within 12 months of surgery [42]. This point is illustrated by a fascinating case report of a young *non-obese* diabetic woman who underwent BPD to treat chylomicronaemia. Due to an unrestricted high fat and carbohydrate post-operative diet, she actually *put on* weight, but her plasma insulin and blood glucose returned to normal within 3 months [86].

If reduced food intake was the sole explanation for improved diabetes control, purely restrictive procedures such as laparoscopic gastric banding and VBG should be as effective as Roux-en-Y gastric bypass. There is no doubt that laparoscopic banding and VBG do indeed appear to ameliorate diabetes, but unfortunately there are no randomized trials comparing these techniques with gastric bypass. The few small observational studies available report resolution of diabetes in 38–66% of patients undergoing banding and sleeve gastrectomy [69,72,75,87,88], a somewhat less impressive outcome than that reported after gastric bypass and BPD/DS. Gastric bypass has been reported to abolish the requirement for medical treatment in 82–95% of type 2 diabetic patients [9,60,76–78], and (within the limitations outlined earlier) results after BPD/DS are even more spectacular (100% diabetes remission) [63,79].

Perhaps the most striking argument against weight loss being the most important factor in promoting diabetes control is the rapidity with which serum glucose returns to normal after gastric bypass, BPD and DS. This dramatic onset of euglycaemia sometimes occurs within days of surgery, and long before there is any significant weight loss [9,42,63,89]. In contrast, resolution of diabetes is not usually seen until about 6–18 months after purely restrictive operations such as laparoscopic banding [72].

A common feature of gastric bypass, BPD and DS operations is that food is diverted away from the hormonally active proximal small bowel. Studies in non-obese diabetic rats [90] and humans [91] have shown that even when the entire stomach is preserved (thus allowing early resumption of a normal diet), bypass of the foregut dramatically improves glucose tolerance independent of weight loss and calorie restriction. Observations such as these have led to the concept that malabsorptive surgery disturbs a complex neurohumoral signalling mechanism within the antrum, duodenum and proximal jejunum, which modulates the production and metabolism of insulin. The implication is that type 2 diabetes may, in fact, be a disease of the foregut rather than the pancreas.

Diabetes as a foregut disease

The gut is a powerful endocrine organ intimately involved in the control of appetite, weight and glucose homeostasis and so it is easy to speculate that the clinical effects of bariatric surgery might at least in part be due to modulation of gut hormones.

Infusions of gut hormones such as PYY, glucagon-like peptide-1 (GLP-1) and oxyntomodulin reduce food intake in both lean and obese individuals [92,93] and the fact that levels of all three hormones are elevated after Roux-en-Y gastric bypass could provide an explanation for the anorectic effect so frequently seen after this operation [94–96]. However, gut hormones may also play a more direct role in improving glucose homeostasis in obese diabetics. GLP-1, glucagons and glucose-dependant insulinotropic peptide act as incretins, gut hormones that stimulate beta cell production of insulin in response to food (especially carbohydrate) entering the foregut [97–100]. Any disturbance of this 'enteroinsular axis' following surgical diversion of food into the more distal small intestine could therefore affect glucose homeostasis and possibly lead to changes in insulin resistance.

Pories and colleagues proposed that hyperinsulinaemia in type 2 diabetes is the result of over stimulation of the islet cells by an abnormal incretin signal from the gut, a stimulus which is abolished by re-routing food away from the duodenum and upper jejunum [101]. Although plausible, Rubino and Gagner have extended this argument and proposed the presence of as-yet unidentified 'anti-incretin' factors secreted by the duodenum, which would act as a homeostatic counterbalance to the effect of incretins (Figure 11.6). They speculate that type 2 diabetes occurs when there is an imbalance due to a relative excess of anti-incretin activity, leading to a delayed insulin response to ingested carbohydrate and thus glucose intolerance. If anti-incretins also blocked the actions of insulin at a receptor or post-receptor level, insulin resistance with secondary hyperinsulinaemia would result [82].

DIABETES

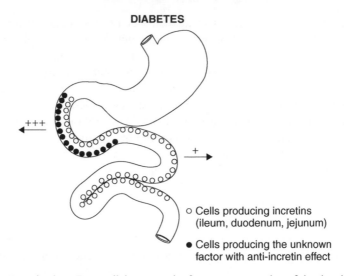

Figure 11.6   Hypothesis 1. Type 2 diabetes results from overexpression of duodenal anti-incretins causing imbalances with secretion of incretins by the foregut. This would lead to delayed insulin response to food and impaired insulin action. With permission from Lippincott Williams & Wilkins

By diverting food away from the duodenum, both gastric bypass and BPD may avoid excessive stimulation of incretins (as proposed by Pories) or anti-incretins (as proposed by Rubino and Gagner), which would have the effect of lowering plasma insulin and/or glucose. These hypotheses do not fully explain the excellent resolution of type 2 diabetes seen after the DS procedure, in which at least 2–5 cm of proximal duodenum is retained (Figure 11.5), but all three operations (particularly BPD and DS) result in chyme entering the distal small bowel at a much earlier phase of digestion than normal. Stimulation of the terminal ileum by nutrients releases GLP-1, a powerful incretin, which could improve the action of insulin, promoting euglycaemia (Figure 11.7). GLP-1 also delays gastric emptying, and probably explains the marked early satiety noted after BPD and DS.

There is certainly some experimental evidence to substantiate aspects of the hypothesis that surgery improves diabetes via modulation of the enteroinsular axis, as jejuno-ileal bypass (an operation abandoned in the early 1980s) and BPD have both been associated with raised levels of the incretins GIP and enteroglucagon (an old name for what is almost certainly GLP-1), which can persist for over 20 years after surgery [102,103]. Exogenous GLP-1 infusion in type 2 diabetics has been shown to have an anti-diabetogenic effect [99] and the GLP-1 analogue exanatide not only produces weight loss, but augments the effects of sulfonylureas [104].

One obvious implication of these data is that the long-term control of diabetes after malabsorptive surgery results from increased endogenous GLP-1 production. This has led to the suggestion that surgical transposition of a segment of ileum into the more proximal jejunum would be an ideal operation for treatment of type 2 diabetes, as it would maximize GLP-1 release [105,106], without the need for

GASTRIC BYPASS

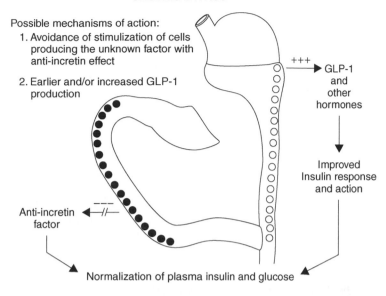

Possible mechanisms of action:
1. Avoidance of stimulization of cells producing the unknown factor with anti-incretin effect

2. Earlier and/or increased GLP-1 production

+++ → GLP-1 and other hormones

Improved Insulin response and action

Anti-incretin factor

Normalization of plasma insulin and glucose

Figure 11.7   Hypothesis 2. Mechanisms responsible for rapid control of diabetes after gastric bypass. With permission from Lippincott Williams & Wilkins

extensive malabsorption. This technique is being pioneered in humans by surgeons in Brazil [107], but well-planned studies of ileal transposition in obese and non-obese type 2 diabetics are required to evaluate safety and clinical efficacy before this experimental approach can be widely recommended [106].

Changes in serum lipids and insulin resistance

As mentioned earlier, when obese diabetics undergo malabsorptive bariatric surgery, enhancement of insulin sensitivity and glucose tolerance occurs well before any major effect on body weight is noted. BPD and DS cause marked lipid malabsorption and it has been suggested that the reduction in plasma lipids these operations induce may play a major role in reversal of insulin resistance [86].

Abnormal fat deposition in skeletal muscle has been identified as a mechanism for obesity-related insulin resistance and it is proposed that lipid deprivation may deplete intramyocellular fat, thereby reversing insulin resistance. Greco and colleagues studied quadriceps muscle biopsies in morbidly obese patients before and after BPD or a low calorie diet. After BPD, insulin resistance was fully reversed within 6 months. Even though most patients were still obese at this stage, intramyocellular lipids had decreased, whereas after non-surgical weight loss, only very modest changes in insulin sensitivity and myocellular lipids were noted [108].

An alternative suggestion implicates decreased hepatic clearance of insulin (causing hyperinsulinaemia) as a cause of insulin resistance. It is proposed that increased free fatty acids in portal blood [109] and/or increased free fatty acid oxidation [110] (which in turn inhibits glucose oxidation), prevents effective handling of glucose and insulin by the liver, an effect which is reversed by the decrease in lipid absorption and reduced intra-abdominal adipose tissue seen after BPD/DS.

11.6 Conclusions

Is surgery helpful in controlling type 2 diabetes?

There is a wealth of non-randomized clinical evidence to support the view that the majority of patients with type 2 diabetes experience greatly improved glycaemic control and reduced insulin resistance after bariatric surgery. This effect appears to be independent of weight loss, and probably results from a combination of reduced calorie intake, foregut bypass, increased intestinal secretion of GLP-1, and lipid malabsorption.

Which is the best operation for diabetes control?

Due to a lack of published randomized trials, it is not possible to recommend any particular surgical procedure as the optimum choice for diabetic patients, but it would appear that Roux-en-Y gastric bypass, BPD and DS produce more complete and rapid resolution of type 2 diabetes compared with simple restrictive procedures such as laparoscopic banding and VBG.

Which type 2 diabetics should be offered bariatric surgery?

Although randomized trials looking at diabetes-specific end-points are awaited, observational studies show that gastric bypass, BPD and DS are associated with diabetes remission in 80–100% of patients. Perhaps of even more importance, Pories and Albrecht also showed surgery is linked to reduced mortality. Over a 10 year period of follow-up, diabetic patients submitted to gastric bypass had a 1% chance of dying compared to a mortality rate of 4.5% in a matched group of diabetics who did not undergo bariatric surgery [101].

However, Pories reported a small number of patients whose diabetes appeared to be resistant to bariatric surgery [9]. Some of these were due to failures in operative technique, but most were older patients who had suffered with diabetes for longer and others whose type 2 diabetes was sufficiently severe to require insulin, presumably as a result of well-established islet secretory failure. It follows that it may be advisable to offer weight reduction surgery to younger diabetics and those at an earlier stage in their disease, before insulin secretory failure becomes irreversible.

Should non-obese type 2 diabetics be offered bariatric surgery?

The advent of minimally invasive laparoscopic surgical approaches to banding, gastric bypass, BPD and even DS operations will almost certainly increase the acceptability of surgery, but it should be remembered that enthusiasm for a more aggressive surgical approach needs to be tempered by an awareness of the small but significant risks of death and complications.

The current recommendation is that only diabetics with a BMI > 35 should be offered surgery. However, there is published evidence of 90% diabetes remission in a group of patients with only moderate obesity (mean BMI 33) [80]. As earlier intervention may be more likely to successfully control plasma glucose and insulin, there is an argument for lowering the BMI threshold for surgical intervention in type 2 diabetes. This is supported by the observation that insulin resistance increases with increasing obesity, but only up to a BMI of 30, after which it plateaus [111]; thus patients with a BMI of 30 are likely to have a similar degree of insulin resistance to heavier individuals, which could justify including a metabolic surgical option in the treatment paradigm offered to such patients.

Unfortunately, at the present time, we have no randomized evidence with which to interrogate the hypothesis that surgical intervention at a BMI of 30 will prove safe and cost-effective. A multidisciplinary consensus meeting held in Rome, March 2007 is due to publish eagerly awaited recommendations for clinical and research practice later in 2008.

References

1. Kral, J.G. (1985) Morbid obesity and related health risks. *Annals of Internal Medicine*, **103**, 1043.
2. IFSO (1997) Statement on patient selection for bariatric surgery. *Obesity Surgery*, **7**, 41.
3. Pi-Sunyer, F.X. (1993) Medical hazards of obesity. *Annals of Internal Medicine*, **119**, 655–60.
4. Perry, I.J., Wannamethee, S.G., Walker, M.K. *et al.* (1995) Prospective study of risk factors for development of non-insulin dependant diabetes in middle-aged British men. *British Medical Journal*, **310**, 560–4.
5. Colditz, G.A., Willett, W.C., Ronitzky, A. *et al.* (1995) Weight gain as a risk factor for clinical diabetes mellitus in women. *Annals of Internal Medicine*, **122**, 481–6.
6. Kral, J. (2001) Morbidity of severe obesity. *Surgical Clinics of North America*, **81**, 1039–61.
7. Sjostrom, C.D., Lissner, L., Wedel, H. *et al.* (1999) Reduction in incidence of diabetes, hypertension and lipid disturbances after intentional weight loss induced by bariatric surgery: the SOS Intervention Study. *Obesity Research*, **7**, 477–84.
8. Mason, E.E., Renquist, K. and Jiang, D. (1992) Predictors of two obesity complications: diabetes and hypertension. *Obesity Surgery*, **2**, 231–7.
9. Pories, W.J., Swanson, M.S., MacDonald, K.G. *et al.* (1995) Who would have thought it? An operation proves to be the most effective therapy for adult-onset diabetes mellitus. *Annals of Surgery*, **222**, 339–52.

10. Cowan, G.S.M., Jr and Buffington, C.K. (1998) Significant changes in blood pressure, glucose and lipids with gastric bypass surgery. *World Journal of Surgery*, **22**, 987–92.

11. Gleysteen, J.J., Barboriak, J.J. and Sasse, E.A. (1990) Sustained coronary risk factor reduction after gastric bypass surgery for morbid obesity. *American Journal of Clinical Nutrition*, **51**, 774–8.

12. Wittgrove, A.C., Clark, W., Schubert, K.R. *et al.* (1996) Laparoscopic gastric bypass, Roux en Y: technique and results in 75 patients with 3–30 months follow-up. *Obesity Surgery*, **6**, 500–04.

13. Noya, G., Cossu, M.L., Coppola, M. *et al.* (1998) Biliopancreatic diversion for treatment of morbid obesity: experience in 50 cases. *Obesity Surgery*, **8**, 61–6.

14. Lean, M.E.J., Powrie, J.K., Anderson, A.S. *et al.* (1990) Obesity, weight loss and prognosis in type 2 diabetes. *Diabetic Medicine*, **7**, 228–33.

15. Tuomilehto, J., Lindstrom, J., Eriksson, J.G. *et al.* (2001) Prevention of type 2 diabetes mellitus by changes in lifestyle among subjects with impaired glucose tolerance. *New England Journal of Medicine*, **344**, 1390–2.

16. Knowler, W.C., Barrett-Connor, E., Fowler, S.E. *et al.* (2002) Reduction in the incidence of type 2 diabetes with lifestyle intervention or metformin. *New England Journal of Medicine*, **346**, 393–403.

17. Hanefeld, M. and Weck, M. (1989) Very low calorie diet therapy in obese non-insulin dependent diabetes patients. *International Journal of Obesity*, **13** (suppl 2), 33–7.

18. Fukuda, M., Tahara, Y., Yamamoto, Y. *et al.* (1989) Effects of very low calorie diet weight reduction on glucose tolerance, insulin secreitn, and insulin resistance in obese non-insulin dependent diabetics. *Diabetes Research and Clinical Practice*, **7**, 61–9.

19. Di Biase, G., Mattioli, P.L., Contaldo, F. and Mancini, M. (1981) A very low calorie formula diet (Cambridge Diet) for the treatment of diabetic-obese patients. *International Journal of Obesity*, **5**, 319–24.

20. Wing, R.R., Marcus, R.D., Salata, R. *et al.* (1991) Effects of a very low calorie diet on long term glycaemic control in obese type 2 diabetic subjects. *Archives of Internal Medicine*, **151**, 1334–40.

21. Rotella, C.M., Cresci, B., Mannucci, E. *et al.* (1994) Short cycles of very low calorie diet in the therapy of obese type 2 diabetes mellitus. *Journal of Endocrinological Investigation*, **17**, 171–9.

22. Wing, R.R., Blair, E., Marcus, M. *et al.* (1994) Year-long weight loss treatment for obese patients with type II diabetes: does including an intermittent very low calorie diet improve outcomes? *American Journal of Medicine*, **97**, 354–62.

23. Capstick, F., Brokks, B.A., Burns, C.M. *et al.* (1997) Very low calorie diet (VLCD): A useful alternative in the treatment of the obese NIDDM patient. *Diabetes Research and Clinical Practice*, **36**, 105–11.

24. Williams, K.V., Mullen, M.L., Kelley, D.E. and Wing, R.R. (1998) The effect of short periods of caloric restriction on weight loss and glycemic control in type 2 diabetes. *Diabetes Care*, **21**, 2–8.

25. Wing, R.R., Epstein, L.H., Paternostro-Bayles, M. *et al.* (1988) Exercise in a behavioral weight control programme for obese patients with type 2 (non-insulin dependent diabetes). *Diabetologia*, **31**, 902–9.

26. Zilli, F.C.M., Croci, M., Tufano, A. and Caviezel, F. (2000) The compliance of hypocaloric diet in type 2 diabetic obese patients: a brief term study. *Eating and Weight Disorders*, **5**, 217–22.

27. Balsiger, B.M., Poggio, J.L., Mai, J. *et al.* (2000) Ten and more years after vertical banded gastroplasty as primary operation for morbid obesity. *Journal of Gastrointestinal Surgery*, **4**, 598–605.

28. Capella, J.F. and Capella, R.F. (1996) The weight reduction operation of choice: Vertical banded gastroplasty or gastric bypass? *American Journal of Surgery*, **171**, 74–9.

29. Deitel, M. (1997) Staple disruption in vertical banded gastroplasty (commentary). *Obesity Surgery*, **7**, 139–41.
30. MacLean, L.D., Rhode, B.M. and Forse, R.A. (1990) Late results of vertical banded gastroplasty for morbid and superobesity. *Surgery*, **107**, 20–7.
31. Svenheden, K., Akesson, L., Holmdahl, C. *et al.* (1997) Staple disruption in vertical banded gastroplasty. *Obesity Surgery*, **7**, 136–8.
32. Toppino, M., Morino, M., Capuzzi, P. *et al.* (1999) Outcome of vertical banded gastroplasty. *Obesity Surgery*, **9**, 51–4.
33. Fobi, M.A.L. and Fleming, A.W. (1986) Vertical banded gastroplasty vs gastric bypass in the treatment of obesity. *Journal of the National Medical Association*, **78**, 1091–6.
34. Deitel, M., Jones, B.A., Petrov, I. *et al.* (1986) Vertical banded gastroplasty: results in 233 patients. *Canadian Journal of Surgery*, **29**, 322–4.
35. Maclean, L.D., Rhode, B. and Shizgal, H.M. (1987) Nutrition after vertical banded gastroplasty. *Annals of Surgery*, **208** (5), 555–63.
36. Hell, E. and Miller, K.A. (2000) Comparison of vertical banded gastroplasty and adjustable silicone gastric banding, in *Update: Surgery for the Morbidly Obese Patients* (eds M. Deitel and S.M. Cowan, Jr), FD Communications Inc, Toronto, pp. 379–86.
37. O'Brien, P.E., Brown, W.A., Smith, A. *et al.* (1999) Prospective study of a laparoscopically placed, adjustable gastric band in the treatment of morbid obesity. *British Journal of Surgery*, **85**, 113–8.
38. Fielding, G.A., Rhodes, M. and Nathanson, L.K. (1999) Laparoscopic gastric banding for morbid obesity: surgical outcome in 335 cases. *Surgical Endoscopy*, **13**, 550–4.
39. Belachew, M., Legrand, M., Vincent, V. *et al.* (1998) Laparoscopic adjustable gastric banding. *World Journal of Surgery*, **22**, 955–63.
40. Favretti, F., Cadiere, G.B., Segato, G. *et al.* (1995) Laparoscopic placement of adjustable silicone gastric banding: early experience. *Obesity Surgery*, **5**, 71–3.
41. Scopinaro, N., Adami, G.F., Marinari, G.M. *et al.* (2000) Biliopancreatic diversion: two decades of experience, in *Update: Surgery for the Morbidly Obese Patients* (eds M. Deitel and S.M. Cowan, Jr), FD Communications Inc, Toronto, pp. 227–58.
42. Scopinaro, N., Adami, G.F., Marinari, G.M. *et al.* (1998) Biliopancreatic diversion. *World Journal of Surgery*, **22**, 936–46.
43. Marceau, P., Hould, F.S., Potvin, M. *et al.* (1999) Biliopancreatic diversion (duodenal switch procedure). *European Journal of Gastroenterology & Hepatology*, **11**, 99–103.
44. Marceau, P., Hould, F.S., Simard, S. *et al.* (1998) Biliopancreatic diversion with duodenal switch. *World Journal of Surgery*, **22**, 947–54.
45. Deitel, M., Crosby, R.D. and Gagner, M. (2008) The First International Consensus Summit for Sleeve Gastrectomy (SG) New York City, October 25–27, 2007. *Obesity Surgery*, **18**, 487–96.
46. Fruhbeck, G., Diez-Caballero, A., Gil, M.J. *et al.* (2004) The decrease in plasma ghrelin concentrations following bariatric surgery depends on the functional integrity of the fundus. *Obesity Surgery*, **14**, 606–12.
47. Cohen, R., Uzzan, B., Bihan, H. *et al.* (2005) Ghrelin levels and sleeve gastrectomy in super-super obesity. *Obesity Surgery*, **15**, 1501–2.
48. Pereferrer, F.S., Gonzalez, M.H., Rovira, A.F. *et al.* (2008) Influence of sleeve gastrectomy on several experimental models of obesity: metabolic and hormonal implications. *Obesity Surgery*, **18**, 97–108.
49. Kotidis, E.V., Koliakos, G., Papavramidis, T.S. *et al.* (2006) The effect of biliopancreatic diversion with pylorus-preserving sleeve gastrectomy and duodenal switch on fasting serum ghrelin, leptin and adiponectin levels: is there a hormonal contribution to the weight reducing effect of this procedure? *Obesity Surgery*, **16**, 554–9.

50. Cummings, D.E. and Shannon, M.H. (2003) Ghrelin and gastric bypass: Is there a hormonal contribution to surgical weight loss? *Journal of Clinical Endocrinology and Metabolism*, **88**, 2999–3002.

51. Skroubis, G., Sakellaropoulos, G., Pouggouras, K. *et al.* (2002) Comparison of nutritional deficiencies after Roux-en-Y gastric bypass and after biliopancreatic diversion with Roux-en-Y gastric bypass. *Obesity Surgery*, **12**, 551–8.

52. Paiva, D., Bernardes, L. and Suretti, L. (2002) Laparoscopic biliopancreatic diversion: technique and initial results. *Obesity Surgery*, **12**, 358–61.

53. Scopinaro, N., Marinari, G.M. and Camerini, G. (2002) Laparoscopic standard biliopancreatic diversion: technique and preliminary results. *Obesity Surgery*, **12**, 362–5.

54. Baltasar, A., Bou, R., Miro, J. *et al.* (2002) Laparoscopic biliopancreatic diversion with duodenal switch: technique and initial experience. *Obesity Surgery*, **12**, 245–8

55. Rabkin, R.A., Rabkin, J.M., Metcalf, B. *et al.* (2003) Laparoscopic technique for performing duodenal switch with gastric reduction. *Obesity Surgery*, **13**, 263–8.

56. Champion, J.K., Hunt, T. and DeLisle, N. (1999) Laparoscopic vertical banded gastroplasty and Roux-en-Y gastric bypass in morbid obesity. *Obesity Surgery*, **9**, 123.

57. Gagner, M., Garcia-Ruiz, A., Arca, M.J. *et al.* (1999) Laparoscopic isolated gastric bypass for morbid obesity. *Surgical Endoscopy*, **S19**, 6.

58. Higa, K.D. Boone, K.B. *et al.* (2000) Laparoscopic Roux-en-Y gastric bypass for morbid obesity: technique and preliminary results in our first 400 patients. *Archives of Surgery (Chicago, Ill: 1960)*, **135**, 1029–33.

59. Wittgrove, A.C. and Clark, W. (1999) Laparoscopic gastric bypass: a five-year prospective study of 500 patients followed from 3–60 months. *Obesity Surgery*, **9**, 123–43.

60. DeMaria, E.J., Sugerman, H.J., Kellum, J.M. *et al.* (2002) Results of 281 consecutive total laparoscopic Roux-en-Y gastric bypasses to treat morbid obesity. *Annals of Surgery*, **235**, 640–5.

61. MacLean, L.D., Rhode, B.M. and Nohr, C.W. (2000) Late outcome of isolated gastric bypass. *Annals of Surgery*, **231**, 524–8.

62. Feng, J.J. and Gagner, M. (2002) Laparoscopic biliopancreatic diversion with duodenal switch. *Seminars in Laparoscopic Surgery*, **9**, 125–9.

63. Hess, D.S. and Hess, D.W. (1998) Biliopancreatic diversion with a duodenal switch. *Obesity Surgery*, **8**, 267–82.

64. Pories, W.J., MacDonald, K.G., Jr, Flickinger, E.G. *et al.* (1992) Is type II diabetes mellitus (NIDDM) a surgical disease? *Annals of Surgery*, **215**, 633–42.

65. Baltasar, A., Bou, R., Bengochea, M. *et al.* (2001) Duodenal switch: an effective therapy for morbid obesity –intermediate results. *Obesity Surgery*, **11**, 54–8.

66. MacDonald, K.G., Long, S.D., Swanson, M.S. *et al.* (1997) The gastric bypass operation reduces the progression and mortality of non-insulin-dependent diabetes mellitus. *Journal of Gastrointestinal Surgery*, **1**, 213–20.

67. Sjostrom, C.D., Peltonen, M., Wedel, H. *et al.* (2000) Differentiated long-term effects of intentional weight loss on diabetes and hypertension. *Hypertension*, **36**, 20–5.

68. Bacci, V., Basso, M.S., Greco, F. *et al.* (2002) Modifications of metabolic and cardiovascular risk factors after weight loss induced by laparoscopic gastric banding. *Obesity Surgery*, **12**, 77–82.

69. Dixon, J.B. and O'Brien, P.E. (2002) Health outcomes of severely obese type 2 diabetic subjects 1 year after laparoscopic adjustable gastric banding. *Diabetes Care*, **25**, 358–63.

70. Abu-Abeid, S., Keidar, A. and Szold, A. (2001) Resolution of chronic medical conditions after laparoscopic adjustable silicone gastric banding for the treatment of morbid obesity in the elderly. *Surgical Endoscopy*, **15**, 132–34.

71. Haciyanli, M., Erkan, N., Bora, S. *et al.* (2001) Vertical banded gastroplasty in the Aegean region of Turkey. *Obesity Surgery*, **11**, 482–6.

72. Dolan, K., Bryant, R. and Fielding, G. (2003) Treating diabetes in the morbidly obese by laparoscopic gastric banding. *Obesity Surgery*, **13**, 439–43.

73. Mittermair, R.P., Weiss, H., Nehoda, H. *et al.* (2003) Laparoscopic Swedish adjustable gastric banding: 6-year follow-up and comparison to other laparoscopic bariatric procedures. *Obesity Surgery*, **13**, 412–17.

74. Angrisani, L., Furbetta, F., Doldi, S.B. *et al.* (2002) Results of the Italian multicenter study on 239 super-obese patients treated by adjustable gastric banding. *Obesity Surgery*, **12**, 846–50.

75. O'Brien, P.E., Dixon, J.B., Brown, W. *et al.* (2002) The laparoscopic adjustable gastric band (Lap-Band): a prospective study of medium-term effects on weight, health and quality of life. *Obesity Surgery*, **12**, 652–60.

76. Smith, S.C., Edwards, C.B. and Goodman, G.N. (1996) Changes in diabetic management after Roux-en-Y gastric bypass. *Obesity Surgery*, **6**, 345–8.

77. Dhabuwala, A., Cannan, R.J. and Stubbs, R.S. (2000) Improvement in comorbidities following weight loss from gastric bypass surgery. *Obesity Surgery*, **10**, 428–35.

78. Schauer, P.R., Ikramuddin, S., Gourash, W. *et al.* (2000) Outcomes after laparoscopic Roux-en-Y gastric bypass for morbid obesity. *Annals of Surgery*, **232**, 515–29.

79. Scopinaro, N., Gianetta, E., Adami, G.F. *et al.* (1996) Biliopancreatic diversion for obesity at eighteen years. *Surgery*, **119**, 261–8.

80. Noya, G., Cossu, M.L., Coppola, M. *et al.* (1998) Biliopancreatic diversion preserving the stomach and pylorus in the treatment of hypercholesterolaemia and diabetes type II: results in the first 10 cases. *Obesity Surgery*, **8**, 67–72.

81. Dietel, M. (2000) Diabetes and bariatric surgery. *Obesity Surgery*, **10**, 285.

82. Rubino, F. and Gagner, M. (2002) Potential of surgery for curing type 2 diabetes mellitus. *Annals of Surgery*, **236**, 554–9.

83. Sugarman, H.J., Kellum, J.M., Engle, K.M. *et al.* (1992) Gastric bypass for treating severe obesity. *American Journal of Clinical Nutrition*, **55**, 560S–6.

84. Weiner, M.F. (1980) Rapid weight gain due to overinsulinisation. *Obesity & Bariatric Medicine*, **9**, 118–19.

85. Woods, W.C., Decke, E. and Vaselli, J.R. (1974) Metabolic hormones and regulation of body weight. *Physiological Reviews*, **81**, 26–43.

86. Mingrove, G., De Gaetano, A., Greco, A.V. *et al.* (1997) Reversibility of insulin resistance in obese diabetic patients: role of plasma lipids. *Diabetologia*, **40**, 599–605.

87. Buchwald, H., Avidor, Y., Braunwald, E. *et al.* (2004) Bariatric Surgery: a systematic review and meta-analysis. *Journal of the American Medical Association*, **292**, 1724–37.

88. Silecchia, G., Boru, C., Pecchia, A. *et al.* (2006) Effectiveness of laparoscopic sleeve gastrectomy (first stage of biliopancreatic diversion with duodenal switch) on co-morbidities in super-obese high-risk patients. *Obesity Surgery*, **16**, 1138–44.

89. Pies, W.J. and Albrecht, R.J. (2001) Etiology of type II diabetes mellitus: role of the foregut. *World Journal of Surgery*, **25**, 527–31.

90. Rubino, F. and Marescaux, J. (2004) Effect of duodenal-jejunal exclusion in a non-obese animal model of type 2 diabetes: a new perspective for an old disease. *Annals of Surgery*, **239**, 1–11.

91. Cohen, R.V., Schiavon, C.A., Pinheiro, J.S. *et al.* (2007) Duodenal-jejunal bypass for the treatment of type 2 diabetes in patients with BMI 22–34: a report of two cases. *Surgery for Obesity and Related Diseases*, **3**, 195–7.

92. Batterham, R.L., Cohen, M.A., Ellis, S.M. *et al.* (2003) Inhibition of food intake in obese subjects by peptide YY3-36. *New England Journal of Medicine*, **349** (10), 941–8.

93. Cohen, M.A., Ellis, S.M., Le Roux, C.W. *et al.* (2003) Oxyntomodulin suppresses appetite and reduces food intake in humans. *Journal of Clinical Endocrinology and Metabolism*, **88**, 4696–701.

94. Korner, J., Bessler, M., Cirilon, L.J. *et al.* (2005) Effects of Roux-en-Y gastric bypass surgery on fasting and postprandial concentrations of plasma ghrelin, peptide YY, and insulin. *Journal of Clinical Endocrinology and Metabolism*, **90**, 359–65.

95. Borg, C.M., le Roux, C.W., Ghatei, M.A., Bloom, S.R. *et al.* (2006) Progressive rise in gut hormone levels after Roux-en-Y gastric bypass suggests gut adaptation and explains altered satiety. *British Journal of Surgery*, **93**, 210–15.

96. le Roux, C.W., Aylwin, S.J., Batterham, R.L., Borg, C.M. *et al.* (2006) Gut hormone profiles following bariatric surgery favor an anorectic state, facilitate weight loss, and improve metabolic parameters. *Annals of Surgery*, **243**, 108–14.

97. Holst, J.J. (1994) Glucagon-like peptide 1: a newly discovered gastrointestinal hormone. *Gastroenterology*, **97**, 1848–55.

98. Kellum, J.M., Kuemmerle, J.F., O'Dorisio, T.M. *et al.* (1990) Gastrointestinal hormone responses to meals before and after gastric bypass and vertical stapled gastroplasty. *Annals of Surgery*, **211**, 763–7.

99. Gutnaik, M., Orskov, C., Holst, J.J. *et al.* (1992) Antidiabetogenic effect of glucagon-like peptide-1 (7–36) amide in normal subjects and patients with diabetes mellitus. *New England Journal of Medicine*, **326**, 1316–22.

100. Creutzfeldt, W. and Nauck, M. (1992) Gut hormones and diabetes mellitus. *Diabetes-Metabolism Reviews*, **8**, 149–77.

101. Pories, W.J. and Albrecht, R.J. (2001) Etiology of type II diabetes mellitus: role of the foregut. *World Journal of Surgery*, **25**, 527–531

102. Sarson, D.L., Scopinaro, N. and Bloom, S.R. (1981) Gut hormone changes after jejunoileal (JIB) or biliopancreatic (BPB) bypass surgery for morbid obesity. *International Journal of Obesity*, **5**, 471–80.

103. Naslund, E., Backman, L., Holst, J.J. *et al.* (1998) Importance of small bowel peptides for the improved glucose metabolism 20 years after jejunoileal bypass for obesity. *Obesity Surgery*, **8**, 253–60.

104. Poon, T., Nelson, P., Shen, L., Mihm, M. *et al.* (2005) Exenatide improves glycemic control and reduces body weight in subjects with type 2 diabetes: a dose-ranging study. *Diabetes Technology & Therapeutics*, **7** (3), 467–77.

105. Strader, A.D., Vahl, T.P., Jandacek, R.J. *et al.* (2005) Weight loss through ileal transposition is accompanied by increased ileal hormone secretion and synthesis in rats. *American Journal of Physiology. Endocrinology and Metabolism*, **288**, E447–E453.

106. Mason, E.E. (1999) Ileal transposition and enteroglucagon/GLP-1 in obesity (and diabetic?) surgery. *Obesity Surgery*, **9**, 223–8.

107. De Paula, A.L., Macedo, A.L., Prudente, A.S. *et al.* (2006) Laparoscopic sleeve gastrectomy with ileal interposition ('neuroendocrine brake'): pilot study of a new operation. *Surgery for Obesity and Related Diseases*, **2**, 464–7.

108. Greco, Av., Mingrove, G., Giancaterini, A. *et al.* (2002) Insulin resistance in morbid obesity: reversal with intramyocellular fat depletion. *Diabetes*, **51**, 144–51.

109. Stromblad, G. and Bjorntorp, P. (1986) Reduced hepatic insulin clearance in rats with dietary-induced obesity. *Metabolism: Clinical and Experimental*, **35**, 323–7.

110. Randle, P.J., Garland, P.B., Newsholme, E.A. *et al.* (1965) The glucose fatty acid cycle in obesity and maturity onset diabetes mellitus. *Annals of the New York Academy of Sciences*, **31**, 324–33.

111. Elton, C.W., Tapscott, E.B., Pories, W.J. *et al.* (1994) Effect of moderate obesity on glucose transport in human muscle. *Hormone and Metabolic Research*, **26**, 181–83.

12
Childhood obesity and type 2 diabetes

Krystyna A. Matyka
Clinical Sciences Research Institute, Walsgrave Hospital, Coventry, UK

12.1   Introduction

In the last 10 to 20 years childhood obesity has emerged as a disease of major public health significance. It has implications for the physical and emotional well-being of affected children as well as having potential longterm consequences on adult health. The aetiology is complex and attempts at both prevention and intervention have proved extremely challenging. This chapter aims to explore some of the issues surrounding obesity in childhood based on currently available evidence.

12.2   Childhood is a time of change

The scope of this chapter cannot cover childhood evolution in any great detail. However, some background is essential as there are implications for the definition, aetiology, potential consequences as well as management of this complex disorder in children of different ages.

The first years of life can be divided into three distinct periods: infancy, childhood and adolescence. Growth and body mass during these periods are determined by genetic, intra-uterine, nutritional, environmental and endocrine influences which vary in importance depending on the developmental stage of the child. Growth velocity is at its greatest during infancy, decelerates during childhood and increases again during the pubertal growth spurt [1]. During infancy, growth is predominantly nutritionally driven but by the third year of life the endocrine system becomes more important. Growth hormone is the main mediator of growth during childhood and during puberty the

Obesity and Diabetes, Second Edition   Edited by Anthony H. Barnett and Sudhesh Kumar
© 2009 John Wiley & Sons, Ltd

actions of growth hormone are augmented by sex steroids, testosterone and oestrogen. Body mass index (BMI) changes dramatically during this time. Body fat increases steeply during the first year of life leading to an increase in BMI, falls to a nadir in mid-childhood and then starts to rise again after about 7 years of age [2]. It has been suggested that the timing of this so-called 'adiposity rebound' is critical to the development of later obesity with children at greater risk if the timing is early, before 5.5 years of age [3]. During puberty BMI increases further and there are gender dependent differences with girls accumulating more fat mass and boys more lean muscle mass during this time [4].

Caloric requirements of growing children are extremely high. Average caloric requirements during the first few months of life are around 110 kcal/kg/day compared to approximately 90 kcal/kg/day during childhood and 50 kcal/kg/day during puberty. These calories are used to promote normal growth as well as cover energy expenditure through activity. The composition of this diet changes considerably throughout the early years. The almost exclusively milk-based diet during infancy is high in both fat and sugar, breast milk has approximately 60% fat, but this changes to a more adult type of diet by adolescence. As a result of all these changes, assessing the aetiology and predicting the consequences and hence the significance of obesity in children at different stages of development is very difficult.

It is also important to remember environmental influences. Infants and children will be totally dependent on their parents for food provision. Even adolescents who are striving for independence will still rely on their parents to do the shopping and make the family food choices. When considering an approach to the assessment and management of obese and overweight children the developmental stage of the child should always be considered and the importance of the family never underestimated.

12.3 The problem of size

The definition of childhood obesity should be based on a measure that not only reflects body fatness but also delineates those who are at risk of increased morbidity and mortality. This measure should be easy to perform, be reproducible and population specific normative data should be available. This is a problematic area in childhood for a number of reasons. Tremendous changes occur in body habitus during normal growth and maturation as already described, suggesting that one measure may not be adequate for all stages of development. In addition, although the metabolic complications of obesity can be seen in childhood they are uncommon and the greatest risks of childhood obesity occur in adult life. Finally, although paediatric centile charts are available for a number of growth parameters in many countries no centile charts are available for minority ethnic groups who appear to be at special risk of the complications of obesity in childhood [5].

A variety of measures for the assessment of childhood obesity have been proposed [6]. Skinfold thickness is an assessment of subcutaneous fat and can be measured along the trunk, subscapular and iliac regions, or in the extremities, triceps region. Skinfold thickness correlates reasonably well with total body adiposity and an adverse cardiovascular risk profile. Studies have demonstrated a link between skinfold thickness and adverse lipid and insulin profiles [7]; however, these associations do vary with age and gender [8,9]. The assessment of skinfold thickness is relatively easy but is poorly reproducible and as a result it is not routinely used in clinical practice.

Waist circumference can also be performed. Waist circumference is easier to measure, reproducible and centile charts are available. Waist and hip circumference are good predictors of abdominal fat and are often expressed as a ratio, waist–hip ratio (WHR) [10]. Abdominal fat is related to adverse health outcomes such as dyslipidaemia and glucose intolerance in obese children [11,12]. Studies suggest that waist circumference alone is a more powerful predictor of an adverse cardiovascular risk profile than WHR in children [7]. This may be due to the fact that there is a proportionately greater increase in hip circumference during normal childhood growth than waist circumference [13].

BMI is currently the measure of choice for defining overweight and obesity in children over 2 years of age [14–16]. It is easy to measure, reproducible and centile charts are available. Definitions for both overweight and obesity have been proposed based on centiles but there has been little consensus internationally. In the United States the definitions are based on a weight over the 85th centile for overweight and 98th centile for obesity but the 85th centile is not plotted on United Kingdom centile charts. Recently, the International Obesity Task Force has provided BMI cut-offs based on the adult definition of $25 \, kg/m^2$ for overweight and $30 \, kg/m^2$ for obesity [15]. Although these measures are not ideal they do provide some international consensus and provide some continuity when moving from paediatric to adult care. Recent guidelines from the National Institute for Clinical Excellence (NICE) in England also recommend the use of BMI for highlighting those children in whom further evaluation and management may be necessary. NICE recommend that children with a BMI over the 91st centile should be offered tailored intervention whilst those with a BMI greater than 98th centile should be assessed for co-morbidities [16].

One of the reasons for the lack of uniformity is that the *clinical* relevance of any of these cut-offs in childhood is not clear [17]. None of the measures described accurately highlights those most at risk of obesity related complications. In addition as children grow they may move across centiles and the longterm implications of obesity in for example a two-year-old are still far from clear.

12.4 The size of the problem

Given the difficulties of defining obesity it is not surprising that attempts to compare prevalence of childhood obesity internationally have been problematic. In addition studies of both adults and children suggest that the 'pathological' definition of obesity may need to be different in individuals from different ethnic backgrounds to reflect an increased risk of weight related metabolic complications. The most recent global survey by Wang and Lobstein suggests that the prevalence of obesity is not only high but also rising in most parts of the world (Figure 12.1). Data are more robust from developed parts of the world and prevalence is highest, approximately 20–30% of

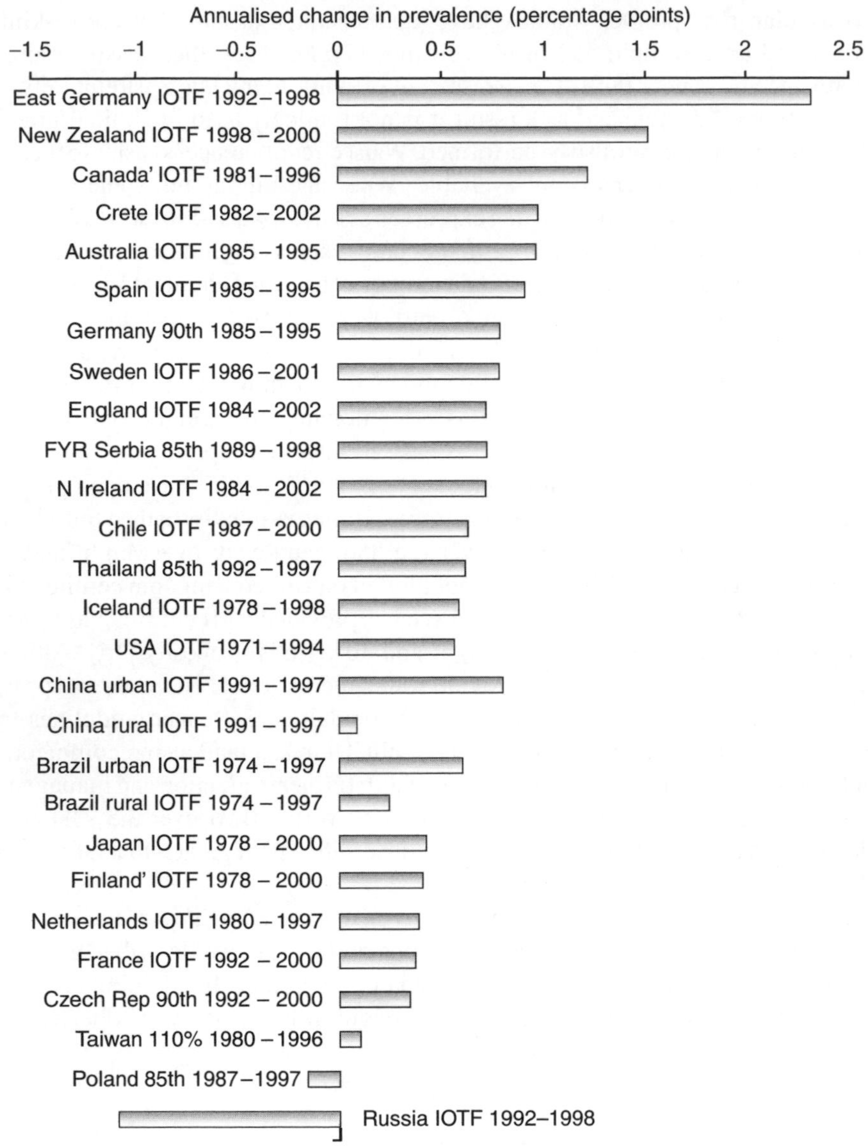

Annualised change in prevalence (percentage points)

−1.5	−1	−0.5	0	0.5	1	1.5	2	2.5

East Germany IOTF 1992–1998

New Zealand IOTF 1998 – 2000

Canada' IOTF 1981–1996

Crete IOTF 1982– 2002

Australia IOTF 1985 – 1995

Spain IOTF 1985 – 1995

Germany 90th 1985 – 1995

Sweden IOTF 1986 – 2001

England IOTF 1984 – 2002

FYR Serbia 85th 1989 – 1998

N Ireland IOTF 1984 – 2002

Chile IOTF 1987 – 2000

Thailand 85th 1992 – 1997

Iceland IOTF 1978 – 1998

USA IOTF 1971–1994

China urban IOTF 1991–1997

China rural IOTF 1991 – 1997

Brazil urban IOTF 1974 – 1997

Brazil rural IOTF 1974 – 1997

Japan IOTF 1978 – 2000

Finland' IOTF 1978 – 2000

Netherlands IOTF 1980 – 1997

France IOTF 1992 – 2000

Czech Rep 90th 1992 – 2000

Taiwan 110% 1980 – 1996

Poland 85th 1987–1997

Russia IOTF 1992–1998

• Self-reported data

Figure 12.1 Change in combined prevalence of overweight and obesity among school-age children in surveys since 1970. The chart shows country, method of measurement and period of assessment. Reprinted by the permission of the publisher (Taylor and Francis Group http://www.informaworld.com) [18]

children, in North America, Europe and parts of the western Pacific. Prevalence rates are lowest in South-east Asia and sub-Saharan Africa with countries in South and Central America, northern Africa and the Middle East somewhere in between. Rates have also been rising by 200–300% since the 1970s and the predictions for 2010 are frightening with estimates of overweight of 46% of school children in America and 38% in Europe [18].

12.5   What causes obesity in childhood?

Pathological causes of obesity

Genetic and endocrine abnormalities are rare causes of obesity in childhood. However, they are important to mention as parents of obese children may be concerned that their child has an underlying 'hormonal' problem and this belief can be a significant barrier to the lifestyle changes that need to be made when tackling childhood obesity. The clinical features of these genetic and endocrine disorders are highlighted in Table 12.1. Children with simple obesity tend to be tall for their age as excess nutrition supplements the growth hormone drive to growth. They are also more likely to develop early puberty. Obese children with short stature, poor growth, delayed puberty or developmental problems should raise concern as they are more likely to have an underlying disorder for which they should be screened.

   Although the majority of children are likely to develop problems with their weight as a result of environmental factors it is likely that genetic factors will contribute to obesity risk. Family studies suggest that heritable factors contribute 45–75% of BMI variation [19,20] and our understanding of the polygenic contribution to obesity is increasing (for review see [21]). In addition a number of single gene defects including leptin deficiency, leptin receptor deficiency, melanocortin-4 receptor deficiency and pro-opiomelanocortin deficiency have been described in children but are extremely rare [22]. These children have defects in central control of appetite leading to a variable degree of lack of satiety and develop severe early-onset obesity usually in the first two years of life. Although these conditions are rare they have enabled us to gain valuable insight in to the potential mechanisms involved in human weight control with potential implications for the development of effective pharmacological interventions in obesity management.

Environmental causes of obesity

Obesity is an energy balance disorder and is likely to occur if energy intake is too high, energy expenditure is too low or a combination of the two. This equation is easy to understand and discuss with families but despite a great deal of data on the possible causes of the rapidly increasing tide of obesity among young children we are still remarkably ignorant of the most likely reasons [23]. This is important as it is difficult to tackle a problem if we do not know the cause. A failing of a large number of epidemiological studies is that they are not longitudinal or if they are they are of short duration only. Studies have also tended to focus on either nutrition or physical activity and it is likely to be a combination of many factors including genetic susceptibility, sleep and so on [24].

Table 12.1 Pathological causes of obesity in childhood

Genetic disorders	Clinical findings
Prader–Willi	Short stature
	Hypotonia in early infancy
	Hypogonadotrophic hypogonadism
Bardet–Biedl	Mental deficiency
	Polydactyly
	Retinitis pigmentosa
	hypogonadism
Alstrom	Retinitis pigmentosa
	Type 2 diabetes
	Cardiomyopathy
	Deafness
Cohen	Hypotonia
	Mental deficiency
	Prominent incisors
Single gene defects	Early onset severe obesity (<2 years)
	Uncontrollable appetite
Endocrine disorders	
Hypothyroidism	Goitre
	Poor linear growth
Growth hormone deficiency	Short stature
	Poor linear growth
	Cherubic facies
Hypothalamic damage due to tumour	History of intracranial tumour
Cushing's syndrome	Moon facies
	Hirsutism
	Violaceous striae
	Hypertension
	Poor linear growth
Pseudohypoparathyroidism	Hypocalcaemia
	Hyperphosphataemia
	Short fourth metacarpal

In addition, given the pervasive nature of the problem it is likely that our environment per se may contribute to obesity risk. The provision of lifts, labour-saving devices in the home, good central heating, replacement of manual labour by more sedentary tasks, increasing variety of foods and portion sizes may all have contributed to any one person's risk. Although individuals may have some control over their own personal environment that is have their own 'personal choice' there are a large number of socio-environmental barriers which may prevent them from being successful in terms of weight management. For an interesting discussion of this dilemma please see Nuffield Council on Bioethics, Public Health: Ethical Issues, Chapter 5: Obesity.

12.6 Does obesity in childhood matter?

Obese children appear to be at risk of the same complications of obesity as are obese adults (Table 12.2). However, no data exist which correlate definitions of childhood obesity based on BMI cut-offs with the risk of adverse health outcomes in childhood. Instead BMI criteria are used to highlight those who may be at greater risk and who would benefit from assessment and intervention [16]. Currently the greatest concern is the development of type 2 diabetes, the emergence of which has changed the face of paediatric diabetes practice over the last 5–10 years.

Gastrointestinal

Non-alcoholic fatty liver disease (NAFLD) is increasingly recognized as a metabolic complication of obesity. There are no population-based studies of prevalence but clinic based reports of children attending weight management services suggest that up to 80% of children with clinical obesity have the biochemical markers of hepatic fatty

Table 12.2 Consequences of obesity

	Consequence	Clinical features
Metabolic	Insulin resistance	Acanthosis nigricans
	Type 2 diabetes	Polyuria
		Polydipsia
		Glycosuria $\pm$ ketonuria
	Hypertension	
	Dislipidaemia	
Gynaecological	Polycystic ovary syndrome	Menstrual irregularity
		Hirsutism
Respiratory	Obesity hypoventilation syndrome	Sleep apnoea
		Snoring
		Burning headaches
		Daytime sleepiness
Gastrointestinal	Non-alcoholic steatotic hepatitis	Abdominal pain
		Raised serum transaminases
	Gallstones	Abdominal pain
Orthopaedic	Slipped femoral epiphysis	Limp
		Joint pain
		Limitation of abduction/internal rotation
Neurological	Benign intracranial hypertension	Headache
		Vomiting
		Papilloedema
Psychological	School bullying	
	Depression	
	Low self esteem	

infiltration [25,26]. Children may present with abdominal pain although they are usually asymptomatic. Raised liver aminotransferases on biochemical testing suggest the diagnosis but fatty infiltration of the liver may be present in the absence of biochemical evidence of inflammation. The ideal plan of investigation for obese children with raised liver transaminases remains unclear. An ultrasound may show fat deposition in the liver but a liver biopsy is the only way to accurately differentiate this condition from other hepatic inflammation and is also necessary to assess the degree of steatosis and liver damage. Autoimmune hepatitis, Wilson's disease, infectious hepatitis and alpha-1 antitrypsin deficiency can all present with raised liver enzymes and are potentially treatable conditions so are important conditions to exclude.

NAFLD is fast becoming the most common cause of liver disease in childhood yet the natural history and ideal management remain unclear. Gradual weight loss through diet and physical activity has resulted in clinical benefits [27,28]. In addition, pilot data using insulin sensitizers such as metformin or anti-oxidants such as vitamin E have been promising and further more definitive studies are under way.

Gynaecological

Polycystic ovarian syndrome (PCOS) involves a triad of symptoms: obesity, menstrual irregularity and hirsutism. The precise aetiology of this complex disorder and whether obesity is a primary or secondary phenomenon is not known [29]. However, hyperinsulinaemia, such as occurs during puberty, has been suggested as being a prerequisite for the development of PCOS [30]. Recognized therapeutic options exist making it an important condition to diagnose and treat [31]. Metformin is beneficial in improving menstrual irregularities although the data regarding the effects on weight loss or hirsutism are inconsistent.

Orthopaedic

Slipped upper femoral epiphysis is a recognized complication of obesity and presents as a limp or joint pain, often knee pain [32]. Clinical findings include limitation of abduction and internal rotation at the hip joint. Referral to an orthopaedic surgeon is necessary. Blount's disease, involving bowing of the tibia, and flat feet have also been described in childhood obesity [33].

Neurological

Benign intracranial hypertension is an uncommon complication of obesity, particularly in children [34,35]. Patients present with symptoms of raised intracranial pressure and may need therapeutic lumbar puncture. Symptoms are said to improve with weight loss but ongoing ophthalmological assessment is essential as some children may have residual visual problems.

Psychological

It is beyond the scope of this chapter to provide a comprehensive overview of the psychological consequences of obesity in childhood. Psychological issues may be an aetiological factor in the development of obesity and can be significant barriers to successful intervention [36]. Bullying at school is almost universal and needs to be addressed as school often provides the only source of physical activity for these children. Professional help may be necessary and is likely to involve the entire family.

Respiratory

Obstructive sleep apnoea (OSA) has been widely reported among adults with obesity and is felt to be due to an increase in parapharyngeal fat pads or visceral neck fat. Data from paediatric studies suggest that young children who are overweight may be less at risk with adenotonsillar hypertrophy being more problematic than excess weight although this may change as children go through adolescence [37]. Interestingly OSA itself may predispose to problems with weight. OSA leads to disrupted sleep and sleep deprivation which is linked to both adult and childhood obesity. It may also cause daytime behavioural problems including alterations in diet and physical activity. Snoring is a non-specific symptom but those children with a history of respiratory pauses during sleep, burning headaches or excessive daytime sleepiness or should be referred for further evaluation [38].

Renal

Renal complications are also included in the list of obesity-related problems. One study reported seven African–American children with severe obesity and proteinuria who were found to have focal segmental glomerulosclerosis on renal biopsy [39]. One child improved with weight reduction whilst another progressed to end-stage renal disease.

Cardiovascular disease risk factors

A number of cohort studies have examined cardiovascular disease (CVD) risk profiles in children [8,9,40–42]. One impressive study is the Bogalusa Heart Study which began in 1973 and is a cross sectional and longitudinal study of the early natural history of atherosclerosis [43]. The survey has included school age children and young adults in a biracial (one third African–American) cohort. This study has published a number of papers that have highlighted the link between overweight and obesity and an abnormal CVD risk profile even in young children. This includes changes in lipid, blood pressure and insulin profiles [41,44]. The Bogalusa Heart Study demonstrated that insulin resistance tracked strongly from childhood to adulthood and resulted in a 36-fold increase in the prevalence of obesity, a 2.5-fold increase in hypertension and a threefold increase in dyslipidaemia in those with persistently elevated fasting insulin [44]. Childhood obesity *per se* is also a powerful predictor of the metabolic syndrome in young adulthood and this relationship remains significant even after adjusting for fasting insulin values [45]. An autopsy study of children who died during the course of the survey has confirmed this link with early histological changes in coronary artery architecture [46]. Despite these findings the majority of CVD risk prevention programmes are targeted almost exclusively at adults. However, in North America the concerns are so great that the American Heart Association has recently published a consensus statement on cardiovascular health in childhood highlighting childhood obesity as a significant risk factor for adult cardiovascular disease [47].

More recent studies have highlighted the difficulties of assessing CVD risk in childhood. One thousand adolescents were assessed for 'metabolic syndrome' using a variety of diagnostic criteria (American Heart Association criteria, AHA paediatric criteria and IDF criteria) at baseline and then reviewed three years later. The authors found that over 50% of adolescents 'lost' their metabolic diagnosis and new cases were also found during the course of the study with a cumulative incidence rate from 3.8–5.2%. [48]. The suggestion that metabolic abnormalities may be inconsistent features in childhood obesity does present a dilemma when considering management or designing interventional studies. Furthermore, measures which assess physical fitness, and which are not routinely used in clinical practice, have been suggested as useful physiological markers: physical fitness providing a degree of cardiovascular protection even in the presence of obesity [49].

Type 2 diabetes mellitus (T2DM)

An emerging epidemic
It is probably true to say that the emergence of T2DM as a well-described disease of childhood has taken the paediatric community by surprise. Cases have been reported since the 1970s mainly in Pima Indians but it is probably over the last 5–10 years that the disease has emerged as a paediatric entity of great concern.

Diagnosis
Up until recently children presenting with T1DM had a classic clinical presentation of polyuria, polydipsia and weight loss in a slim, ketotic child. T2DM also has some 'classical' features of a more insidious presentation and may be found on routine testing, but children may also have weight loss and present with ketonuria, although ketoacidosis is rare. A systematic approach to the differential diagnosis of diabetes type, including laboratory tests such as C-peptide concentrations and antibody tests, has been proposed [50]. Often the correct diagnosis may not be obvious at presentation but become more obvious with time: it is usually safer to start insulin treatment where there is diagnostic uncertainty and adjust the 'diagnosis' once the clinical course becomes more obvious.

Epidemiology

Good population-based studies of the prevalence of T2DM in childhood are scarce. Data are available from a small number of studies looking at children attending weight loss services or from national diabetes registers that may well just represent the tip of an iceberg. It is therefore difficult to predict which child may be at greatest risk of T2DM.

Table 12.3 summarizes some of the larger studies that are apparent in the literature since 2000. The population based studies predictably show lower rates of impaired glucose tolerance and diabetes than clinic-based or register-based studies. Of interest are the Japanese data: over 7 million young people have undergone urine screening and those with persistent glycosuria have undergone blood glucose testing [51]. Over a twenty year period the prevalence of T2DM increased 10-fold in young children from 6 to 12 years old and doubled among adolescents from 7.3 to 13.9/100 000. Interestingly, recent data suggest that this epidemic is slowing down: possibly due to a decrease in the prevalence of obesity among young children in Japan [52]. One study suggested that ethnic background influenced diabetes risk: in young people aged 10–19 years the prevalence of T2DM varied from 6% in the non-Hispanic whites to 76% among the American Indians [53].

Risk factors

The lack of good population-based studies means that we have no robust data on risk factors for T2DM within communities and hence no guidelines as to who may benefit from screening. Studies of the clinical characteristics of children who have been diagnosed with T2DM do provide some indicators of who may be at greatest risk of metabolic complications in childhood.

Ethnicity.   Most children with T2DM come from an ethnic minority background. In an Australian study of 128 children with T2DM 29% were Caucasian, 22% were Indigenous Australians, 22% Asian, 12% North African or Middle Eastern and 10% Maori or Polynesian [54]. In a recent case study report from the UK prevalence rates of T2DM were 3.9/100 000 Black and 1.25/100 000 South Asians compared to 0.35/100 000 White [55].

Studies of South Asians suggest that risk is associated with a tendency to deposit adipose tissue more centrally and may not be related to total adiposity. This process starts early; although Indian babies are lighter at birth their fat mass is preserved and there is a tendency to truncal or central adiposity even during intrauterine development [56]. By 8 years of age these lower birth weight babies already have abnormalities in blood pressure, fasting plasma insulin, skinfold ratios and cholesterol concentrations [57].

Alterations in body composition are related to metabolic risk in adults and there are data which suggest that this is also true in childhood. Magnetic resonance spectroscopy studies have demonstrated excessive hepatic fat accumulation in Caucasian and Hispanic adolescents compared to African Americans [58]. Obese Hispanic adolescents have greater intramyocellular lipid content than Caucasians and African–Americans, of comparable weight, age and gender. These data suggest that ethnicity plays an important role in the amount of lipid accumulated in skeletal muscle and liver, and hence metabolic risk, which occur independently of the degree of obesity.

Table 12.3 Studies of the epidemiology of type 2 diabetes in childhood

Country	Study period	Population	Age (years)	Comment
Population-based				
Germany [95]	2007	721 school leavers. Fasting glucose	15.5 mean	2.5% IFG, IGT, T2DM
Japan [52]	1975–2000	School based urine glucose screening programme		Incidence – 3.0/100 000/year
US [53]	2001	Population based observational six-centre study	<20 yr	0.18% prevalence of diabetes overall. 0–9 year >80% T1DM. 10–19 year 6% (non-Hispanic white) to 76% (American Indian) had T2DM
Turkey [96]	2004	Population-based study of 1647 adolescents. Fasting plasma glucose.		1.96% IGT, none had T2DM
Taiwan [97]	1999	3 million students: fasting blood glucose if persistent glycosuria	6–18 yr	Prevalence of undiagnosed diabetes (all types) 9.0/100 000 boys and 15.3/100 000 girls
US [64,104]	1988–1994	2867 adolescents as part of 3rd NHANES	12–19	0.4% had diabetes – 31% of these had Type 2 diabetes. 1.8% had IFG
Case series				
UK [55]	2004–2005	Monthly reporting of cases by paediatricians	<17	67 cases reported
Clinic based				
Argentina [98]	2005	Clinic population – 427 obese children	10.7 ± 3.5 yr	7% IGT, 1.6% T2DM
Germany [99]	2004	520 obese children from weight management clinic – OGTT	14.0 ± 2.0 yr	1.5% T2DM, IFG in 3.7%, IGT in 2.1%

Diabetes registers			
Australia, New South Wales [54]	2001–2006	Australasian Paediatric Endocrine Group NSM Diabetes Register	<19 yr	11% of incident cases of diabetes. Annual incidence of 2.5/100 000 person years.
Western Australia [100]	1990–2002	Prospectively recorded diabetes database	<17 yr	43 patients with T2DM with average annual increase 27%
Austria [101]	1999–2001	Nationwide diabetes register	<15	8 cases of T2DM. 0.25/100000 incidence
US – Wyoming [102]	1999–2001	Review of diabetes cases among American Indian Youth	<20	Annual prevalence 0.7/1000 T1DM and 1.3/1000 T2DM. 53% of prevalent cases and 70% of incident cases
Hong Kong [103]	1984–1996	Register of all diabetes cases in Hong Kong	<15	18 cases of T2DM. Incidence of T1DM 1.4/100 000 vs. 0.1/100 000 T2DM

Puberty. The majority of children with T2DM are pubertal at the time of presentation. There is a 30% reduction in insulin action during adolescence which is felt to be mediated by the increased secretion of growth hormone during this time of rapid growth and development [59]. Recent studies suggest that young people may demonstrate *transient* deteriorations in glucose tolerance. A study from the Yale weight management clinic showed that 33 of 117 subjects had IGT at baseline testing. At two years eight of these subjects had developed T2DM yet 15 subjects had reverted to normal glucose tolerance [60]. These data have significant implications for the management of these young people.

Family history. T2DM runs very strongly in families and the majority of children with diagnosed diabetes have a family history of the condition [55,61]. Data from adult studies suggest that defects in insulin sensitivity may be inherited but families also share similar lifestyles which may also have a significant impact on the development of T2DM [62].

Complications

Although there are few studies that have examined the development of both micro- and macrovascular complications of childhood T2DM the available data suggest that it does appear to be a more severe form of childhood diabetes. For a comprehensive review of the subject see [63].

Microvascular complications can be present at diagnosis and progress more rapidly that in children with T1DM. Twenty-two percent of Pima Indians have evidence of microalbuminuria at presentation [64] and 18% of Korean children with T2DM had persistent microalbuminuria compared to 11% of children with T1DM despite similar (poor) glycaemic control [65]. The prevalence of retinopathy is lower among adolescent patients with T2DM versus those with T1DM yet the disease duration is often strikingly shorter [66].

Macrovascular complications are reported frequently. Hypertension is eight times more common in young people with T2DM than in young people with T1DM at diagnosis [67]. A large multicentre study from North America of almost 300 young people with T2DM highlighted that 33% had elevated total cholesterol, 24% had elevated low-density lipoprotein-cholesterol, 29% had high triglyceride concentrations and 44% had low concentrations of high-density lipoprotein-cholesterol [68].

12.7   Management of childhood obesity

Prevention

A Cochrane review has examined the efficacy of obesity prevention strategies in childhood [69]. The authors commented that 'the mismatch between the prevalence and significance of the condition and the knowledge base from which to inform preventive activity, is remarkable and an outstanding feature of this review'. Only seven 'long-term' randomized controlled studies, lasting 12 months, were identified and three short-term studies of 3 months duration were therefore included. The studies used a number of interventions and it was difficult to generalize the findings. One study examined the effect of dietary education aimed at young children, 3–9 years old. A significant reduction in prevalence of overweight and obesity was reported in the group of children who were given 'multimedia' information regarding healthy eating which included the use of qualified staff to underline health messages [70]. No significant changes were seen in the control group and also in a group of children who were given written information only. Four long-term studies examined the effect of a combination of dietary education and physical activity intervention. The results of these have been disappointing. The APPLES study in the UK assessed the impact of a school-based intervention including teacher training, modification of school meals and action plans tackling physical activity in the school curriculum [71]. Six hundred and thirty four children aged 7–11 years old took part. Although the programme had a beneficial effect on changing the healthy living ethos of the schools involved it had little impact on children's behaviour other than a small increase in the consumption of vegetables. Children, especially young children, have a limited amount of influence on the family food and activity choices and a programme aimed exclusively at children rather than involving the whole family may be of limited success. Another group did examine the effect of behavioural and educational messages regarding diet and activity given to 1640 children aged 5–7 years *and* their parents [72]. At one year there were no changes in BMI although there were significant differences in body fat mass, as assessed by skinfold thickness, in the intervention group.

The results from these studies are disappointing. However, given the complexity of the aetiology of the current epidemic of obesity it seems unlikely that a focused approach aimed exclusively at children is likely to succeed, especially in the short term. Instead, the approach to the prevention of obesity in childhood should be seen as part of a bigger picture of social and environmental change which can only be achieved by governments. Changes will need to be accomplished in collaboration with the public health service, the food industry, advertisers and public transport providers, to name but a few, with the aims of changing the behaviour of the general population [73]. The epidemic has evolved over a prolonged period of time and realistic longterm goals need to be developed to protect the health of nations.

Intervention

Aims

North American guidelines recommend that interventions for childhood obesity should begin early [14]. Yet, data suggest that overweight children are referred less aggressively than underweight children [74]. Childhood is a time of constant growth and development and any childhood obesity intervention must not compromise this process. The aims of obesity interventions in growing children will therefore be different to those for adults and adolescents who have achieved final adult height [14]. Adequate nutritional intake to maintain normal linear growth is essential and severe caloric restriction is inappropriate in young children. Weight loss is difficult to achieve in a growing child and instead the focus should be on a reduction in BMI. This can be achieved by weight maintenance or a reduction in rate of weight gain whilst allowing normal linear growth.

Diet and exercise

There have been a number of childhood obesity intervention studies [75]. Almost exclusively the main outcome measure has been weight change: either weight loss or reduction in weight for height. The great majority of studies has involved only a small number of children and these have been of relatively short duration. Furthermore, most studies have been performed in specialized child obesity centres, mainly in North America, and the appropriateness of generalizing the results to other clinical contexts remains unclear. Although a large number of studies have been performed only randomized controlled studies will be considered in this section.

Few randomized controlled studies have been performed and these have recently been reviewed for the Cochrane Collaboration [76]. Only one study examined the effect of dietary counselling and found no significant difference between a group of 50 prepubertal children who were given dietary counselling and a group who were 'untreated' controls [77]. Other studies focused on physical activity as a means of weight change. In these studies a variety of methods were employed. In one of a number of studies by Epstein, prepubertal children were assigned to either diet alone or diet plus exercise which was provided in the form of an 8 week intensive programme followed by 10 monthly maintenance sessions [78]. Percent overweight, described as percent weight for height, was reduced in both intervention groups but was only significantly different at 6 months but not at 12 months following initiation of the intervention.

Epstein has also examined the benefit of a reduction in sedentary behaviour versus an increase in physical activity [79]. The rationale for this approach, often called 'lifestyle activity', is that increasing energy expenditure through normal daily living is potentially a more sustainable form of physical activity than participating in more structured exercise programmes. Statistically significant differences in percent overweight were found in children in both groups at both 6 and 12 months of treatment. However, at 24 months the lifestyle group had maintained their relative weight changes whereas children in the physical activity group had returned to baseline levels [79].

Behavioural interventions have also been examined. A variety of techniques has been employed and has been shown to be effective compared to conventional treatment, usually dietary advice and medical follow up. Cognitive behavioural therapy, relaxation therapy and family therapy all appear to be effective [80–83]. There is also the suggestion that therapies involving the parents as the main motivators of change are more effective than treatments which are predominantly child focused. However, it is important to note that the great majority of these studies have involved younger children

and it is uncertain whether these results could be extrapolated to emotionally challenging adolescents with weight problems.

It would appear from these studies that weight loss is both difficult to achieve and to
sustain. It is therefore important to know if weight loss, or even a physical activity
intervention *per se*, may have health benefits in children as in adults. A weight
reduction of 10% from baseline in adults has been shown to have significant benefits
on cardiovascular morbidity [84]. Recent studies have also shown a dramatic impact
of weight loss on the risk of diabetes. The Finnish Diabetes Prevention Study and the
American Diabetes Prevention Program have both shown that intensive lifestyle
intervention in obese patients with impaired glucose tolerance (IGT) led to a
reduction in the risk of progression to Type 2 diabetes of 58% [85,86]. This was
achieved with an average reduction in weight of only 4 kg over the 3–4 year period of
the studies. Unfortunately, none of the randomized controlled studies quoted above
appear to have examined the health benefits of weight loss in childhood. Smaller
studies have suggested that weight management in children does provide some health
benefits especially with respect to CVD risk factors.

Pharmacological therapy

Pharmacological interventions are increasingly being used in the management of
childhood obesity. Recent NICE guidelines suggest that drug treatment should be
considered only if multicomponent dietary, exercise and behavioural approaches have
been started and evaluated. NICE goes on to say that drug treatment is not generally
recommended in children under the age of 12 years but may be prescribed in
exceptional circumstances such as severe life-threatening comorbidities. Children
over the age of 12 years can be prescribed treatment if there are severe comorbidities.

Data from a large ($n = 539$) randomized controlled trial in North America suggest
that orlistat, a pancreatic lipase inhibitor, may be useful as part of a weight loss
intervention in adolescents as part of a healthy lifestyle intervention [87]. Yet only
26.5% of the study group achieved a BMI reduction of greater than 5% and 13.3%
achieved a reduction in BMI of 10% over the 12 month period although this was
associated with a reduction in waist circumference. It is likely that only a carefully
selected small subgroup of young people attending weight management services will
respond well to Orlistat but for these the benefits may be significant.

Sibutramine is a noradrenaline and serotonin reuptake inhibitor and acts to inhibit
appetite. A large multicentre, randomized, double blind controlled trial has been
performed in teenagers aged from 12 to 16 years of age [88]. Almost 500 young people
took part in the 12 month study (Figure 12.2). Those in the sibutramine group performed
better than placebo with a change from baseline in BMI ($-2.9 \, \text{kg/m}^2$ [95% CI, -3.5 to
$-2.2 \, \text{kg/m}^2$]) and body weight ($-8.4 \, \text{kg}$ [CI, -9.7 to $-7.2 \, \text{kg}$]) ($p < 0.001$). In addition
those in the sibutramine group had greater improvements in triglyceride levels, high-
density lipoprotein cholesterol levels, insulin levels, and insulin sensitivity ($p < 0.001$).
Interestingly, 24 and 38% of the sibutramine and placebo groups, respectively, did not
complete follow-up.

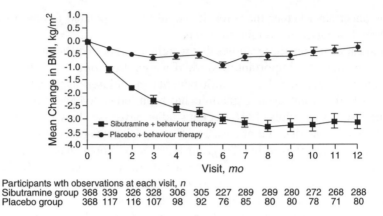

Participants wth observations at each visit, *n*
Sibutramine group 368 339 326 328 306 305 227 289 289 280 272 268 288
Placebo group   368 117 116 107   98   92 76 85   80 80 78 71 80

Figure 12.2 Mean (± SEM) changes in BMI from baseline to each visit. Reprinted with permission from the Annals of internal medicine [88]

Surgery

Recent NICE guidelines suggest that bariatric surgery may be a treatment option for some young people with severe obesity. There are significant clinical and ethical considerations when pursuing such an option. The impact of a degree of malnutrition in a developing child is a concern as well as the ability of a child to make an informed decision with respect to a procedure that is life long. Data from studies of adults do suggest that bariatric surgery carries immense benefits [89]. It is likely that children will benefit as well but there are no good data at present. Studies of bariatric surgery in childhood are now being performed that show that surgery is effective in managing weight, but there can be significant complications, including serious vitamin deficiencies and death [90]. Yet for those children with severe obesity of long standing and with associated comorbidities surgery may be the only effective way of preventing early death.

Summary

Although the data for the effectiveness of obesity interventions for childhood are poor there are some suggestions that family based approaches to changes in diet and physical activity may be beneficial. The main goals of management will depend on the age of the child and an age-based, step-wise approach should be pursued. Advice needs to be given on an individual basis but the aim should be to introduce small but sustainable lifestyle changes in diet and physical activity to achieve a gradual improvement in BMI [14]. The whole family should be involved and needs to provide support for their child during this process. The role of pharmacological intervention and surgery is still ill-defined.

12.8   Management of T2DM

Although T2TM has increased in frequency the number of young people with this condition remained relatively small and it has been difficult to conduct good randomized controlled studies of interventions for diabetes management. A consensus statement from the American Diabetes Association recommends diet and exercise as the initial approach to treatment, although they acknowledge that the majority of patients will require pharmacological intervention [91]. Successful treatment with lifestyle is defined as a cessation of excessive weight gain whilst maintaining normal linear growth, near-normal fasting glucose values and a glycosylated haemoglobin value less that 7%. Metformin is the drug of choice if lifestyle is unsuccessful. In a placebo controlled study Jones *et al.*, found that metformin was useful in managing childhood T2DM over a 16 week period [92]. The study was small with approximately 40 children in each study arm and the groups were not well matched. Treatment with metformin led to a reduction in HbA1c with a difference from placebo of $-1.2 \pm 0.2\%$ [92].

Second-line treatment is less clear and there is currently no recommended treatment algorithm. A number of agents have been tried including sulfonylureas, meglitinides and insulin although these obviously carry the side effects of increasing weight gain. A large multicentre study is about to start sponsored by the National Institutes of Health with three treatment arms: metformin alone versus metformin and rosiglitazone versus metformin and an intensive lifestyle programme. This will hopefully provide advice regarding a more structured approach to management [93].

It is likely that education will also be extremely important. A fascinating study from Skinner examined weight perceptions of 104 adolescents with T2DM and their adult carers attending a paediatric diabetes service [94]. The mean BMI was 36.4 kg/m^2 and 87% had a BMI over the 95th centile. Of these 40% of parents and 55% of adolescents felt the weight of the adolescent was 'about right'. These misperceptions led to significant decrements in approaches to a healthy lifestyle: family education about the risks of excess weight is paramount.

12.9   Conclusions

Obesity is common in childhood and can lead to significant morbidity as well as premature adult mortality. Of greatest concern is the spectre of juvenile onset T2DM with its devastating consequences on cardiovascular health. Primary prevention has to be the key aim but this cannot be achieved without a huge investment of public and political will. In the meantime overweight and obese children need to be managed by a dedicated multidisciplinary team which ideally would span both the hospital and community health networks. Greater investment of resources for both treatment and prevention of childhood obesity need to be made if a public health disaster is to be avoided.

References

1. Clayton, P.E. and Gill, M.S. (2001) Normal growth and its endocrine control, in *Clinical Paediatric Endocrinology* (eds C.G.D. Brook and P.C. Hindmarsh), Blackwell Science, Oxford.
2. Cole, T.J., Freeman, J.V. and Preece, M.A. (1995) Body mass index reference curves for the UK 1990. *Archives of Disease in Childhood*, **73**, 25–9.
3. Dietz, W.H. (1997) Periods of risk in childhood for the development of adult obesity – what do we need to learn? *Journal of Nutrition*, **127**, 1884S–6S.
4. Hergenroeder, A.C. and Klisch, W.J. (1990) Body composition in adolescent athletes. *Pediatric Clinics of North America*, **37**, 1057–80.
5. Whincup, P., Gilg, J., Papacosta, O. *et al.* (2002) Early evidence of ethnic differences in cardiovascular risk: cross-sectional comparison of British South Asian and white children. *British Medical Journal*, **324**, 635–8.
6. Cole, T.J. and Rolland-Cachera, M.F. (2002) Measurement and definition, in *Child and Adolescent Obesity* (eds W. Burniat, T. Cole, I. Lissau and E. Poskitt), Cambridge University Press, Cambridge.
7. Freedman, D.S., Serdula, M.K., Srinivasan, S.R. and Berenson, G.S. (1999) Relation of circumferences and skinfold thicknesses to lipid and insulin concentrations in children and adolescents: the Bogalusa Heart Study. *American Journal of Clinical Nutrition*, **69**, 308–17.
8. Morrison, J.A., Barton, B.A., Biro, F.M. *et al.* (1999) Overweight, fat patterning and cardio-vascular disease risk factors in black and white boys. *Journal of Pediatrics*, **135**, 451–7.
9. Morrison, J.A., Sprecher, D.L., Barton, B.A. *et al.* (1999) Overweight, fat patterning and cardiovascular disease risk factors in black and white girls: the National Heart, Lung and Blood Institute Growth and Health Study. *Journal of Pediatrics*, **135**, 458–64.
10. Goran, M.I., Gower, B.A., Treuth, M. and Nagy, T.R. (1998) Prediction of intra-abdominal and subcutaneous abdominal adipose tissue in healthy prepubertal children. *International Journal of Obesity*, **22**, 549–58.
11. Caprio, S., Hyman, L.D., Limb, C. *et al.* (1995) Central adiposity and its metabolic correlates in obese adolescent girls. *American Journal of Physiology*, **269**, E118–E126.
12. Caprio, S., Hyman, L.D., McCarthy, S. *et al.* (1996) Fat distribution and cardiovascular risk factors in obese adolescent girls: importance of the intra-abdominal fat depot. *American Journal of Clinical Nutrition*, **64**, 12–17.
13. Weststrate, J.A., Deurenberg, P. and van Tinteren, H. (1989) Indices of body fat distribution and adiposity in Dutch children from birth to 18 years of age. *International Journal of Obesity*, **13**, 456–77.
14. Barlow, S.E. and Dietz, W.H. (1998) Obesity evaluation and treatment: Expert Committee Recommendations. *Pediatrics*, **102** (3), e29.
15. Cole, T.J., Bellizzi, M.C., Flegal, K.M. and Dietz, W.H. (2000) Establishing a standard definition for child overweight and obesity worldwide: international survey. *British Medical Journal*, **320**, 1240–3.
16. National Institute for Health and Clinical Excellence. Obesity, guidance on the prevention, identification, assessment and management of overweight and obesity in adults and children. NICE clinical guideline 43. London: NICE, December, 2006.
17. Kelishadi, R., Cook, S.R., Motlagh, M.E. *et al.* (2008) Metabolically obese normal weight and phenotypically obese metabolically normal youths: the CASPIAN Study. *Journal of the American Dietetic Association*, **108**, 82–90.
18. Wang, Y. and Lobstein, T. (2006) Worldwide trends in childhood overweight and obesity. *International Journal of Pediatric Obesity*, **1**, 11–25.
19. Sorensen, T.I., Price, R.A., Stunkard, A.J. and Schulsinger, F. (1989) Genetics of obesity in adult adoptees and their biological siblings. *British Medical Journal*, **298**, 87–90.

20. Stunkard, A.J., Harris, J.R., Pedersen, N.L. and McClearn, G.E. (1990) The body mass index of twins who have been reared apart. *New England Journal of Medicine*, **322**, 1483–7.

21. Farooqi, I.S. and O'Rahilly, S. (2007) Genetic factors in human obesity. *Obesity Reviews*, **8**, 37–40.

22. Farooqi, I.S. and O'Rahilly, S. (2005) New advances in the genetics of early onset obesity. *International Journal of Obesity*, **29**, 1149–52.

23. Reilly, J.J., Ness, A.R. and Sherriff, A. (2007) Epidemiological and physiological approaches to understanding the etiology of pediatric obesity: finding the needle in the haystack. *Pediatric Research*, **61**, 646–52.

24. Must, A. and Tybor, D.J. (2005) Physical activity and sedentary behaviour: a review of longitudinal studies of weight and adiposity in youth. *International Journal of Obesity*, **29**, S84–S96.

25. Lobstein, T. and Jackson-Leach, R. (2006) Estimated burden of paediatric obesity and co-morbidities in Europe. Part 2. Numbers of children with indicators of obesity-related disease. *International Journal of Pediatric Obesity*, **1**, 33–41.

26. Papandreou, D., Rousso, I. and Mavromichalis, I. (2007) Update on non-alcoholic fatty liver disease in children. *Clinical Nutrition*, **26**, 409–15.

27. Vajro, P., Fontanella, A., Perna, C. *et al.* (1994) De Vincenzo A. Persistent hyperamino-transferasemia resolving after weight reduction in obese children. *Journal of Pediatrics*, **125**, 239–41.

28. Tock, L., Prado, W.L., Caranti, D.A. *et al.* (2006) Non-alcoholic fatty liver disease in obese adolescents after multidisciplinary therapy. *European Journal of Gastroenterology and Hepatology*, **18**, 1241–5.

29. Franks, S. (1995) Polycystic Ovary Syndrome. *New England Journal of Medicine*, **333**, 853–61.

30. Utiger, R.D. (1996) Insulin and the polycystic ovary syndrome. *New England Journal of Medicine*, **335**, 657–8.

31. Iourno, M.J. and Nestler, J.E. (1999) The polycystic ovary syndrome: treatment with insulin sensitizing agents. *Diabetes, Obesity and Metabolism*, **1**, 127–36.

32. Loder, R.T., Aronson, D.D. and Greenfield, M.L. (1993) The epidemiology of bilateral slipped capital femoral epiphysis. *Journal of Bone and Joint Surgery*, **75**, 1141–7.

33. Dietz, W.H., Jr, Gross, W.L. and Kirkpatrick, J.A., Jr (1982) Blount disease (tibia vara): another skeletal disorder associated with childhood obesity. *Journal of Pediatrics*, **101**, 735–7.

34. Stevenson, S.B. (2008) Pseudotumor cerebri: yet another reason to fight obesity. *Journal of Pediatric Health Care*, **22**, 40–3.

35. Rangwala, L.M. and Liu, G.T. (2007) Pediatric idiopathic intracranial hypertension. *Survey of Ophthalmology*, **52**, 597–617.

36. Erikson, S.J., Robinson, T.N., Haydel, K.F. and Killen, J.D. (2000) Are overweight children unhappy? Body mass index, depressive symptoms, and overweight concern in elementary school children. *Archives of Pediatric and Adolescent Medicine*, **154**, 931–5.

37. Ievers-Landis, C.E. and Redline, S. (2007) Pediatric sleep apnea. *American Journal of Respiratory Critical Care Medicine*, **175**, 436–41.

38. Gaultier, C. (1995) Obstructive sleep apnoea syndrome in infants and children: established facts and unsettled issues. *Thorax*, **50**, 1204–10.

39. Adelman, R.D., Restaino, I.G., Alon, U.S. and Blowey, D.L. (2001) Proteinuria and focal segmental glomerulosclerosis in severely obese adolescents. *Journal of Pediatrics*, **138**, 481–5.

40. Daniels, S.R., Morrison, J.A., Sprecher, D.L. *et al.* (1999) Association of fat distribution and cardiovascular risk factors in children and adolescents. *Circulation*, **99**, 541–5.

41. Freedman, D.S., Dietz, W.H., Srinivasan, S.R. and Berenson, G.S. (1999) The relation of overweight to cardiovascular risk factors in children and adolescents: the Bogalusa Heart Study. *Pediatrics*, **103**, 1175–82.

42. Sinaiko, A.R., Donahue, R.P., Jacobs, D.R. and Prineas, R.J. (1999) Relation of weight and rate of increase in weight during childhood and adolescence to body size, blood pressure, fasting insulin, and lipids in young adults. *Circulation*, **99**, 1471–76.

43. Berenson, G.S., McMahan, C.A., Voors, A.W. *et al.* (1980) *Cardiovascular Risk Factors in Children: The Early Natural History of Atherosclerosis and Essential Hypertension*, Oxford University Press, New York, NY.

44. Bao, W., Sathanur, R., Srinivasan, S.R. and Berenson, G.S. (1996) Persistent elevation of plasma insulin levels is associated with increased cardiovascular risk in children and young adults. The Bogalusa Heart Study. *Circulation*, **93**, 54–9.

45. Srinivasan, S.R., Myers, L. and Berenson, G.S. (2002) Predictability of childhood adiposity and insulin for developing insulin resistance syndrome (syndrome X) in young adulthood. The Bogalusa Heart Study. *Diabetes*, **51**, 204–9.

46. Berenson, G.S., Srinivasan, S.R., Bao, W. *et al.* (1998) Association between multiple cardiovascular risk factors and atherosclerosis in children and young adults. *New England Journal of Medicine*, **338**, 1650–8.

47. Daniels, S.R., Arnett, D.K., Eckel, R.H. *et al.* (2005) Overweight in children and adolescents: pathophysiology, consequences, prevention, and treatment. *Circulation*, **111**, 1999–2012.

48. Goodman, E., Daniels, S.R., Meigs, J.B. and Dolan, L.M. (2007) Instability in the diagnosis of metabolic syndrome in adolescents. *Circulation*, **115**, 2316–2322.

49. Eisenmann, J.C., Welk, G.J., Ihmels, M. and Dollman, J. (2007) Fatness, fitness, and cardiovascular disease risk factors in children and adolescents. *Medicine & Science in Sports & Exercise*, **39**, 1251–6.

50. Porter, R. and Barrett, T.G. (2004) Acquired non-type 1 diabetes in childhood: subtypes, diagnosis, and management. *Archives of Disease in Childhood*, **89**, 1138–44.

51. Kitagawa, T., Owada, M., Urakami, T. and Yamanchi, K. (1998) Increased incidence of non-insulin dependent diabetes mellitus among Japanese school-children correlates with an increased intake of animal protein and fat. *Clinical Paediatrics*, **37**, 111–16.

52. Urakami, T., Morimoto, S., Nitadori, Y. *et al.* (2007) Urine glucose screening program at schools in Japan to detect children with diabetes and its outcome-incidence and clinical characteristics of childhood type 2 diabetes in Japan. *Pediatric Research*, **61**, 141–45.

53. SEARCH for Diabetes in Youth Study Group, Liese, A.D., D'Agostino, R.B., Jr, Hamman, R.F. *et al.* (2006) The burden of diabetes mellitus among US youth: prevalence estimates from the SEARCH for Diabetes in Youth Study. *Pediatrics*, **118**, 1510–18.

54. Craig, M.E., Femia, G., Broyda, V. *et al.* (2007) Type 2 diabetes in indigenous and non-indigenous children and adolescents in New South Wales. *Medical Journal of Australia*, **186**, 497–9.

55. Haines, L., Wan, K.C., Lynn, R. *et al.* (2007) Rising Incidence of Type 2 Diabetes in Children in the U.K. *Diabetes Care*, **30**, 1097–101.

56. Yajnik, C.S., Lubree, H.G., Rege, S.S. *et al.* (2002) Adiposity and hyperinsulinaemia in Indians are present at birth. *Journal of Clinical Endocrinology and Metabolism*, **87**, 5575–80.

57. Bavdekar, A., Yajnik, C.S., Fall, C.H. *et al.* (1999) Insulin resistance syndrome in 8-year-old Indian children: small at birth, big at 8 years, or both? *Diabetes*, **48**, 2422–9.

58. Liska, D., Dufour, S., Zern, T.L. *et al.* (2007) Interethnic differences in muscle, liver and abdominal fat partitioning in obese adolescents. *PLoS One*, **2**, e569.

59. Amiel, S., Sherwin, R., Simonson, D. *et al.* (1986) Impaired insulin action in puberty: a contributing factor to poor glycaemic control in adolescents with diabetes. *New England Journal of Medicine*, **315**, 215–19.

60. Weiss, R., Taksali, S.E., Tamborlane, W.V. *et al.* (2005) Predictors of changes in glucose tolerance status in obese youth. *Diabetes Care*, **28**, 902–9.

61. Rodriguez-Moran, M. and Guerrero-Romero, F. (2006) Hyperinsulinemia in healthy children and adolescents with a positive family history for type 2 diabetes. *Pediatrics*, **118**, e1516–e1522.

62. Petersen, K.F., Dufour, S., Befroy, D. *et al.* (2004) Impaired mitochondrial activity in the insulin-resistant offspring of patients with type 2 diabetes. *New England Journal of Medicine*, **350**, 664–71.

63. Pinhas-Hamiel, O. and Zeitler, P. (2007) Acute and chronic complications of type 2 diabetes mellitus in children and adolescents. *Lancet*, **369**, 1823–31.

64. Fagot-Campagna, A., Knowler, W.C. and Pettit, D.J. (1998) Type 2 diabetes in Pima Indian children: cardiovascular risk factors at diagnosis and 10 years later. *Diabetes*, **47** (suppl), A155.

65. Yoo, E.G., Choi, I.K. and Kim, D.H. (2004) Prevalence of microalbuminuria in young patients with type 1 and type 2 diabetes mellitus. *Journal of Paediatric Endocrinology and Metabolism*, **17**, 1423–27.

66. Eppens, M.C., Craig, M.E., Cusumano, J. *et al.* (2006) Prevalence of diabetes complications in adolescents with type 2 compared with type 1 diabetes. *Diabetes Care*, **29**, 1300–1306.

67. Zdravkovic, V., Daneman, D. and Hamilton, J. (2004) Presentation and course of type 2 diabetes in youth in a large multi-ethnic city. *Diabetic Medicine*, **21**, 1144–8.

68. Kershnar, A.K., Daniels, S.R., Imperatore, G. *et al.* (2006) Lipid abnormalities are prevalent in youth with type 1 and type 2 diabetes: The search for diabetes in youth study. *Journal of Pediatrics*, **149**, 314–19.

69. Campbell, K., Waters, E., O'Meara, S. *et al.* (2002) Interventions for preventing obesity in children Cochrane Review, in *The Cochrane Library, Issue 4*, Update Software, Oxford.

70. Simonettei D'Arca, A., Tarsitani, G., Cairella, M. *et al.* (1986) Prevention of obesity in elementary and nursery school children. *Public Health*, **100**, 166–73.

71. Sahota, P., Rudolf, M.C.J., Dixey, R. *et al.* (2001) Randomised controlled trial of primary school based intervention to reduce risk factors for obesity. *British Medical Journal*, **323**, 1029–32.

72. Mueller, M.J., Asbeck, I., Mast, M. *et al.* (2001) Prevention of obesity – more than an intention. Concept and first results of the Kiel Obesity Prevention Study (KOPS). *International Journal of Obesity*, **25** (suppl 1), S66–S74.

73. Crawford, D. (2002) Population strategies to prevent obesity. *British Medical Journal*, **325**, 728–9.

74. Miller, L.A., Grunwald, G.K., Johnson, S.L. and Krebs, N.F. (2002) Disease severity at time of referral for paediatric failure to thrive and obesity: time for a paradigm shift? *Journal of Pediatrics*, **141**, 121–4.

75. Epstein, L.H., Myers, M.D., Raynor, H.A. and Saelens, B.E. (1998) Treatment of pediatric obesity. *Pediatrics*, **101**, 554–70.

76. Summerbell, C.D., Ashton, V., Campbell, K.J. *et al.* (2003) Interventions for treating obesity in children. *Cochrane Database of Systematic Reviews*, (3), Art. No.: CD001872. DOI: 10.1002/14651858.CD001872.

77. Flodmark, C.E., Ohlsson, T., Ryden, O. and Sveger, T. (1993) Prevention of progression to severe obesity in a group of obese schoolchildren treated with family therapy. *Pediatrics*, **91**, 880–4.

78. Epstein, L.H., Wing, R.R., Penner, B.C. and Kress, M.J. (1985) Effect of diet and controlled exercise on weight loss in obese children. *Journal of Pediatrics*, **107**, 358–61.

79. Epstein, L.H., Wing, R.R., Koeske, R. and Valoski, A. (1985) A comparison of lifestyle exercise, aerobic exercise and callisthenics on weight loss in obese children. *Behaviour Therapy*, **16**, 345–56.

80. Warschburger, P., Fromme, C., Petermann, F. *et al.* (2001) Conceptualisation and evaluation of a cognitive-behavioural training programme for children and adolescents with obesity. *International Journal of Obesity*, **25** (suppl 1), S93–S95.

81. Duffy, G. and Spence, S.H. (1993) The effectiveness of cognitive self management as an adjunct to a behavioural intervention for childhood obesity: a research note. *Journal of Child Psychology and Psychiatry*, **34**, 1043–50.

82. Epstein, L.H., Wing, R.R., Woodall, K. *et al.* (1985) Effects of family-based behavioural treatment on obese 5–8 year old children. *Behaviour Therapy*, **16**, 205–12.

83. Senediak, C. and Spence, S.H. (1985) Rapid versus gradual scheduling of therapeutic contact in a family based behavioural weight control programme for children. *Behaviour Psychotherapy*, **13**, 265–87.

84. Krebs, J.D., Evans, S., Cooney, L. *et al.* (2002) Changes in risk factors for cardiovascular disease with body fat loss in obese women. *Diabetes, Obesity & Metabolism*, **4**, 379–87.

85. Tuomilehto, J., Lindstrom, J., Eriksson, J.G. *et al.* (2001) Prevention of type 2 diabetes mellitus by changes in lifestyle among subjects with impaired glucose tolerance. *New England Journal of Medicine*, **344**, 1343–50.

86. Diabetes Prevention Program Research Group (2002) Reduction in the incidence of Type 2 diabetes with lifestyle intervention or metformin. *New England Journal of Medicine*, **346**, 393–403.

87. Chanoine, J.P., Hampl, S., Jensen, C. *et al.* (2005) Effect of orlistat on weight and body composition in obese adolescents: a randomized controlled trial. *Journal of the American Medical Association*, **293**, 2873–83.

88. Berkowitz, R.I., Fujioka, K., Daniels, S.R. *et al.* Sibutramine Adolescent Study Group (2006) Effects of sibutramine treatment in obese adolescents: a randomized trial. *Annals of Internal Medicine*, **145**, 81–90.

89. Buchwald *et al.* (2004) Bariatric surgery: a systematic review and meta-analysis. *Journal of the American Medical Association*, **292**, 1724–37.

90. Lawson, M.L., Kirk, S., Mitchell, T. *et al.* Pediatric Bariatric Study Group (2006) One-year outcomes of Roux-en-Y gastric bypass for morbidly obese adolescents: a multicenter study from the Pediatric Bariatric Study Group. *Journal of Pediatric Surgery*, **41**, 137–43.

91. American Diabetes Association (2000) Type 2 diabetes in children and adolescents. *Diabetes Care*, **23**, 381–9.

92. Jones, K.L., Arslanian, S., Peterokova, V.A. *et al.* (2002) Effect of metformin in pediatric patients with type 2 diabetes: a randomized controlled trial. *Diabetes Care*, **25**, 89–94.

93. The TODAY Study Group, Zeitler, P., Epstein, L., Grey, M. *et al.* (2007) Treatment options for type 2 diabetes in adolescents and youth: a study of the comparative efficacy of metformin alone or in combination with rosiglitazone or lifestyle intervention in adolescents with type 2 diabetes. *Pediatric Diabetes*, **8**, 74–87.

94. Skinner, A.C., Schlundt, D., Weinberger, M. *et al.* (2008) Accuracy of perceptions of overweight and relation to self-care behaviours among adolescents with Type 2 diabetes and their parents. *Diabetes Care*, **31**, 227–9.

95. Herder, C., Schmitz-Beuting, C., Rathmann, W. *et al.* (2007) Prevalence of impaired glucose regulation in German school-leaving students. *International Journal of Obesity*, **31**, 1086–8.

96. Uckun-Kitapci, A., Tezic, T., Firat, S. *et al.* (2004) Calikolu AS. Obesity and type 2 diabetes mellitus: a population-based study of adolescents. *Journal of Pediatric Endocrinology*, **17**, 1633–40.

97. Wei, J.-N., Sung, F.-C., Lin, C.-C. *et al.* (2003) National Surveillance for Type 2 Diabetes Mellitus in Taiwanese Children. *Journal of the American Medical Association*, **290**, 1345–50.

98. Mazza, C.S., Ozuna, B., Krochik, A.G. and Araujo, M.B. (2005) Prevalence of type 2 diabetes mellitus and impaired glucose tolerance in obese Argentinean children and adolescents. *Journal of Pediatric Endocrinology*, **18**, 491–8.

99. Wabitsch, M., Hauner, H., Hertrampf, M. *et al.* (2004) Type II diabetes mellitus and impaired glucose regulation in Caucasian children and adolescents with obesity living in Germany. *International Journal of Obesity & Related Metabolic Disorders*, **28**, 307–313.

100. McMahon, S.K., Haynes, A., Ratnam, N. *et al.* (2004) Increase in type 2 diabetes in children and adolescents in Western Australia. *Medical Journal of Australia*, **180**, 459–61.

101. Rami, B., Schober, E., Nachbauer, E., Waldhor, T., Austrian Diabetes Incidence Study Group (2003) Type 2 diabetes mellitus is rare but not absent in children under 15 years of age in Austria. *European Journal of Pediatrics*, **162**, 850–2.

102. Moore, K.R., Harwell, T.S., McDowall, J.M. *et al.* (2003) Three-year prevalence and incidence of diabetes among American Indian youth in Montana and Wyoming, 1999 to 2001. *Journal of Pediatrics*, **143**, 368–71.

103. Huen, K.F., Low, L.C., Wong, G.W. *et al.* (2000) Epidemiology of diabetes mellitus in children in Hong Kong: the Hong Kong childhood diabetes register. *Journal of Pediatric Endocrinology*, **13**, 297–302.

104. Fagot-Campagna, A., Saaddine, J.B., Flegal, K.M. and Beckles, G.L.A. (2001) Diabetes, impaired fasting glucose, and elevated HbA1c in US adolescents: the Third National Health and Nutrition Examination Survey. *Diabetes Care*, **24**, 834–7.

13

Obesity and PCOS

Diana Raskauskiene and Richard N. Clayton
Department of Endocrinology, School of Medicine, Keele University, Stoke-on-Trent, UK

13.1 Definition of the syndrome

Polycystic ovary syndrome (PCOS) is the most [1] commonly diagnosed female endocrinopathy and it is the commonest cause of anovulatory infertility affecting about 5% of women in the reproductive age group [2]. It is considered to be a syndrome not a disease that manifests with heterogeneous clinical features. The most common features of PCOS are irregular menstrual cycles (oligomenorrhoea or amenorrhoea leading to chronic anovulation and subfertility), and signs of androgen excess (hirsutism, acne, alopecia). Obesity is a frequent accompaniament although not a diagnostic criterion. The diagnosis of PCOS is problematic as there are three differing sets of criteria following those from the 1990 NIH-NICHHD (National Institutes of Health – National Institutes of Child Health and Human Development) conference: ovulatory dysfunction, clinical evidence of hyperandrogenism and/or hyperandrogenaemia and exclusion of related disorders such as congenital adrenal hyperplasia, hyperprolactinaemia, or Cushing's syndrome [3]. These were North American criteria and did not include the morphological appearance of the ovaries, which is surprising since the original description of the syndrome by Stein & Leventhal included anatomical criteria. European and Australasian groups have always allowed morphological appearance of the ovary as one criterion and this has been formalized at a consensus meeting of the European Society for Human Reproduction and the American Society for Reproductive Medicine, known as the Rotterdam criteria [4]. The Androgen Excess Society has also defined the syndrome [5] attempting to integrate the NIH and Rotterdam criteria. Table 13.1 shows the three sets of criteria. However, the presence of polycystic ovaries on ultrasound scan, which is defined by presence of eight or more subcapsular follicular cysts ≤ 10 mm in diameter and increased ovarian stroma, in the absence of other clinical features is not sufficient alone to diagnose PCOS. Polycystic ovaries are present in

Obesity and Diabetes, Second Edition   Edited by Anthony H. Barnett and Sudhesh Kumar
© 2009 John Wiley & Sons, Ltd

Table 13.1 Criteria for diagnosis of PCOS

NIH (1990): includes all of the following
1. Hyperandrogenism and/or hyperandrogenaemia
2. Oligo-ovulation
3. Exclusion of 'secondary' causes
ESHRE/ARMS: to include two of the following plus exclusion of 'secondary' [2] disorders
1. Oligo-anovulation
2. Clinical and/or biochemical signs of hyperandrogenism
3. Polycystic ovaries.
Androgen Excess Society: to include all of the following (2006)
1. Hirsuitism and/or hyperandrogenaemia
2. Oligo-anovulation and/or polycystic ovaries
3. Exclusion of 'secondary' disorders

ESHRE/ARMS, European Society for Human Reproduction and the American Society for Reproductive Medicine.

20–25% of randomly selected women with little or no clinical features [6]. Thus, this feature is neither sufficient nor necessary to make the clinical diagnosis of PCOS. It is evident that data from studies adopting different sets of diagnostic criteria will be difficult to compare because of the considerable patient heterogeneity both within and between studies. The problems this poses for clinical practice and research have been highlighted by Barth *et al.* [7]. These authors highlight the imprecision in definition of clinical hyperandrogenism; its poor validation, dubious reproducibility, and considerable subjectivity. Biochemical hyperandrogenism is even more imprecise as numerous physiological and analytical factors influence serum testosterone levels, the only androgen worth measuring is serum total testosterone. Ascertainment of chronic anovulation is less contentious based on careful menstrual history and serum progesterone values. Even the morphological diagnosis of polycystic ovaries on ultrasound is highly observer dependent with only 50% consensus between observers. Barth *et al.* [7] propose that definitions are more precisely defined so that studies can be reliably compared. Thus meaningful conclusions about the epidemiology, pathophysiology and long-term consequences of 'PCOS', particularly in the context of metabolic and vascular sequelae as discussed in this chapter should be regarded as preliminary.

Two recent studies have subdivided PCOS cohorts according to the Rotterdam criteria, producing greater homogeneity within groups. At one end of the spectrum is the 'classic' PCOS phenotype of PCO morphology, hyperandrogenism and anovulation, at the other end PCO morphology with menstrual irregularity and no features of hyperandrogenism. The subgroup with classic PCOS were the most obese, most insulin resistant and had highest androgen levels, even after accounting for the obesity. Those at the 'mild' end of the spectrum had androgen levels and metabolic profile no different from controls. The group with hyperandrogenism, PCO, but normal ovulation lay in between the other subgroups [8,9]. In the Boston study only the subgroup with the classic PCOS phenotype had an increased frequency of metabolic syndrome (approx 25% of patients). These studies reinforce the importance of clear patient stratification for genetic and epidemiological long-term risk studies. Moreover, the effect of body mass index (BMI) as a/the major determinant of clinical manifestations is reemphasized.

13.2 Genetics of PCOS

Several studies have suggested that PCOS is a familiar disorder and various features of the syndrome may be differentially inherited [10]. It is further suggested that the morphological appearance of polycystic ovaries is inherited as an autosomal dominant trait, though no single gene has been identified as causal. However, the heterogeneous clinical characteristics of this syndrome indicate the complex interaction between genetic and environmental factors to be causal [11]. Several approaches have been adopted in the search for genetic predisposition markers. These fall into two broad categories: (1) family linkage analysis studies, though here there is an inherent problem in not being able to assign a robust male phenotype. The most useful approach here is the sib-pair analysis; (2) association studies comparing cases and controls for association with polymorphisms in 'candidate' genes. The list of candidate genes examined is long and includes those involved in insulin secretion and action, obesity, gonadotrophins and receptors, steroidogenic enzymes, sex hormone binding globulin (SHBG) and other ovarian proteins. There is poor reproducibility between these many studies due to small numbers and patient heterogeneity. The limitations for both approaches has been highlighted by Menke and Strauss [12].

The latest studies with large cohorts of patients defined by the old NIH criteria of anovulation and hyperandrogenaemia performed linkage analysis in families and sib-pair analysis. Linkage was established to a region of chromosome 19 and association with fibrillin, a glycoprotein associated with transforming growth factor-β signalling is proposed. Fibrillin 3 is found in ovarian stroma. In one study [13] there was association of the chromosome 19 variant with markers of insulin resistance raising the possibility of a common genetic susceptibility between PCOS and weight gain. The relative contribution of genetic predisposition and environmental factors to development of the PCOS phenotype is still unclear. Thus, one can imagine the scenario of a slim young woman with genetic predisposition to polycystic ovary morphology who gains weight, especially central adiposity, progressing from little/no clinical manifestations to the full-blown picture of PCOS. The challenge is to develop a simple way of identifying such women so as to target preventative measures to this cohort.

Because most women, both lean and obese, have evidence of insulin resistance early genetic studies focussed on genes involved in insulin secretion and action. Molecular studies of the insulin receptor gene in women with PCOS have not shown linkage to distinct polymorphisms or functional mutations in the gene leading to any disturbance of receptor function [14]. The observation that insulin resistance is reversible by weight reduction in obese women with PCOS led to investigation of the insulin gene in the pathogenesis of PCOS. Waterworth *et al.* [15] reported an association between PCOS and allelic variation at the INS VNTR (insulin gene variable number of tandem repeats) locus in three different populations. They showed that class III alleles and especially

III/III genotypes are associated with PCOS and are most strongly associated with anovulatory PCOS. The group of women with one or two class III alleles had significantly higher fasting insulin levels and higher mean body mass index than women with I/I genotype [15]. Since there is evidence that insulin gene VNTR class III alleles were found to be associated with type 2 diabetes, the conclusion was that this genotype can be related to anovulatory PCOS as well as the concomitant risk for development of type 2 diabetes mellitus [16]. Recently it was confirmed that among women with polycystic ovaries, increasing severity of clinical phenotype was associated with decreasing insulin sensitivity and related to paternally transmitted insulin gene VNTR class III alleles [17]. Despite these encouraging early data there are no confirmatory reports so allelic variation in the insulin gene does not seem to be the link between insulin resistance and PCOS.

There is increasing evidence for genetic predisposition to obesity in the general population. Studies in adopted children showed a strong correlation between weight classes and BMI of the biological parents, but no correlation with the BMI of their adoptive parents [18]. Genetic factors are estimated to explain 30–50% of the heritability of obesity. The human obesity map is now very complex and expanding, with full details from the 2005 update found in Rankinen *et al.* [19].

13.3   Scope of the chapter

Obesity is a feature in between 35 and 60% of women with PCOS and associated with a greater severity of clinical manifestations than non-obese women with the syndrome. Increased insulin resistance (IR) is a cardinal feature of obesity and overweight in PCOS and may play a pathogenetic role [20]. Present data strongly support an association between PCOS and several long-term diseases such as type 2 diabetes, dyslipidaemia, hypertension and cardiovascular disease risk. This emphasizes the need for early diagnosis of the syndrome and adequate treatment strategies.

This review will analyse pathogenetic mechanisms underlying the relationship between obesity and PCOS, survey clinical features of obese women with the syndrome and their management.

13.4   Pathogenetic mechanisms underlying the relationship between obesity and PCOS (Table 13.2)

Insulin/insulin resistance

The observation of insulin resistance and hyperinsulinaemia in a subset of women with PCOS has added a new dimension to the understanding of the pathogenesis of PCOS, as well as recognition that the syndrome has substantial metabolic as well as reproductive implications. Burghen *et al.* first reported the presence of hyperinsulinaemia in a group

Table 13.2 Main pathogenic mechanisms in PCOS

Genetic predisposition	Familial clustering of syndrome PCO morphology may be inherited in autosomal dominant manner
Abnormal feedback/regulation of gonadotrophin secretion	Altered GnRH pulse frequency/amplitude
	Increased bio/immuno ratio of LH chronic hyperoestrogenaemia inhibits FSH secretion
Increased androgen production	Increased ovarian response to LH (dysregulation of 17–20 lyase) Increased adrenal androgens (11b hydroxysteroid dehydrogenase Dysregulation leading to ACTH) High intraovarian androgens inhibit folliculogenesis
Insulin resistance/ hyperinsulinaemia	Amplifies LH-stimulated androgen production in ovary and ACTH action in adrenals Reduces SHBG levels leading to high free androgen index Associated with metabolic complications, and dyslipidaemia

of obese PCOS subjects and showed significant correlation with raised serum testosterone, androstendione and insulin [21]. Since then, there have been many reports confirming the presence of insulin resistance and consequent hyperinsulinaemia in obese and non-obese subjects with PCOS. Studies have demonstrated insulin resistance in PCOS unrelated to body weight and composition, though obese PCOS women have consistently been shown to have a greater degree of insulin resistance compared to weight-matched control. Interestingly, euglycemic glucose clamp studies have shown significant and substantial decreases ($\sim$35–40%) in insulin-mediated glucose disposal in PCOS which is of similar magnitude to that to seen in patients with type 2 diabetes [22,23]. As mentioned above, insulin resistance is consistently accompanied by hyperinsulinaemia. Barbieri *et al.* first reported the effect of insulin and insulin-like growth factors on ovarian androgen production in ovarian tissue obtained from hyperandrogenic and normal cycling women [24]. At the ovarian level, insulin is able to stimulate steroidogenesis both in granulosa and thecal cells by increasing 17α-hydroxylase and 17–20 lyase activity (both components of the P450c17 enzyme system) [25] and stimulates the expression of 3β-hydroxysteroid dehydrogenase in human luteinized granulosa cells [26]. In addition, insulin appears to increase the sensitivity of pituitary gonadotropes to gonadotropin releasing hormone (GnRH) action and potentiate the ovarian steroidogenic response to gonadotropins, by mechanisms probably related to an increase of the luteinizing hormone (LH) receptor number [27]. It has been shown that insulin lowers SHBG levels thus increasing the circulating, biologically available, androgens particularly free testosterone which by inhibiting follicular maturation, may initiate the sequence of events leading to PCOS [28]. Moreover, insulin is able to inhibit both hepatic and ovarian IGF binding protein-1

(IGFBP-1) to regulate ovarian growth and cyst formation [29]. *In vitro* studies have shown that insulin may also increase 17α-hydroxylase and 17–20 lyase activity in the adrenal gland directly [30] or potentiates the responsivity of the enzymes to adrenocorticotropic hormone (ACTH) stimulation [31].

Some aspects of insulin action in obesity are similar to those seen in PCOS. Obesity, especially the abdominal type of the disorder, has a strong relationship to insulin resistance and hyperinsulinaemia. The mechanisms by which obesity may induce insulin resistance have being extensively investigated over last two decades. To sum up, enlargement of adipose tissue increases availability of several metabolites such as free fatty acids, lactate, which can affect insulin secretion and its peripherial action [32]. Obesity can be related to insulin resistance by increased production of leptin and tumour necrosis factor-α (TNF-α) in adipose tissue. TNF mediates serine phosphorylation of insulin receptor substrate-1, which then interferes with insulin action by inhibiting insulin receptor and type 1 IGF receptor tyrosine kinases and by stimulating IGF binding protein production [33]. TNF can also inhibit signalling through peroxisome proliferator-activated receptor-γ (PPAR-γ). Leptin may contribute to insulin resistance of obesity via mechanisms similar to TNF [34]. Therefore obesity is an important factor, and it appears that this has a more pronounced effect on insulin action in PCOS than in control women. In PCOS women the degree of insulin resistance and hyperinsulinaemia is greater than accounted for by obesity alone [35].

Growth hormone/IGF

Abnormalities of growth hormone (GH) secretion and/or altered IGF-I concentrations may play a pathogenetic role in PCOS as *in vitro* and *in vivo* evidence supports a stimulatory role of GH in early and later stages of folliculogenesis and ovulation [36]. Therefore reduced GH secretion may contribute to impaired follicular development and anovulation in PCOS. Abdominal obesity, which can exacerbate insulin resistance and reproductive features of the PCOS, is associated with profoundly reduced and disorderly GH secretion [37]. Plasma GH concentrations in PCOS have been reported as reduced, normal or increased [38]. The majority of studies in PCOS have evaluated the status of the somatotropic axis on the basis of acute secretagogue-stimulated GH release and reported a blunted GH response in women with PCOS compared with weight-matched controls [39,40]. Recently a profound reduction of daily basal (62%) and pulsatile (76%) GH release in obese women with PCOS compared to healthy lean controls was reported but none of these parameters differed from those in the BMI-matched controls. Total GH secretion in obese PCOS, lean and obese control women correlated strongly and negatively with percent body fat. The conclusion is therefore that altered GH secretory dynamics are related to obesity and *not* PCOS *per se*.

The effects of IGF-I and IGF-II on ovarian function are well known. They exert their action through activation of two types of receptors, I and II, which are present in granulosa, thecal and stromal cells of ovary [38]. Both IGFs are able to stimulate ovarian progesterone and oestradiol secretion and increase aromatase activity and androgen production in granulosa-luteal and thecal cells [41]. Activation of IGF receptors has also been associated with a reduction of IGF binding proteins which may be related to an increase bioavailability of IGF. Insulin regulates IGF and IGF binding proteins system by increasing number of IGF type I receptors and by inhibiting IGF binding protein-I production. Thus, hyperinsulinemia may lead to a self-perpetuating cycle of events resulting in exaggeration of the effects of both insulin and IGF at an ovarian level. No differences in serum IGF-I and IGF-II levels between PCOS and control women have been found, regardless of body weight, but obese PCOS women have lower serum IGF binding protein-1 level than lean PCOS. This probably represents an insulin-related effect, as a negative correlation between insulin and IGF binding protein-1 has been found [27].

In summary, IGF-I and IGF-II may be involved in the pathogenesis of hyperandrogenism in the PCOS. In normal-weight PCOS women IGF biovailability seems to be increased by various mechanisms such as insulin-induced hepatic and ovary IGF binding protein-1 suppression and GH-induced stimulation [43]. Conversely, in obese PCOS IGF-1 biovailability seems to be reduced in comparison to normal-weight PCOS but relatively higher than in non-affected women because of combination of low GH and high insulin level. Therefore IGF/IGF binding protein system in obese PCOS women seems to be differently expressed compared to normal-weight PCOS, suggesting a different pathogenetic impact.

SHBG

SHBG is a glycoprotein produced in the liver as a carrier for different sex hormones with high binding affinity for testosterone and dihydrotestosterone (DHT) and a lower affinity for oestradiol [44]. The concentrations of SHBG are stimulated by various factors such as oestrogens, cortisol, iodothyronines and GH, and decreased by androgens, insulin, prolactin and IGF-I. Decreased basal concentrations are detected in PCOS, with a more significant reduction in obese PCOS, and insulin is thought to lower serum SHBG levels by acting directly to reduce hepatic SHBG synthesis. An inverse correlation between insulin sensitivity and free testosterone index in obese PCOS has been found and it is probably secondary to the inverse correlation of SHBG and serum insulin. Furthermore, a significant inverse correlation of SHBG with BMI in both obese PCOS and obese controls also was shown. This indicates that hyperinsulinaemia in obese PCOS lowers the SHBG levels and hence enhances the expression of hyperandrogenaemia [28]. Recently, a prospective study has proposed that measurement of serum SHBG concentration is useful and adequate to identify women with PCOS. They even proposed threshold SHBG level <37 nmol/l which had a sensitivity of 87.5%, a specificity of 86.8%, a positive likelihood ratio 6.63 and negative likelihood ratio 0.14 for the diagnosis of PCOS [45]. In summary, obesity may directly worsen hyperandrogenism in women with PCOS by reducing SHBG concentration and therefore increasing levels of free androgens.

Androgens

Polycystic ovary syndrome is characterized by chronic anovulation. Raised androgens (testosterone and/or androstendione) is the most consistent biochemical abnormality in PCOS. This supports the hypothesis that, despite the multifactoral and multiorgan nature of the syndrome, it appears that an underlying disorder in androgen biosynthesis or metabolism may be the central event suppressing ovarian folliculogenesis and giving rise to the disorder. The exact nature of this abnormality in androgen secretion/metabolism is however still unknown. An important stage of androgen synthesis is activity of the P450c17 enzyme, which is located in the ovarian theca-interstitial cells and in the adrenal zona reticularis. Expression and activation of the P450c17 gene in ovary and/or adrenal cortex is regulated by a number of hormones and growth factors such as LH, ACTH, insulin and IGF. Hyperactivity of P450c17 enzyme represents a major mechanism leading to ovarian hyperandrogenism [46]. Whether hyperactivity of the P450c17 enzyme system is a primary event or secondary to other central or peripheral factors is unclear. Interestingly, phosphorylation of serine residues of the insulin receptor, which may be a factor leading to insulin resistance and compensatory hyperinsulinaemia in PCOS has been suggested as increasing the activity of the P450c17 enzyme system. Therefore, the serine phosphorylation of both the P450c17 enzymes and the insulin receptor may represent a single primary disorder which could explain the association between insulin resistance and hyperandrogenism in women with PCOS [20].

Other factors, such as the follicule stimulating hormone (FSH)-inducible inhibin–follistatin–activin system, produced by the granulosa cell acting on the theca cell, may be implicated in the dysregulation of ovarian steroidogenesis in PCOS because some *in vitro* studies have demonstrated that inhibin stimulates ovarian androgen production [47].

Increased secretion of androgens by the adrenal often coexists with ovarian hyperandrogenism. The secretion of dehydroepiandrosterone sulfate, an exclusive adrenal steroid, is increased in up to 50% of subjects with PCOS, both basally and in response to ACTH. As adrenal androgen production is ACTH dependent, central factors may induce a pituitary hyper-responsiveness to corticotropin releasing hormone. Several peripheral factors have been considered as enhancing adrenal androgen production. As was mentioned, insulin may increase the activity of 17α-hydroxylase and 17–20 lyase in the adrenal both directly and through ACTH stimulation. Interleukin-6 has also been proposed to modulate intra-adrenal steroidogenesis by the ability of this cytokine to increase dehydroepiandrostenedione secretion [48]. Rodin *et al.* demonstrated dysregulation of 11β hydroxysteroid dehydrogenase, either primary or secondary, leading to increased ACTH-stimulated androgen production in some women with PCOS [49]. The increased oxidation of cortisol to cortisone (an inactive metabolite) in PCOS may result in compensatory overstimulation of the hypothalamic–pituitary–adrenal axis, which can lead to increased adrenal androgen secretion. Similar altered cortisol metabolism has been reported in obese patients [50]. Obesity especially abdominal type of the disorder seems to amplify the degree of hyperandrogenism in PCOS. Previous studies reported that obese PCOS women have higher total and free testosterone levels compared with non-obese PCOS [51].

Hyperandrogenism per se may enhance insulin resistance and lead to hyperinsulinemia which plays a role in development of abdominal type of obesity in PCOS women. In fact, androgens may induce insulin resistance through the activation of the lipolytic cascade, leading to increase free fatty acid release and this phenomenon has been mainly observed in the visceral fat depot due to the high androgen receptor density present at this site [52].

Oestrogens

Elevated levels of oestrone and of free oestradiol have been detected in women with PCOS and it may be a result of reduced concentration of SHBG. Moreover, since androstendione is aromatized to oestrone in fat tissue, this is more marked in obese PCOS subjects. Therefore PCOS women are not oestrogen deficient, rather oestrogen replete and are not at risk of osteoporosis despite oligo/amenorrhoea. Increased oestrogen concentrations may lead to positive feedback on LH secretion and a negative feedback on FSH secretion and therefore may impact on the LH/FSH ratio. The elevated levels of LH substantially contribute to the development of hyperplasia of the ovarian stroma and thecal cells, further increasing androgen production and in turn providing more substrate for extraglandular aromatization and chronic anovulation. Obesity is a condition of hyperoestrogenaemia and oestrogen production correlates with body weight and amount of body fat [53]. Oestrogen metabolism is also altered in obese women. There is less formation of inactive oestradiol metabolites, such as 2-hydroxyoestrogens, and a higher production of oestrone sulphate, with concomitant increase in active oestrogens levels in obese women [54].

Neuroendocrine factors

Perturbations of gonadotropin secretion are one of the hallmarks of PCOS. The most commonly described abnormality is an elevated serum LH or an elevated LH/FSH ratio, an increased LH pulse frequency and increased LH pulse amplitude, an exaggerated response of LH to GnRH, and altered diurnal LH pulse frequency [54,55]. However, serum LH levels may be normal in up to 40% of women with PCOS [56]. On the other hand, Lobo et al. reported that bioactive/immunoreactive LH ratio is elevated in PCOS which means that increased LH bioactivity may be responsible for enhanced androgen production in the ovary of women with the syndrome [57]. It is a matter of debate whether the increase of gonadotropins, when present, is a primary abnormality of the hypothalamic–pituitary axis or the cause is dysregulation of the feedback signalling. Recent studies have revealed decreased sensitivity of the GnRH pulse generator to inhibition by ovarian steroids, particularly progesterone. This abnormality is reversed by the androgen receptor antagonist flutamide, suggesting that elevated androgen levels may alter the sensitivity of the hypothalamic GnRH pulse generator to steroid inhibition and lead to enhanced LH secretion. As such, women with PCOS require higher levels of progesterone to slow the frequency of GnRH pulsatility, resulting in inadequate FSH synthesis and persistent LH stimulation of ovarian androgens [58]. In fact, both spontaneous ovulation or exogenous progesterone administration are associated with normalization of LH secretion in PCOS women [55]. Obesity may to some extent exaggerate the abnormal LH secretory pattern. A negative correlation between LH and body weight in PCOS has been found and obese PCOS women are characterized by significantly lower LH concentrations than non-obese PCOS women. Interestingly, in very obese PCOS women LH concentrations frequently resemble the normal range [59]. Potential factors involved in the different LH secretion between obese and non-obese PCOS women may be elevated insulin concentrations, since significant correlations between LH and insulin has been found in PCOS women.

Dietary factors

There are theoretical possibilities that dietary composition may play a role in the development of the obesity in PCOS since there are data suggesting that women eating vegetarian-rich and fibre-rich diet may have lower serum androgen concentrations compared to those following typical Western diets [60]. Moreover, a very high lipid intake has been described in PCOS and significant negative correlation has been found between lipid intake and SHBG values [61].

13.5   Clinical features of obese PCOS women

Metabolic abnormalities

Insulin resistance/impaired beta-cell function

PCOS is characterized by several metabolic abnormalities, which are strongly influenced by presence of obesity. Insulin resistance is a common co-morbidity in women with PCOS and is associated with increased risk for hypertension and cardiovascular disease. Studies have shown that 25–35% of obese women with PCOS, by 30 yr of age, will have either impaired glucose tolerance or type 2 diabetes [62]. The studies examining insulin resistance in obese and non-obese women with PCOS have shown that obese PCOS women had significantly lower insulin sensitivity than non-obese women with PCOS. On the other hand, non-obese women with PCOS may demonstrate insulin resistance in the presence of completely normal glucose tolerance. Nevertheless, both fasting and glucose-stimulated insulin concentrations are in fact significantly higher in obese than non-obese PCOS women [63]. Acanthosis nigricans (AN) is a common sign of severe insulin resistance and often occurs in patients with insulin receptor defects. Mild to moderate AN is commonly present in obese PCOS women, but it is not a clinical feature of non-obese counterparts. Moreover, it has been shown that there is no significant difference in prevalence of AN in obese PCOS women compared with weight-matched controls [64].

The percentage of obese women with PCOS is high and this subgroup of PCOS affected women is characterized by increased prevalence of glucose intolerance ranging from 20 to 40%. In contrast, impaired glucose tolerance in non-obese women with PCOS has been found only occasionally, consistent with the synergistic negative effect of obesity and PCOS on glucose tolerance [20]. It has been reported that postmenopausal women with history of PCOS has a 15% prevalence of type 2 diabetes which is much higher than in the general population [65]. In the presence of peripheral insulin resistance, pancreatic beta cell insulin secretion increases but impaired glucose tolerance and type 2 diabetes mellitus develops when the compensatory increase in insulin secretion is no longer able to maintain euglycaemia. Ehrmann *et al.* recently documented that insulin secretory dysfunction in women with PCOS contributed significantly to the observed glucose intolerance with up to 40% of women demonstrating either IGT or type 2 diabetes mellitus [66]. Norman *et al.* performed a follow-up study of women with PCOS seeking to establish the frequency of change of IGT and type 2 diabetes over an average period of 6.2 years. They reported 9% of normoglycaemic women at baseline developed IGT and 8% were diagnosed having diabetes, and 54% of women with IGT at baseline had diabetes at follow-up. In the group converting to IGT or diabetes, there was significantly greater BMI, weight, waist circumference and waist–hip ratio gain compared with those who remained normoglycaemic [67]. This observation may indicate that obesity and further weight gain play a crucial role in developing IGT and diabetes in PCOS.

Dyslipidaemia and vascular risk

Women with PCOS would be predicted to be the high risk for dyslipidaemia because they are often obese and have elevated androgen levels [68]. Moreover, insulin resistance and hyperinsulinaemia tend to increase risks for dyslipidaemia associated with insulin resistance. A number of studies have shown that obese women with PCOS have lower high-density lipoprotein (HDL) and/or HDL2 levels as well as higher levels of cholesterol, triglyceride, apolipoprotein B and free fatty acids than their lean counterparts and BMI proved to be the best predictor of these alterations on multiple regression analysis [69,70]. The largest study (557 pts vs. 295 controls), using the Rotterdam criteria for definition, reports higher total cholesterol and LDL levels and lower HDL and apolipoprotein A1 levels in PCOS women after correction for age and BMI [71]. Both PCOS and hyperandrogenism were independent determinants of the differences, with the obese hyperandrogenic subgroup having the most adverse lipid profile. It has also been reported that PCOS women have higher concentration and proportion of small, dense low density lipoprotein (LDL III) cholesterol [72,73]. These findings indicate that women with PCOS accompanied by increased concentration of LDL III are at increased risk for cardiovascular morbidity and mortality, independent of total LDL concentration [74]. PCOS women also have impaired fibrinolytic activity with significantly increased tissue plasminogen activator antigen (t-PA) compared to weight-matched control women and t-PA correlated with BMI and inversely correlated with insulin sensitivity index in both PCOS and controls. These findings suggest that elevated t-PA and dysfibrinolysis may be a factor in increased cardiovascular morbidity seen in PCOS [75].

The largest retrospective survey of PCOS in the UK [76] could not confirm an increased mortality and morbidity from coronary heart disease among women with PCOS. One explanation might be that the number of deaths was quite small (70 out of 700) and longer follow-up might be required to show the effects of increased vascular risk factor prevalence on mortality. Nevertheless, even this study has confirmed that women with PCOS had higher levels of several cardiovascular risk factors such as diabetes, hypertension, hypercholesterolaemia, hypertriglyceridaemia and increased waist–hip ratio and more prevalent history of cerebrovascular disease [76]. Neverthe-less, there are no prospective studies showing an increase in coronary events in PCOS women. The best evidence for a link between PCOS and vascular mortality is indirect and comes from a cohort study of 82 439 nurses in USA followed up for 14 years. Solomon and colleagues [77] found that women who had usually irregular menses or very irregular menses at age 20–35 had an age-adjusted relative risk for CHD end points of 1.25–1.67 compared to women with regular menses. In the subgroup with very irregular menses the relative risk was 1.5 after adjustment for BMI, age, smoking, parity and menopausal status. The same authors [78] reported a twofold increased risk of type 2 diabetes in the Nurses Health Study 2 in women with very irregular menses, again BMI adjusted. Given that the most common cause of very irregular menses in young women is PCOS these data provide indirect evidence for a link between PCOS and increased vascular events.

Other studies have investigated subclinical atherosclerosis among women with PCOS by ultrasound examination of carotid arteries. A significantly higher mean carotid intima-media wall thickness (IMT) and plaque number has been shown in affected women compared to controls. It has also been shown that in the total cohort and in the age group <45 years several cardiovascular risk factors such as age, BMI, blood pressure, waist–hip ratio, and triglycerides are significantly associated with IMT. Conversely, in women ≥45 years old PCOS was a highly significant predictor of IMT but BMI, LDL, insulin, systolic blood pressure, and triglycerides were also significant predictors [79]. Recently another study investigated macrovascular and microvascular function in PCOS women. Pulse wave velocity (PWV) at the level of the brachial artery was found to be significant elevated in the PCOS group but PWV measured in the aorta did not differ from controls. Microvascular function was studied by wire myography, by measuring the concentration responses to norepinephrine (noradrenaline, NE) before and after incubation with insulin (100 and 1000 pM). In vessels from control subjects, insulin reduced the contraction response to NE but there was no change in maximum contraction in the PCOS group using different doses of insulin. This study demonstrated an increased vascular stiffness and a functional defect in the vascular action of the insulin *ex vivo* in patients with PCOS [80].

Direct assessment of coronary atherosclerosis is provided by coronary artery calcification (CAC)scores that detect calcification in atheromatous plaques. CAC is an independent predictor of all cause mortality in asymptomatic subjects after controlling for age, gender, ethnicity and cardiac risk factors [81]. CAC shows increased prevalence in PCOS women compared to controls [82–84]. Although the age ranges of women varied in these studies that of Shroff *et al.* comprised the youngest (mean age 32 years) all with BMI >30 and demonstrated a fivefold higher prevalence of CAC in patients (33% vs. 8%). This could not be accounted for by increase in traditional cardiovascular disease risk factors, measures of insulin resistance, or body fat distribution. Cardiovascular risk has also been linked to chronic low-grade inflammation [85] and levels of C-reactive protein are reportedly increased in PCOS women [86–88], although some of the increase may be related to obesity. The study of CAC by Shroff *et al.* [84] found no difference between CRP levels, or those of other proinflammatory cytokines TNF-α or interleukin-6, in those women with CAC vs. those without, suggesting no link to inflammation. The preliminary conclusion is that PCOS is an independent risk factor for atherosclerosis in young women.

Endothelial function in PCOS
Obesity and insulin resistance are associated with blunted endothelium-dependent but not endothelium-independent vasodilation [89], with failure of hyperinsulinaemia to augment endothelium-dependent vasodilation [90]. This indicates that obesity is associated with endothelial dysfunction and endothelial resistance to the enhancing effect of insulin on endothelium-dependent vasodilation. Endothelial dysfunction might therefore contribute to the increased risk of atherosclerosis in obese insulin-resistant subjects, such as those with PCOS. Insulin resistance has been proposed as a central metabolic basis for the clustering of risk factors in the metabolic syndrome. However, Pinkney *et al.* [91] have argued that the central problem may be endothelial dysfunction rather than insulin resistance. In resistance vessels, the endothelium regulates blood flow and blood pressure through the production of powerful vasoactive substance such as NO, endothelin-1 and thromboxane A2 [92]. Endothelial dysfunction can lead to defective vasodilation and disturbance of the balance of vasoactive substances favouring vasoconstriction and development of hypertension. The vascular endothelium is a key regulator of haemostasis and fibrinolysis, controlling the activities of the intrinsic pathway, the fibrinolytic and protein-C anticoagulant pathways, as well as influencing platelet activation and adhesion. Endothelial dysfunction can account for the increased levels of plasminogen activator inhibitor-1 observed in patients with the 'insulin resistance syndrome'. Insulin-resistant subjects have reduced skeletal muscle capillarization [93,94], which, together with failure of the endothelial vasodilator response to insulin, results in delayed delivery of insulin to the interstitial fluid [95,96]. Although the interstitial insulin concentration is not the main determinant of insulin action, in the dynamic state transendothelial insulin transport is a rate-limiting step before insulin binding to tissue receptors [97]. Thus, the metabolic syndrome is a marker of peripheral small-vessel endothelial dysfunction.

Central large-vessel endothelial dysfunction plays a major role in atherogenesis. The presence of systemic endothelial dysfunction (large and small vessel) is a plausible explanation for the observed association between atherosclerotic macrovascular disease and metabolic syndrome. Nevertheless, Mather *et al.* [98] recently reported normal endothelium-dependent vasodilatation in women with PCOS despite insulin resistance and obesity. In contrast, impairment in metacholine-induced (endothelium-dependent) leg blood flow in obese PCOS women compared with obese controls was recently reported [99], as was a reduced vasodilator response to insulin. Endothelium-dependent vasodilation was inversely correlated with free testosterone concentration, which was an independent predictor of leg blood flow, as well as with BMI.

Abnormalities of menstrual cycle and infertility

PCOS is the commonest cause (78%) of anovulatory infertility [100]. It was demonstrated that menstrual abnormalities are more frequent in obese than non-obese PCOS women [101]. In addition, it was shown that a reduced incidence of pregnancy and inadequate response to pharmacological treatments to induce ovulation is more common in obese PCOS women [102]. It has been found that obese PCOS women tend to have lower ovulation responses to pulsatile GhRH analogue administration than non-obese counterparts [103]. In the recent studies of PCOS women conceiving after *in vitro* fertilization or intracytoplasmic sperm injection, it was observed that those with obesity had higher gonadotropin requirement during stimulation [104]. In conclusion, obese women with PCOS demonstrate more pronounced irregularity of menstrual cycles and infertility, which requires a special approach for their treatment.

13.6   Treatment of obese women with PCOS (Table 13.3)

Weight reduction by lifestyle modification

There is long-standing clinical evidence concerning the efficacy of weight reduction on clinical and endocrinological features of obese women presenting with PCOS. It has been reported that weight loss may improve menstrual abnormalities and both ovulation and fertility rate. Moreover, it was confirmed that hirsutism and AN were significantly improved in most patients following weight loss. Reduction of hyperandrogenaemia appears to be the key factor responsible for these effects since peripheral testosterone,

Table 13.3   Principal elements in treatment of PCOS

1. Lifestyle modifications of weight reduction and exercise
2. Drugs to reduce insulin resistance for example:
   metformin, thiazolidinediones, ? D-chiro-inositol
3. Treatment of specific clinical/metabolic features as required:
   hirsuitism/acne/alopecia
   anovulation/subfertility
   dyslipidaemia
   IGT/type 2 diabetes

androstenedione and dehydroepiandrostenedione sulfate values were significantly reduced after weight loss in obese PCOS women [105]. These findings were subsequently confirmed by Kiddy *et al.* in women who obtained even moderate weight loss after long-term calorie restriction. They reported an improvement in menstrual pattern, endocrine profile and fertility in obese women (BMI > 25) with PCOS if they lost more than 5% of their body weight. Conversely, no significant benefit was observed in women who lost less, maintained their excess body weight or increased it [106]. An important beneficial effect of weight loss is the subsequent reduction of the degree of hyperinsulinaemia and insulin resistance state. Changes in testosterone and insulin (basal and glucose-stimulated) concentrations may be significantly correlated, regardless of body weight variations [105]. Diet-induced reduction of insulin levels has been shown to decrease P450c17α enzyme activity and consequently ovarian androgen production [107]. A lifestyle modification programme for obese PCOS women was performed in one recent study and included a diet and exercise programme for 6 months. Obese women with PCOS were classified as responders to the intervention if they regained ovulation during the study. As a result of intervention, responders showed 11% reduction in central fat, 71% improvement in insulin sensitivity index, a 33% fall in fasting insulin levels, and a 39% reduction in LH levels, but none of these parameters changed significantly in obese PCOS who failed to restore ovulation pattern [108]. An interventional study of 12 weeks of energy restriction followed by 4 weeks of weight maintenance prescribing a high protein or low protein diet for obese PCOS women was performed by Moran *et al.* They reported that pregnancies, improvements in menstrual cyclicity, lipid profile, and insulin resistance as well as decrease in weight (7.5%) and abdominal fat (12.5%) occurred independently of diet composition. Improvements in menstrual cyclicity were associated with greater decreases in insulin resistance and fasting insulin. On the low protein diet, HDL decreased 10% and free androgen index increased 44%, which could suggest that high protein weight loss diet may result in minor differential metabolic improvements [109]. Recently it was reported that a short-term (7 days) very low calorie restriction diet (4.2 MJ/day) prescribed for obese PCOS women reduced plasma glucose (18%), insulin (75%), total testosterone (23%) and leptin (50%), whereas serum oestrogens, SHBG and androstenedione concentrations remained unchanged. Contrary to expectation, calorie restriction enhanced basal and pulsatile LH secretion, further pointing to anomalous feedback control of pituitary LH release in PCOS [110]. To summarize, the principal effects of weight loss on both clinical and endocrinological features in women with obesity and PCOS include not only reduction of total and particularly visceral fat, but also improved menstrual cycles and fertility rate, reduced androgen and insulin concentrations, and improved insulin sensitivity.

Insulin-lowering medications

Agents that lower insulin levels by improving insulin sensitivity may provide a new therapeutic modality for obese PCOS women. Metformin acts mainly by suppressing hepatic glucose production, and its insulin-sensitizing actions are primarily mediated through the weight loss that frequently occurs during therapy. Velasquez *et al.* first demonstrated that metformin administration to obese PCOS women was not only able to significantly improve insulin levels, but also to decrease LH and testosterone concentrations, regardless of changes in body weight, with a significant improvement in menstrual abnormalities in most patients [111]. Glueck *et al.* reported that following metformin treatment 91% of previously amenorrhoeic women with PCOS resumed normal menses independently of metformin dose and duration of treatment. They also observed a significant decrease of BMI, fasting insulin, testosterone and increased oestradiol in metformin treated PCOS women [112]. Another study has demonstrated an improvement in insulin action and significant increases in levels of SHBG and decreased testosterone and androstenedione in obese PCOS women following 6 months treatment with metformin. Although no changes were recorded in body weight they observed a significant improvement in menstrual cyclicity [113]. Further, a study by Moghetti and coworkers demonstrated long-term efficacy of metformin treatment in obese women with PCOS. Their findings demonstrated marked improvement in menstrual cyclicity and ovulation and a significant reduction in serum androgens and LH. These effects were maintained for the entire 12 months treatment period and suggest that metformin may be appropriate for chronic treatment of this syndrome [114].

However, there are some studies finding no improvement of insulin sensitivity and hyperandrogenism in women with PCOS who were morbidly obese (BMI as high as $50 \, \text{kg/m}^2$) women during metformin treatment [62]. Recently Fleming *et al.* presented the results of a placebo-controlled trial assessing ovarian activity and utility of metformin treatment in obese (mean BMI 34.2) PCOS women. There was greater ovulation frequency and the time to first ovulation was significant shorter compared to the placebo group and the effect of metformin on follicular maturation was rapid, because oestrogen levels increased over the first week of treatment. Also a significant weight loss and increased HDL levels were recorded only in metformin treated group PCOS women, whereas the placebo group actually gained weight. However, metabolic risk factor benefits of metformin treatment were not observed in the morbidly obese subgroup of patients (BMI > 37) and there was an inverse relationship between body mass and treatment efficacy [115]. The latter finding suggests that women with extreme obesity and overwhelming insulin resistance might not respond to metformin therapy. Early studies with metformin were observational. Indeed the metaanalysis by Lord *et al.* [116], which concluded that metformin-enhanced ovulation rates either alone or in combination with clomiphene citrate were based on small trials, not all of them double blinded. A large Dutch randomized controlled trial (RCT) showed that addition of metformin to clomiphene neither enhanced ovulation nor pregnancy rates or reduced miscarriage rates [117]. Another multicentre RCT in USA [118] reached the same conclusion viz: either as monotherapy or in combination with clomiphene metformin was ineffective. Further, an RCT in very obese PCOS women (mean BMI 38) combining life-style modification plus/minus metformin showed an increase in menstrual cycles in those who lost significant weight irrespective of metformin treatment

[119]. The conclusion about metformin is that it is largely ineffective for ovulation induction, any benefit that is derived is due to the weight reduction.

Insulin-sensitizing drugs belonging to the class of thiazolidindiones, which are selective ligands for PPAR-γ, a member of the nuclear receptor superfamily of ligand-activated transcription factors have been investigated for PCOS treatment. Troglitazone showed promise but had to be withdrawn from the market [120–122]. Pioglitazone and rosiglitazone have been tried in small trials but as with metformin these have not been blinded and are underpowered statistically. They have not been shown to be beneficial in large RCTs.

Among other insulin-sensitizing agents, the potential use of D-chiro-inositol in PCOS treatment is under investigation. Inositol glycans have been described as mediating insulin action on thecal steroidogenesis. In the placebo-controlled trial by Nestler *et al.* D-chiro-inositol was administered to 22 obese women with PCOS for a total of 6–8 weeks. Administration of this drug resulted in a 55% decrease in serum free testosterone and increased ovulation rate up to 86% in women with PCOS. Furthermore, the treatment with D-chiro-inositol significantly reduced insulin levels during oral glucose tests, reduced systolic and diastolic blood pressure and decreased triglyceride levels without side effects or toxicity among treated women [123]. In conclusion, knowing that insulin resistance with accompanying hyperinsulinaemia has a key role in pathogenesis of PCOS, insulin-sensititizing drugs should theoretically be helpful. However, rigorously evaluated results have been disappointing and these agents cannot be recommended for the treatment of anovulation or other androgenic symptoms in PCOS women [124].

Antiandrogens

Several studies have demonstrated that antiandrogens may significantly decrease insulin resistance and hyperinsulinaemia in women with PCOS as well as reducing androgen levels. These effects have been observed regardless of the type of drug used, similar results being obtained for spironolactone [125], flutamide, and finasteride [53]. Nevertheless, there is no data investigating the effect of pure antiandrogens on fat distribution or impact on weight reduction in obese women with PCOS.

Oral contraceptives

Over the years oral contraceptives have been used in women with PCOS in order to avoid the risk of developing endometrial hyperplasia. The gestagen component decreases the frequency of GnRH pulses and LH secretion, thus reducing ovarian androgen production, while oestrogen increases SHBG concentration. Investigating the long-term effects of oral contraceptive therapy on metabolism and body composition in women with PCOS Pasquali *et al.* have found a significant reduction of waist circumference and waist–hip ratio, as well as of basal insulin levels and an improvement of glucose tolerance in some patients [126]. Although controversy still exists regarding benefits of oral contraceptive in treatment of obese PCOS women, these findings indicate a potential benefit in body composition and the glucose–insulin system in PCOS women.

13.7 Conclusions

This chapter has briefly reviewed the main data supporting the view that obesity is the single most important factor in metabolic and endocrine alterations defining PCOS. Obese women with PCOS are significantly more insulin resistant and have higher insulin levels than weight-matched controls or non-obese affected women. The primary role of insulin resistance and hyperinsulinaemia as a pathogenetic factor is supported by evidence that hyperandrogenism and related clinical features can be improved by reducing insulin levels. Obese women with PCOS have a higher risk for cardiovascular disease, atherosclerosis, endothelial dysfunction, and impaired glucose tolerance or type 2 diabetes mellitus than non-obese counterparts. Therefore we emphasize weight loss as a first-line approach in the treatment of obese PCOS women, which significantly improves the clinical features including subfertility, hormonal and metabolic abnormalities of these patients.

References

1. Franks, S. (1995) Polycystic ovary syndrome. *New England Journal of Medicine*, **333**, 853–861.
2. Balen, A. (1999) Pathogenesis of polycystic ovary syndrome – the enigma unravels? *Lancet*, **354**, 966–967.
3. Zawadzki, J.K. and Dunaif, A. (1992) Diagnostic criteria for polycystic ovary syndrome: towards a rational approach, in *Current Issues in Endocrinology and Metabolism. Polycystic Ovary Syndrome* (eds A. Dunaif, J.R. Givens, F. Haseltine and G.R. Merriam), Blackwell, Boston, MA, pp. 377–384.
4. Rotterdam ESHRE/ASRM-sponsored PCOS concensus workshop group (2003) Concensus on diagnostic criteria and long-term health risks related to PCOS. *Human Reproduction*, **19**, 41–47.
5. Azziz, R., Carmina, E., Dewailly, D. *et al.* (2006) Position statement: criteria for defining PCOSas a predominantly hyperandrogenic syndrome: an androgen Excess society Guideline. *Journal of Clinical Endocrinology and Metabolism*, **91**, 4237–4245.
6. Farquhar, C.M., Birdsall, M., Manning, P. *et al.* (1994) The prevalence of polycystic ovaries on ultrasound scanning in a population of randomly selected women. *Australian and New Zealand Journal of, Obstetric and Gynaecology*, **34**, 67–72.
7. Barth, J.H., Yasmin, E. and Balen, A.H. (2007) The diagnosis of polycystic ovary syndrome: the criteria are insufficiently robust for clinical research. *Clinical Endocrinology*, **67**, 811–815.
8. Barber, T.M., Wass, J.A.H., McCarthy, M.I. and Franks, S. (2007) Metabolic characteristics of women with polycystic ovaries and oligo-amenorrhoea but normal androgen levels: implications for management of PCOS. *Clinical Endocrinology*, **66**, 513–517.
9. Welt, C.K., Gudmundsson, J.A., Arason, G. *et al.* (2006) Characterising discrete subsets of PCOS as defined by the Rotterdam criteria: the impact of weight on phenotype and metabolic features. *Journal of Clinical Endocrinology and Metabolism*, **91**, 4842–4848.

10. Franks, S., Gharani, N., Waterworth, D. *et al.* (1997) The genetic basis of polycystic ovary syndrome. *Human Reproduction*, **12**, 2641–2648.

11. Legro, R.S. (1995) The genetics of polycystic ovary syndrome. *American Journal of Medicine*, **98**, (S1A) 9–11.

12. Menke, M.N. and Strauss, J.F. III (2007) Genetic approaches to PCOS. *Current Opinion in Obstetrics and Gynecology*, **19**, 355–359.

13. Urbanek, M., Sam, S. and Legro, R.S. (2007) Identification of a PCOS susceptibility variant in fibrillin-3 and association with metabolic phenotype. *Journal of Clinical Endocrinology and Metabolism*, **92**, 4191–4198.

14. Talbot, J.A., Bicknell, E.J., Rajhkowa, M. *et al.* (1996) Molecular scanning of the insulin receptor gene in women with polycystic ovary syndrome. *Journal of Clinical Endocrinology and Metabolism*, **81**, 1979–1983.

15. Waterworth, D.M., Bennett, S.T., Gharani, N. *et al.* (1997) Linkage and association of insulin gene VNTR regulatory polymorphism with polycystic ovary syndrome. *Lancet*, **349**, 986–990.

16. Ong, K.K., Phillips, D.I., Fall, C. *et al.* (1999) The insulin gene VNTR, type 2 diabetes and birth weight. *Nature Genetics*, **21**, 262–263.

17. Michelmore, K., Ong, K., Mason, S. *et al.* (2001) Clinical features in women with polycystic ovaries: relationship to insulin sensitivity, insulin gene VNTR and birth weight. *Clinical Endocrinology*, **55**, 439–446.

18. Stunkard, A.J., Sorensen, T.I., Hanis, C., Teasdale, T.W. *et al.* (1986) An adoption study of human obesity. *New England Journal of Medicine*, **314**, 193–198.

19. Rankinen, T., Zuberi, A., Chagnon, Y. *et al.* (2006) The human obesity gene map: the 2005 update. Review. *Obesity Research*, **14**, 529–644.

20. Dunaif, A. (1997) Insulin resistance and polycystic ovary syndrome: mechanism and implication for pathogenesis. *Endocrine Reviews*, **18**, 774–800.

21. Burghen, G.A., Givens, J.R. and Kitabchi, A.E. (1980) Correlation of hiperandrogenism with hyperinsulinism in polycystic ovary disease. *Journal of Clinical Endocrinology and Metabolism*, **50**, 113–116.

22. Dunaif, A., Futterweit, W., Segal, K.R. and Dobrjansky, A. (1989) Profound peripheral insulin resistance, independent of obesity, in polycystic ovary syndrome. *Diabetes*, **38**, 1165–1174.

23. Dunaif, A., Segal, K.R., Shelley, D.R. *et al.* (1992) Evidence for distinctive and intrinsic defects in insulin action in polycystic ovary syndrome. *Diabetes*, **41**, 1257–1266.

24. Barbieri, R.L., Makris, A., Randall, R.W. *et al.* (1986) Insulin stimulates androgen accumulation in incubations of ovarian stroma obtained women with hyperandrogenism. *Journal of Clinical Endocrinology and Metabolism*, **62**, 904–909.

25. Nestler, J.E. and Jakubowicz, D.J. (1996) Decrease in ovarian cytochrome P450c17α activity and serum free testosterone after reduction of insulin secretion in polycystic ovary syndrome. *New England Journal of Medicine*, **335**, 617–623.

26. McGee, E., Sawetawan, C., Bird, I. *et al.* (1995) The effects of insulin on 3(-hydroxysteroid dehydrogenase expression in human luteinized granulosa cells. *Journal of the Society for Gynecologic Investigation*, **2**, 535–541.

27. Poretsky, L., Cataldo, N.A., Rosenwaks, Z. and Giudice, L.C. (1999) The insulin related ovarian regulatory system in healthy and disease. *Endocrine Reviews*, **20**, 535–582.

28. Rajkhowa, M., Bicknell, J., Jones, M. and Clayton, R.N. (1994) Insulin sensitivity in obese and non-obese women with polycystic ovary syndrome – relationship to hyperandrogenaemia. *Fertility and Sterility*, **61**, 605–611.

29. Poretsky, L., Cataldo, N.A., Rosenwaks, Z. and Giudice, L.C. (1999) The insulin related ovarian regulatory system in healthy and disease. *Endocrine Reviews*, **20**, 535–582.

30. L'Allemand, D., Penhoat, A., Lebrethon, M.-C. *et al.* (1996) Insulin-like growth factors enhance steroidogenic enzyme and corticotropin receptor messenger ribonucleic acid levels cells. *Journal of Clinical Endocrinology and Metabolism*, **81**, 3892–3894.

31. Moghetti, P., Castello, R., Negri, C. *et al.* (1996) Insulin infusion amplifies 17(-hydroxycorticosteroid intermediates to ACTH in hyperandrogenetic women: apparent relative impairment of 17, 20-lyase activity. *Journal of Clinical Endocrinology and Metabolism*, **81**, 881–885.

32. Vettor, R., Lombardi, A.M., Fabris, R. *et al.* (2000) Substrate competition and insulin action in animal models. *International Journal of Obesity and Related Metabolic Disorders*, **24**, S22–S24.

33. Hotamisiligil, G.S., Peraldi, P., Budavari, A. *et al.* (1996) IRS-1 mediated inhibition of insulin receptor tyrosine kinase activity in TNF-(and obesity-induced insulin resistance. *Science*, **271**, 665–668.

34. Poretsky, L., Cataldo, N.A. and Rosenwaks, Z.L.C. (1999) The insulin related ovarian regulatory system in healthy and disease. *Endocrine Reviews*, **20**, 535–582.

35. Holte, J., Bergh, C., Berglund, L. and Lithell, H. (1994) Enhanced early insulin response to glucose in relation to insulin resistance inwomen with polycyctic ovary syndrome and normal glucose tolerance. *Journal of Clinical Endocrinology and Metabolism*, **78**, 1054–1058.

36. Hull, K.L. and Harvey, S. (2001) Growth hormone: roles in female reproduction. *Journal of Endocrinology*, **168**, 1–23.

37. Pijl, H., Langerdonk, J.G., Burggraaf, J. *et al.* (2001) Altered neuroregulation of growth hormone secretion in viscerally obese premenopausal women. *Journal of Clinical Endocrinology and Metabolism*, **86**, 5509–5515.

38. Katz, E., Ricciarelli, E. and Adashi, E.Y. (1993) The potential relevance of growth hormone to female reproductive physiology and pathophysiology. *Fertility and Sterility*, **59**, 8–34.

39. Wu, X., Sallinen, K., Zhou, S. *et al.* (2000) Androgen excess contributes to altered growth hormone/insulin-like growth factor-1 axis in nonobese women with polycystic ovary syndrome. *Fertility and Sterility*, **73**, 730–734.

40. Villa, P., Soranna, L., Mancini, A. *et al.* (2001) Effect of feeding on growth hormone response to growth hormone-releasing hormone in polycystic ovary syndrome: relation with body weight and hyperinsulinism. *Human Reproduction*, **16**, 430–434.

41. Volitainen, R., Franks, S., Mason, H.D. and Marticainen, H. (1996) Expression of insulin-like growth factors (IGF), IGF-binding protein, and IGF receptor messenger ribonucleic acids in normal and polycystic ovaries. *Journal of Clinical Endocrinology and Metabolism*, **81**, 1003–1008.

42. Nahum, R., Thong, K.J. and Hillier, S.G. (1995) Metabolic regulation of androgen production by human thecal cells *in vitro*. *Human Reproduction (Oxford, England)*, **10**, 75–81.

43. Brismar, K., Ferqvist-Forbes, E., Wahren, J. and Hall, K. (1994) Effect of insulin on the hepatic production of insulin-like growth factor binding protein-1 (IGFBP-1), IGFBP-3 and IGF-1 in insulin- dependent diabetes. *Journal of Clinical Endocrinology and Metabolism*, **79**, 872–878.

44. Hautanen, A. (2000) Synthesis and regulation of sex hormone-binding globulin in obesity. *International Journal of Obesity and Related Metabolic Disorders*, **24**, S64–S70.

45. Escobar-Morreale, H.F., Acuncion, M., Calvo, R.M. *et al.* (2001) Receiver operating characteristic analysis of the performance of basal serum hormone profiles for the diagnosis of polycystic ovary syndrome in epidemiological studies. *European Journal of Endocrinology*, **145**, 619–624.

46. Rosenfield, R.L. (1999) Ovarian and adrenal function in polycystic ovary syndrome. *Emergency Medicine Clinics of North America*, **28**, 265–293.

47. Barner, R.B. (1998) The pathogenesis of polycystic ovary syndrome: lessons from ovarian stimulation studies. *Journal of Endocrinological Investigation*, **21**, 567–579.

48. Rosenfield, R.L. (1999) Ovarian and adrenal function in polycycstic ovary syndrome. *Emergency Medicine Clinics of North America*, **28**, 265–293.

49. Rodin, A., Thakker, H., Taylor, N. and Clayton, R.N. (1994) Hyperandrogenism in polycystic ovary syndrome. Evidence of dysregulation of 11(hydroxysteroid dehydrogenase. *New England Journal of Medicine*, **330**, 460–465.

50. Pasquali, R. and Vicennati, V. (2000) The abdominal obesity phenotype and insulin resistance with abnormalities of the hypothalamic-pituitary-adrenal axis in humans. *Hormone and Metabolic Research*, **32**, 521–525.

51. Holte, J., Bergh, T., Gennarelli, G. and Wide, L. (1994) The independent effects of polycystic ovary syndrome and obesity on serum concentrations of gonadotropins and sex steroids in premenopausal women. *Clinical Endocrinology*, **41**, 473–481.

52. Björntorp, P. (1996) The regulation of adipose tissue distribution in humans. *International Journal of Obesity and Related Metabolic Disorders*, **20**, 291–302.

53. Diamanti-Kadarakis, E., Mitrakou, A., Hennes, M.M.I. *et al.* (1995) Insulin sensitivity and antiandrogenic therapy in women with polycystic ovary syndrome. *Metabolism: Clinical and Experimental*, **44**, 525–531.

54. Soule, A.G. (1996) Neuroendocrinology of the polycystic ovary syndrome. *Baillière's Clinical Endocrinology and Metabolism*, **10**, 205–219.

55. Taylor, A.E., McCourt, B., Martin, K.A. *et al.* (1997) Determinants of abnormal gonadotropin secretion in clinically defined women with polycystic ovary syndrome. *Journal of Clinical Endocrinology and Metabolism*, **83**, 2248–2256.

56. Conway, G.S., Jacobs, H.S., Holly, J.M. and Wass, J.A. (1990) Effects of luteinizing hormone, insulin like growth factor, and insulin like growth factor small binding protein in polycystic ovary syndrome. *Clinical Endocrinology*, **33**, 593–603.

57. Lobo, R.A., Kelzky, O.A., Cmpeau, J.D. and Di Zerga, G.S. (1983) Elevated bioactive luteinizing hormone in women with polycystic ovary syndrome. *Fertility and Sterility*, **39**, 674–678.

58. McCartney, C.R., Eagleson, C.A. and Marshall, J.C. (2002) Regulation of gonadotropin secretion: implications of polycystic ovary syndrome. *Seminars in Reproductive Medicine*, **20** (4), 317–326.

59. Morales, A.J., Laughlin, G.A., Butzow, T. *et al.* (1996) Insulin, somatotropic, and luteinizing hormone axes in non-obese and obese women with polycystic ovary syndrome: common and distinct features. *Journal of Clinical Endocrinology and Metabolism*, **81**, 2854–2864.

60. Hill, P., Garbaczewski, L. and Helman, P. (1980) Diet, lifestyle and menstrual activity. *American Journal of Clinical Nutrition*, **33**, 1192–1198.

61. Wild, R.A., Painter, P.C. and Coulson, R.B. (1985) Lipoprotein lipid concentrations and cardiovascular risk in women with polycystic ovary syndrome. *Journal of Clinical Endocrinology and Metabolism*, **61**, 946–951.

62. Ehrmann, D.A., Cavaghan, M.K., Imperial, J. *et al.* (1997) Effects of metformin on insulin secretion, insulin action, and ovarian steroidogenesis in women with polycystic ovary syndrome. *Journal of Clinical Endocrinology and Metabolism*, **82**, 524–530.

63. Morin-Papunen, L.C., Vauhkonen, I., Koivunen, R.M. *et al.* (2000) Insulin sensitivity, insulin secretion, and metabolic and hormonal parameters in healthy women and women with polycystic ovarian syndrome. *Human Reproduction (Oxford, England)*, **15**, 1266–1274.

64. Rajkhowa, M. and Clayton, R.N. (1995) Polycystic ovary syndrome. *Current Obstetrics & Gynaecology*, **5**, 191–200.

65. Dalhgren, E., Johansson, S., Lindstedt, G. *et al.* (1992) Women with polycystic ovary syndrome wedge resected in 1956 to 1965: a long-term follow-up focusing on natural history and circulating hormones. *Fertility and Sterility*, **57**, 505–513.

66. Ehrmann, E., Cavaghan, M.K., Barnes, R.B. *et al.* (1999) Prevalence of impaired glucose tolerance and diabetes in women with polycystic ovary syndrome. *Diabetes Care*, **22**, 141–146.

67. Norman, R.J., Masters, L., Milner, C.R. *et al.* (2001) Relative of conversion from normogly-caemia to impaired glucose tolerance or non-insulin dependent diabetes mellitus in polycystic ovarian syndrome. *Human Reproduction*, **16**, 1995–1998.

68. Wild, R.A. (1995) Obesity, lipids, cardiovascular risk, and androgen excess. *American Journal of Medicine*, **98**, 27S–32S.

69. Robinson, S., Hederson, A.D., Gelding, S.V. *et al.* (1996) Dyslipidaemia is associated with insulin resistance in women with polycystic ovaries. *Clinical Endocrinology*, **44**, 277–284.

70. Rajkhowa, M., Neary, R.H., Kumpatla, P. *et al.* (1997) Altered composition of high density lipoproteins in women with the polycystic ovary syndrome. *Journal of Clinical Endocrinology and Metabolism*, **82**, 3389–3394.

71. Valkenburg, O., Steggers-Thennissen, R.P., Smedts, H.P. *et al.* (2008) A more atherogenic serum lipoprotein profile is present in women with PCOS:a case–control study. *Journal of Clinical Endocrinology and Metabolism*, **93**, 470–476.

72. Dejager, S., Pichard, C., Giral, P. *et al.* (2001) Smaller LDL particle size in women with polycystic ovary syndrome compared. *Clinical Endocrinology*, **54**, 455–462.

73. Pirwani, I.R., Fleming, R., Greer, I.A. *et al.* (2001) Lipids and lipoprotein subfractions in women with PCOS: relationship to metabolic and endocrine parameters. *Clinical Endocrinology*, **54**, 447–453.

74. Gardner, C.D., Fortmann, S.P. and Krauss, R.M. (1996) Association of small LDL particles with the incidence of coronary artery disease in men and women. *Journal of the American Medical Association*, **276**, 875–881.

75. Kelly, C.J.G., Lyall, H., Petrie, J.R. *et al.* (2002) A specific elevation in tissue plasminogen activator antigen in women with polycystic ovary syndrome. *Journal of Clinical Endocrinology and Metabolism*, **87**, 3287–3290.

76. Wild, S., Pierpoint, T., McKeigue, P. and Jacobs, H.S. (2000) Cardiovascular disease in women with polycystic ovary syndrome at long-term follow-up: a retrospective cohort study. *Clinical Endocrinology*, **52**, 595–600.

77. Solomon, C.G., Hu, F.B., Dunaif, A. *et al.* (2002) Menstrual cycle irregularity and risk for future cardiovascular disease. *Journal of Clinical Endocrinology and Metabolism*, **87**, 2013–2017.

78. Solomon, C.G., Hu, F.B., Dunaif, A. *et al.* (2001) Long or highly irregular menstrual cycles as a risk for type 2 diabetes mellitus. *Journal of the American Medical Association*, **286**, 2421–2426.

79. Talbott, E.O., Guzick, D.S., Sutton-Tyrrelli, K. *et al.* (2000) Evidence for association between polycystic ovary syndrome and premature carotid atherosclerosis in middle-aged women. *Atheroscerosis, Thrombosis and Vascular Biology*, **20**, 2414–2418.

80. Kelly, C.J.G., Speirs, A., Gould, G.W. *et al.* (2002) Altered vascular function in young women with polycystic ovary syndrome. *Journal of Clinical Endocrinology and Metabolism*, **87**, 742–746.

81. Budoff, M.J., Shaw, L.J., Liu, S.T. *et al.* (2007) Long-term prognosis associated with coronary calcification: observations from registry of 25 253 patients. *Journal of the American College of Cardiology*, **49**, 1860–1870.

82. Christian, R.C., Dunesic, D.A., Beherenbeck, T. *et al.* (2003) Prevalence and predictors of coronary artery calcification in women with PCOS. *Journal of Clinical Endocrinology and Metabolism*, **88**, 2562–2568.

83. Talbott, E.O., Zborowski, J.V., Boudreaux, M.Y. *et al.* (2004) The relationship between C-reactive protein and carotid intima-media wall thickness in middle aged women with PCOS. *Journal of Clinical Endocrinology and Metabolism*, **89**, 6061–6067.

84. Shroff, R., Kerchner, A., Maifield, M. *et al.* (2007) Young obese women with PCOS have evidence of early coronary atherosclerosis. *Journal of Clinical Endocrinology and Metabolism*, **92**, 4609–4614.

85. Tsimikis, S., Willerson, J.T. and Ridker, P.M. (2006) C-reactive protein and other emerging blood biomarkers to optimise risk stratification of vulnerable individuals. *Journal of the American College of Cardiology*, **47**, C19–31.

86. Kelly, C.C., Lyall, H., Petrie, J.R. *et al.* (2001) Low grade chronic inflammation in women with PCOS. *Journal of Clinical Endocrinology and Metabolism*, **86**, 2453–2455.

87. Boulman, N., Levy, Y., Leiba, R. *et al.* (2004) Increased C-reactive protein levels in PCOS: a marker of cardiovascular disease. *Journal of Clinical Endocrinology and Metabolism*, **89**, 2160–2165.

88. Talbott, E.O., Zborowski, J.V., Rager, J.R. *et al.* (2004) Evidence for an association between metabolic cardiovascular syndrome and coronary and aortic calcification in women with PCOS. *Journal of Clinical Endocrinology and Metabolism*, **89**, 5454–5461.

89. Arcaro, G., Zamboni, M., Rossi, L., Turcato, E. *et al.* (1999) Body fat distribution predicts the degree of endothelial dysfunction in uncomplicated obesity. *International Journal of Obesity*, **23**, 936–942.

90. Steinberg, H.O., Chaker, H., Leaming, R., Johnson, A. *et al.* (1996) Obesity/insulin resistance is associated with endothelial dysfunction. Implications for the syndrome of insulin resistance. *Journal of Clinical Investigation*, **11**, 2601–2610.

91. Pinkney, J.H., Stehouwer, C.D., Coppack, S.W. and Yudkin, J.S. (1997) Endothelial dysfunction: cause of insulin resistance syndrome. *Diabetes*, **46** (Suppl 2), S9–S13.

92. Vane, J.R., Anggard, E.E. and Botting, R.M. (1990) Regulatory functions of vascular endothelium. *New England Journal of Medicine*, **323**, 27–36.

93. Lithell, H., Lindgarde, E., Hellsing, K., Lundqvist, G. *et al.* (1981) Body weight skeletal muscle morphology and enzyme activities in relation to fasting serum insulin concentration and glucose tolerance in 48-year-old men. *Diabetes*, **30**, 19–25.

94. Lillioja, S., Young, A.A., Cutler, C.L., Ivy, J.L. *et al.* (1987) Skeletal muscle capillary density and fiber type are possible determinants of in-vivo insulin resistance in man. *Journal of Clinical Investigation*, **80**, 415–424.

95. Jansson, P.A., Fowelin, J.P., von Schenck, H.P. and Smith, U.P. (1993) Measurement by microdialysis of the insulin concentration in subcutaneous interstitial fluid. *Diabetes*, **42**, 1469–1473.

96. Castillo, C., Bogardus, C., Bergman, R. *et al.* (1994) Interstitial insulin concentration determines glucose uptake rates but not insulin resistance in lean and obese men. *Journal of Clinical Investigation*, **93**, 10–16.

97. Miles, P.D., Levisetti, M., Reichart, D., Khourseed, M. *et al.* (1995) Kinetics of insulin action in vivo: identification of rate limiting steps. *Diabetes*, **44**, 947–953.

98. Mather, K.J., Verma, S., Corenblum, B. and Anderson, T.J. (2000) Normal endothelial function despite insulin resistance in healthy women with polycystic ovary syndrome. *Journal of Clinical Endocrinology and Metabolism*, **85**, 1851–1856.

99. Paradisi, G., Steinberg, H.O., Hempfling, A., Cronin, J. *et al.* (2001) Polycystic ovary syndrome is associated with endothelial dysfunction. *Circulation*, **103**, 1410–1415.

100. Hull, M.G. (1987) Epidemiology of infertility and polycystic ovarian disease: endocrinological and demografic studies. *Gynecological Endocrinology*, **1**, 235–245.

101. Kiddy, D.S., Sharp, P.S., White, D.M. *et al.* (1990) Differences in clinical and endocrine features between obese and non-obese subject with polycystic ovary syndrome: an analysis of 263 consecutive cases. *Clinical Endocrinology*, **32**, 213–220.

102. Galtier-Dereure, F., Pujol, P., Dewailly, D. and Bringer, J. (1997) Choise of stimulation in polycystic ovarian syndrome: the influence of obesity. *Human Reproduction*, **12**, 88–96.
103. Filicori, M., Flamingi, C. and Dellai, P. (1994) Treatment of ovulation with pulsatile gonado-tropin-releasing hormone: prognostic factors and clinical results in 600 cycles. *Journal of Clinical Endocrinology and Metabolism*, **79**, 1215–1220.
104. Fedorsak, P., Dale, P.O., Storeng, R. *et al.* (2001) The impact of obesity and insulin resistance on the outcome of IVF or ICSI in women with polycystic ovary syndrome. *Human Reproduction*, **16**, 1086–1091.
105. Pasquali, R., Antenucci, D., Casimirri, F. *et al.* (1989) Clinical and hormonal characteristics of obese amenorrheic women before and after weight loss. *Journal of Clinical Endocrinology and Metabolism*, **68**, 173–179.
106. Kiddy, D.S., Hamilton-Fairley, D., Buch, A. *et al.* (1992) Improvement in endocrine profile and ovarian function during dietary treatment of obese women with polycystic ovary syndrome. *Clinical Endocrinology*, **36**, 105–111.
107. Jacubowitz, D.J. and Nestler, J.E. (1997) 17α-Hydroxyprogestrone responses to leuprolide and serum androgens in obese women with and without polycystic ovary syndrome after weight loss. *Journal of Clinical Endocrinology and Metabolism*, **82**, 556–560.
108. Huber-Bucholz, M.M., Carey, D.G.P. and Norman, R.J. (1999) Restoration of reproductive potential by lifestyle modification in obese polycystic ovary syndrome: role of insulin sensitivity and luteinizing hormone. *Journal of Clinical Endocrinology and Metabolism*, **84**, 1470–1474.
109. Moran, L.J., Noakes, M., Clifton, P.M. *et al.* (2003) Dietary composition in restoring reproductive and metabolic physiology in overweight women with polycystic ovary syndrome. *Journal of Clinical Endocrinology and Metabolism*, **88**, 812–819.
110. Van Dam, E.W., Roelfsema, F., Veldhuis, J.D. *et al.* (2002) Increase in daily LH secretion in response to short-term calorie restriction in obese women with PCOS. *American Journal of Physiology. Endocrinology and Metabolism*, **282**, 865–872.
111. Velasquez, E.M., Mendoza, S., Hamer, T. *et al.* (1994) Metformin therapy in polycystic ovary syndrome reduced hyperinsulinemia, insulin resistance, hyperandrogenemia, and systolic blood pressure, while facilitating normal menses and pregnancy. *Metabolism: Clinical and Experimental*, **43**, 647–654.
112. Glueck, C.J., Wang, P., Fontaine, R. *et al.* (1999) Metformin-induced resumption of normal menses in 39 of 43 (91%) previously amenorrheic women with polycystic ovary syndrome. *Metabolism: Clinical and Experimental*, **48**, 511–519.
113. Diamanti-Kadarskis, E., Kouli, C., Tsianateli, T. and Bergiele, A. (1998) Therapeutic effects of metformin on insulin resistance and hyperandrogenism in polycystic ovary syndrome. *European Journal of Endocrinology/European Federation of Endocrine Societies*, **138**, 269–274.
114. Mohgetti, P. Castello, R., Negri, C. *et al.* (2000) Metformin effects on clinical, endocrine and metabolic profiles, and insulin sensitivity in polycystic ovary syndrome: a randomised, double-blind, placebo-controlled 6-month trial, followed by open, long-term clinical evaluation. *Journal of Clinical Endocrinology and Metabolism*, **85**, 139–146.
115. Fleming, R., Hopkinson, Z.E., Wallace, A.M. *et al.* (2002) Ovarian function and metabolic factors in women with oligomenorrhea treated with metformin in a randomised double blind placebo-controlled trial. *Journal of Clinical Endocrinology and Metabolism*, **87**, 569–574.
116. Lord, J.M., Flight, I.H. and Norman, R.J. (2003) Insulin-sensitising drugs (metformin, trogli-tazone, rosiglitazone, pioglitazone, D-chiro-inositol) for polycystic ovary syndrome. *Cochrane Database of Systematic Reviews*, (3), CD03053.
117. Moll, E., Bossyut, P.M., Korevaer, J.C. *et al.* (2006) Effect of clomiphene citrate plus metformin and clomiphene citrate plus placebo on induction of ovulation in women with newly diagnosed PCOS: randomised double blind clinical trial. *BMJ (Clinical Research Ed)*, **332**, 1485–1488.

118. Legro, R.S., Bamhart, H.X., Schlaff, W.D. *et al.* (2007) Clomiphene, metformin or both for infertility in PCOS. *New England Journal of Medicine*, **356**, 551–566.

119. Tang, T., Glanville, J., Hayden, C. *et al.* (2006) Combined lifestyle modification and metformin in obese patients with PCOS: a randomised placebo controlled double blind multicentre study. *Human Reproduction*, **21**, 80–89.

120. Dunaif, A., Scott, D., Finegood, D. *et al.* (1996) The insulin-sensiting agent troglitazone improves metabolic and reproductive abnormalities in the plycystic ovary syndrome. *Journal of Clinical Endocrinology and Metabolism*, **81**, 3299–3306.

121. Azziz, R., Ehrmann, D., Legro, R.S. *et al.* (2001) Troglitazone improves ovulation and hirsutism in the polycystic ovary syndrome: a multicenter, double blind, placebo-controlled trial. *Journal of Clinical Endocrinology and Metabolism*, **86**, 1626–1632.

122. Paradisi, G., Steinberg, H.O., Shepard, M.K. *et al.* (2003) Troglitazone therapy improves endothelial function to near normal in women with polycystic ovary syndrome. *Journal of Clinical Endocrinology and Metabolism*, **88**, 576–580.

123. Nestler, J.E., Jacubowicz, D., Reamer, P. *et al.* (1999) Ovulatory and metabolic effects of d-chiro-inositol in the polycystic ovary syndrome. *New England Journal of Medicine*, **340**, 1314–1320.

124. Balen, A.H. (2007) Is metformin the treatment of choice for anovulation in polycystic ovary syndrome? *Nature Clinical Practice Endocrinology & Metabolism*, **3**, 440–441.

125. Moghetti, P., Tosi, F., Castello, R. *et al.* (1996) The insulin resistance in women with hyperandrogenism is partially reversed by antiandrogen treatment: evidence that androgen impair insulin action in women. *Journal of Clinical Endocrinology and Metabolism*, **81**, 952–960.

126. Pasquali, R., Gambineri, A., Anconetani, B. *et al.* (1999) The natural history of the metabolic syndrome in young women with the polycycstic ovary syndrome and the effect of long-term oestrogen–progestagen treatment. *Clinical Endocrinology*, **50**, 517–527.

14

Management of diabesity in primary care: a multidisciplinary approach

Ian W. Campbell

14.1 Prevalence of obesity in primary care

The prevalence of overweight and obesity in adults and children is already at epidemic levels. The Foresight Report published in 2007 by the United Kingdom government predicts that current obesity levels of 24% in men and women would rise to perhaps as many as 60% of adult men and 50% of adult women by the year 2050. The report estimated the financial cost to the National Health Service attributable to overweight and obesity to rise to £10 billion per year by 2050 and the wider costs to society to reach £49.9 billion by the same year [1]. The implications for primary care both now and in the future are immense. Obese patients are 30% more like to acquire an appointment with their GP and will on average account for 30% more in prescription costs. A study of the socioeconomic costs of obesity reveal a catalogue of social deprivation, increased sick leave, higher unemployment and earlier retirement through ill health [2]. This impacts greatly on the ability of primary care to deliver adequate care with limited resources. A review of the health consequences of obesity leaves one in no doubt that primary care is already deeply involved in treating the complications of obesity. Hypertension, coronary heart disease, dyslipidaemia, cancer (colon, breast and prostate), infertility, respiratory and sleep disorders, osteoarthritis and psychological disease can be attributed to some degree, directly or indirectly, to obesity [3]. It is however the metabolic effects of increased insulin resistance and type 2 diabetes that best demonstrate the effect of obesity on the every day life and work of primary care doctors and nurses.

Obesity and Diabetes, Second Edition   Edited by Anthony H. Barnett and Sudhesh Kumar
© 2009 John Wiley & Sons, Ltd

14.2 Current approach to diabetes care in primary care

The management of diabetes has, rightly, been given a high priority within general practice in recent years, with marked improvements in the level of proactive care, reduction in risk factors, and prevention of comorbidities being observed as a result. However it is only recently that the direct relationship between type 2 diabetes and obesity has been accepted by the majority of clinicians. This chapter seeks to describe the way in which overweight type 2 diabetics might be managed in primary care. The distinction between type 1 and type 2 diabetics may be made at a very early stage in treatment, and the criteria for deciding when insulin treatment is required are dealt with elsewhere. It is also assumed that the ongoing management of diabetics, including annual reviews and dealing with complications is not within the remit of this chapter and will also be covered elsewhere in the book.

While up to 80% of an individual's predisposition to developing type 2 diabetes is genetic [4], obesity is now acknowledged as the determining factor in that development, and, conversely, it is quite clear that even a modest reduction in body weight, of between 5 and 10%, can lead to significant improvements in fasting blood glucose and HbA1c [5]. In newly diagnosed type 2 diabetics a reduction in body weight by 10% would lead to a return to normal fasting glucose in half of all cases, and sustained weight loss of 10% would produce a 30% fall in diabetes-related deaths (see table). Faced with this compelling evidence many practitioners now accept that weight management should form an integral part of the management of type 2 diabetes. The difficulty then faced is how to deliver that aspect of care within a primary care setting?

14.3 Early treatment with hypoglycaemic agents

In an already pressured general practice setting it is perhaps too easy to reach for the prescription pad and prescribe hypoglycaemics at an early stage in the management of new diabetics. We are, understandably, concerned with reducing glycaemic levels as quickly as possible, to improve symptomatology, and prevent potentially serious complications. However in the early stages of management, treatment with hypogly-caemic agents is often not necessary, and the judicious with-holding of such medication can have its own benefits. Sulfonylureas have been used extensively to treat type 2 diabetics. However, they can promote weight gain in an individual of, on average 2–4 kg (up to 10 kg) and therefore will adversely affect the underlying cause of the problem [6]. Metformin does not lead to weight gain but can induce side effects of diarrhoea in 10% of cases. On the other hand, within only a few weeks or months the benefits of weight loss can produce dramatic improvements in diabetic control to rival hypoglycaemic drugs. The clinician needs to ask himself at the outset of treatment whether weight loss should be the mainstay of management, at least for the first 3 to 6 months, before con-sidering the introduction of hypoglycaemics as an adjunctive treatment, or in circum-stances where beneficial weight loss has not been achieved.

14.4   Integrating obesity management with diabetes

Within primary care there has been a lot of interest in developing distinctive practice based obesity clinics, often lead by one or two enthusiastic members of the practice team and some achieving excellent results. Many others, however, find the prospects of developing such a stand-alone clinic daunting, citing the lack of time, staff, resources or skill-base as their main concerns. When considering the management of diabetes in primary care however the need for medical management of overweight is inescapably integral to any serious diabetes treatment plan. It must therefore be within the scope and remit of primary care diabetic clinics to provide for the management of overweight. To do otherwise is to fail to recognize and address the root cause of the disease we are trying to control, and thereby miss the perfect opportunity to develop lifelong lifestyle change with all the medical benefits that would confer. This approach does however require an informed and motivated practice team approach, with involvement of a wide variety of professionals to offer the ongoing support and advice necessary for the patient to be encouraged to develop new attitudes to dietary intake and activity levels which are required to produce positive and significant results.

14.5   A multidisciplinary approach

In the management of the overweight diabetic a great strength of primary care is ready access to a multidisciplinary team. The general practitioner, working closely with an enthusiastic practice nurse can, together, deliver high quality care in a familiar and accessible clinical setting. They are ideally placed to take into account the past and present medical history of the patient, and to incorporate proposed lifestyle changes into treatment strategies, tailored to the patients domestic and employment circumstances. The general practitioner and nurse will often, over several years, have built up a significant and important trusting relationship, not only with the patient, but also their family. For the majority of type two diabetics care will be delivered almost exclusively by the general practitioner and the practice nurse. However, management can be greatly enhanced by the involvement of specialists within the primary care setting, both in the early stages of treatment but also when control becomes problematic.

14.6   Dietary treatment of diabetes

Dietary advice will form the backbone of a diabetic's future management and it is therefore crucial to get the right message across from the outset. Poor information delivered early in management can have adverse short- and long-term effects, and should be avoided. The aims of dietary advice should be to minimize symptoms of hyperglycaemia, minimize the risk of hypoglycaemia, and to promote weight loss, while ensuring that any proposed changes are tolerable and sustainable [7]. Remember that in encouraging the patient to make (possibly) substantial changes to their dietary intake you will be asking them to change life-long habits, to stop doing things they enjoy (and perhaps replace with less well received alternatives) and will at first appear to be asking them to make changes that will diminish their ability to socialize with family and friends at the dinner table and on special occasions. For most new diabetics, but depending on the severity of their glycaemia, it is perhaps best to keep the message simple at first, to avoid alienation or confusion.

Dietary changes should modify, rather than totally change the patient's eating pattern. Total calorie intake should be restricted to that needed to achieve and maintain an agreed target weight. At least half the energy intake should be made up of carbohydrate, and from mainly complex carbohydrates, with a high fibre content. At least five portions, and preferably more, of fruit and vegetables should be consumed every day (a portion is 80 g but is most simply measured as one handful), refined carbohydrates in the form of sugary food and drinks should be reduced. Total fat intake should be reduced, and saturated (animal) fats replaced with monounsaturated and polyunsaturated fats commonly found in oily fish and green leafy vegetables [8]. Dietary salt should be reduced, alcohol intake should be in moderation, and special 'diabetic' products which are high in calories are not to be recommended. Much can be achieved from a few simple dietetic changes.

Over the next few appointments, and depending on the symptomatic and glycaemic response, advice can begin to specifically promote weight loss, to include detailed information on reducing portion sizes, reducing calorific intake by 600 kcal (or 20%) daily, calorie calculations for specific and favourite foods, and steps to maximize the potential for a daily intake of at least five portions of fruit and vegetables, an increase in dietary protein and fibre, a reduction of fat intake to less than 10%, and moderation of carbohydrate intake to 50% of calorific intake. Although it may sound rather simplistic, asking the patient to complete a 'food diary' for one week can provide both the clinician and the patient with invaluable information. In the absence of a preprinted diary form, a simple A4 piece of paper, marked off into days of the week will suffice. By the end of the week the patient will usually have begun to make some changes as they confront their previously unrecognized, or unacknowledged habits. Comments such as 'I never realized I ate so much between meals', or 'I wasn't aware that I used so much sugar in my tea over the course of the day' are not unusual when the patient presents the diary. For those patients whose diaries are awash with high sugar, high fat foods, and frequent snacking, it is best to select only a few possible changes to suggest to the patient, the ultimate choice of what to alter resting with the patient. A repeat food diary after a few weeks will present a further opportunity to assist the patient in refining their intake even further. Some patients will want to become expert in managing their diet, to facilitate weight loss, and to exert maximum control of the diabetes. The general practitioner and nurse can be a useful source of information material to aid patient education, by using published healthy eating leaflets and manuals.

For those general practitioners or nurses who lack experience or confidence to advise new diabetics on dietary matters, referral to a community-based dietitian is essential.

An experienced dietitian is ideally placed to provide detailed, but pragmatic dietary advice to facilitate an immediate improvement in symptomatology, but also to promote long-term dietary control of diabetes. Community dietitians are unfortunately an uncommon commodity in practice but when available to the primary care team the value of their contribution can be immense.

The role of the practice receptionist can easily be overlooked. While not directly involved in patient care the receptionist is often closely involved in administering practice based diabetes clinics and annual examination recall systems. An informed and enthusiastic receptionist can play a significant role in both encouraging patients to attend for review and in ensuring patients receive the clinical care they require by being alert to previous non-attendance and under use of regular diabetic medication.

14.7   Clinical assessment

Clinical assessment of patients newly diagnosed with type 2 diabetes should be straight forward. After diagnosis, if not already done, the patient's weight and height should be taken to assess their body mass index (BMI = weight (kg)/height (m^2)). Waist circumference is also a good indicator of excess visceral fat and is independent of height. Measured at the level of the umbilicus a reading of 102 cm or above in men, and 90 cm or above in women, equates to a body mass index of 30 or above and indicates an increased risk of co-morbidity such as coronary heart disease [9]. Body fat analysis equipment, often incorporated into weighing scales, provides a useful indication of body fat mass percentage providing yet another base line measurement to monitor progress on a weight-loss programme. Such equipment, from a reliable manufacturer such as Tanita, is no longer prohibitively expensive and can be acquired by the primary care team. Urinalysis for proteinuria and successive blood pressure readings are mandatory and easily performed in a primary care setting. Biochemical assessment is straightforward. In the process of diagnosis at least one fasting blood sugar and possibly a glucose tolerance test will have been done. Further assessment as first time investigations should include fasting lipid profile, electrolytes, urea and creatinine, thyroid function and sex hormones (when indicated). These results will not only form a baseline from which to assess future changes as weight loss follows, but will also help to reassure the patient that there are no medical reasons why they might not be able to achieve beneficial weight loss. Second line investigations for obesity where indicated might include a chest X-ray, electrocardiogram and a 24 hour cortisol level [6].

14.8   Treatment groups

There is much debate about which obese patients' primary care professionals should invest time and resources to help. However, it should now be beyond dispute that there is a need to assist overweight and obese patients with type 2 diabetes to modify their diet, improve their levels of physical activity and achieve weight loss. Guidelines for obesity management generally advise that medical support and interventions are appropriate in patients with a BMI ≥ 30 in the absence of any comorbid disease but also in those of the BMI ≥ 27 in the presence of comorbidity such as type 2 diabetes, hypertension, coronary heart disease and dyslipidaemia. However, it is clear that even a modest increase in weight over ideal levels confers additional risk of developing type 2 diabetes. Anyone who has type 2 diabetes and whose weight is above the normal BMI range of 18.5–24.9 should be offered an appropriate level of advice and medical support to lose weight. Of course, any weight loss attempts are reliant on patient participation and so while it is ultimately a patient's choice whether to aim for weight loss, the clinician can be influential in providing positive information concerning the desirability and benefit of weight loss and the level of support they are able to offer in order to help the patients make their decision and reach their goal. Patient motivation is commonly in direct proportion to the enthusiasm of the general practitioner and practice nurse.

Within primary care consideration must be given to working with reputable commercial weight loss organizations. These groups can offer patients basic dietary and activity advice to support and encourage a return to a healthier lifestyle and promote weight loss and should be seen as added support, not a threat to primary care workers involved in managing their overweight. They can offer valuable psychological and emotional support with social contact often in out-of-hours meetings and can ease the financial and time constraints of primary care. Practices should make their own assessment of local groups if they wish to 'refer' patients to them. It is important to actively question patients on their use of additional support to lose weight through commercial agencies and not rely on self-supporting, as many will not see them as having a direct bearing on their medical care.

Realistic goals should be set. Obese patients often have overly optimistic expectations of what weight loss can be achieved. One study in a hospital-based overweight clinic found that the average weight loss expected by patients was in excess of 30%. The reality is that in a clinical setting, in primary or secondary care, medically supported weight loss over one year is likely to average between 5 and 10% of body weight. This discrepancy needs to be addressed at the outset as bitter disappointment is likely to follow if not. Patients should be encouraged to work towards a gradual loss of between 0.5 and 1 kg weekly, perhaps for the first 3 to 6 months, following which a period of stability is likely. For some, weight maintenance at this level will be sufficient; for others further weight loss might be achievable in later months. Weight loss is never easy but for those with type 2 diabetes weight loss usually proves to be slower and harder won than for most. Yet in the same group the benefits of sustained weight loss are more substantial and therefore unquestionably worth the effort for both patient and clinician. Patients should be encouraged to attend the practice at least monthly and in the early stages of management, two weekly appointments can prove highly beneficial. A good practice team can work together to provide continuity of care, the patient often alternating between doctor and nurse to optimize successful intervention. As management progresses repeated examination should follow local or national guidelines for diabetes care.

14.9 Physical activity

The health benefits of regular physical activity are great and this must be conveyed to the patient from the outset of treatment. Thirty minutes each day of moderately intense physical activity can be shown to reduce blood pressure, improve lipid profile, decrease cardiovascular risk and improve energy levels and self esteem, all in addition to aiding weight loss and improving diabetes care [10]. Not only does increased physical activity help produce weight loss but individuals who exercise regularly are almost more likely to maintain their weight loss in the long term. Advice on physical activity has not traditionally been seen as the responsibility of the General Practitioner and yet so much can be achieved by a patient motivated to become more active. Before becoming more active it may be helpful for the health professional to discuss with their patient which type and what intensity of activity would be appropriate (see Box 14.1). Patients are often resistant to increasing their activity levels for a variety of reasons. They often perceive that to be beneficial, exercise must be intense and involve frequent gym attendance and exhausting sessions on various types of expensive equipment. They may complain that they are too old, too unfit, embarrassed, too busy, unable to afford it, have no one to go with or simply that they don't want to make the effort. However, for the majority, a careful explanation of the benefits and the type of exercise required may alleviate those fears. In those who are disabled, elderly, suffering from co-morbid disease such as coronary heart disease, or to whom physical activity is a distance memory, more specific advice may be necessary. For those who are significantly challenged a community-based physiotherapist might contribute advice and reassurance about resuming physical activity. For others and for those for the whom the gym is appealing, reassurance by a qualified fitness instructor at a sports club or fitness centre who understands the need to make new activity accessible and achievable and who can recognize the particular needs of the overweight, can be worthwhile. However, not everyone has the financial resources

---

Box 14.1 Choosing the right activity – points to discuss with patients

- What do you want to be able to do?
- How active you've been in the past few months?
- What kind of activity do you enjoy?
- What fits in with your lifestyle?
- What is appropriate for your physical condition?
- What activity is appropriate for your age?
- How quickly do you want to lose weight?
- What activity will you still enjoy in a years time?

or desire to make use of such clubs. Primary Care Trusts have implemented 'exercise on prescription' schemes to encourage inactive people to take up formalized activity under supervision usually at the local sports centre. Further attendance may be offered at a subsidized rate or in specific sessions, for example for the very overweight. Primary Care Trusts need to work closely with local government and may have to put forward strongly the case for increased physical activity as an important contributor to improved health and not just for people with type 2 diabetes but for everyone. Experience however has shown that the effectiveness of such schemes varies. Harland *et al.* [7] found that the most effective form of activity was not formal sports centre based schemes but those that encouraged 'home-based activity', that is, walking. However, for those who are attracted to formal exercise such schemes can provide a welcome introduction to physical activity. The reality, of course, is that for any long-term benefit to be achieved exercise must be regular and frequent. In order to facilitate weight loss, promote dietary control and to improve fitness generally, the patient should be encouraged to find an extra 30 minutes of activity in their daily routine, for example three episodes of 10 minutes each, at least five days each week. Patients can therefore be effectively encouraged to increase activity by, for example, leaving the car at home whenever possible, particularly for any journeys of less than one mile, using stairs and avoiding lifts, getting off the bus a stop or two early and being more active generally around the house. Some primary care teams have even set up links with local rambling groups to facilitate more creative walking activities. Whilst this type of involvement may not be appropriate for every practice it does show what can be achieved by those who are motivated to look beyond the confines of the practice to maximize the potential for walking to health.

14.10 Behavioural change

Behavioural change, encouraging and facilitating changes in habits, is a complex subject in its own right, and not something generally taught to primary care clinicians and nurses. However, it should not be seen as a separate form of management, rather as integral to the whole programme of empowering patient control of their diabetes, dietary habits and attitudes activity. Formal behavioural change, by qualified professionals, can produce sustained benefit, but input needs to be long term and the cost is therefore probably prohibitive in a primary care setting. Much can be achieved, however, by an informed and enthusiastic and patient doctor and nurse, using learned techniques as well as employing patient management skills aquired in practice. An increasing number of dietitians are developing expertise in this area, and their skills can be used to great advantage in helping overweight diabetics. The simplest form of support, deliverable from primary care might involve encouragement of the patient to learn to control unhelpful eating patterns. Advice such as to eat only at the table, to savour eating, and avoid distractions such as watching television simultaneously, to chew longer, to put down the fork back on the plate between mouthfuls, to wait for 20 minutes between courses to avoid over-eating and so on. Continuous positive reinforcement is required, an absence of negative criticism a must, and a willingness to overlook repeated apparent failure essential.

14.11   Use of medication to aid weight loss in primary care

In spite of the best efforts of clinicians and patients, the reality is that many patients will not achieve significant weight loss within the first 6 months of treatment. Many who have achieved a degree of weight loss show a tendency for the weight to plateau after three to six months with subsequent regain not unusual. Obesity should never be regarded as a short-term problem, rather it is a chronic condition with even the most radically motivated patients experiencing times of relapse over months or years after initial treatment. The use of weight loss medication should be considered after 3 to 6 months' compliance to dietary, behaviour and activity advice, a failure to achieve 10% body weight loss or significant reduction in HbA1c, to further reduce markers of comorbidity such as dyslipidaemia and hypertension, and to reduce symptomatology such as joint pain and breathlessness [11]. The role of weight loss medication has often been misunderstood. It should be viewed as an *adjunct* to supported lifestyle change and as an aid to enhance weight loss and in so doing help educate patients towards establishing long-term habit change of improved diet and increased physical activity. Medication should never be seen as an alternative to improved nutrition and increased physical activity.

There are several agents available and currently used by medical practitioners to aid weight loss but there are however only two agents currently recommended and licensed for use within the NHS. These are orlistat (Xenical) and sibutramine (Reductil). Orlistat first became available in 1999 and is classified as a gastrointestinal lipase inhibitor. It reduces absorption of fats, mainly triglycerides, for the small intestine. Sibutramine has been available in some parts of Europe and the USA since 1999 and in the UK since 2001. It is a centrally acting serotonin and noradrenaline reuptake inhibitor. Both orlistat and sibutramine have been shown to be effective in primary care and to convey significant benefit in the treatment of overweight diabetes [8, 12–14]. The National Institute for Health and Clinical Excellence has considered both agents and has given approval of their use within the NHS citing improved rates of weight loss, significant improvements in glycaemia, lipid levels and blood pressure over and above diet and exercise alone. The commonly used hypoglycaemic agent metformin has been shown to have some weight loss effect in diabetics trying to reduce their weight. Its effect on insulin resistance has been utilized in obese non-diabetic subjects to aid weight loss, and in particular in women who are overweight as a result of polycystic ovarian syndrome. Some practitioners have tried to use metformin in combination with orlistat or sibutramine. It does not have any specific licensing arrangements for the treatment of obesity and currently does not have a defined role. The twice daily injection incretin mimetic, Exenatide, has been shown to lower glucose levels and improve diabetes control when used in combination with sulfonylureas and metformin. Additional properties include delayed gastric emptying and reduced appetite which may have beneficial results on overweight patients. For a detailed review of the currently licensed anti-obesity agents, refer to Chapter 10.

14.12   Summary

In recent years the increasing prevalence of type 2 diabetes has been accompanied by an increasing willingness and ability of the primary health care team to deliver evidence-based best practice and diabetes management from primary care. There is clear evidence not only that obesity and overweight are implicated in the development of type 2 diabetes but also that even modest reductions in weight can lead to significantly improved prevention and treatment of diabetes with associated reduction in complications. The motivated general practitioner and practice nurse can equip themselves with the necessary clinical skills and tools to offer effective weight management services within the practice and draw on the support of the specialist skills of allied professional when available and appropriate. Diabesity is a disease of complex aetiology with multisystem pathological results. In order to continue to offer the best possible care to our patients the primary care team needs to engage with effective treatment modalities with enthusiasm and dedication. The multidisciplinary approach to disease management in primary care is an ideal environment to incorporate the management of obesity as an integral part of normal diabetes care.

References

1. Foresight Report, Tackling obesity: future choices (2007).
2. National Audit Office (2001) Tackling Obesity in England. HC 220 Sess. 2000–2001 15 Feb 2001.
3. Jung, R.T. (1997) Obesity as a disease. *British Medical Bulletin*, **53**, 307–21.
4. Frost, G., Masters, K., King, C. *et al.* (1991) A new method of energy prescription to improve weight loss. *Journal of Human Nutrition and Dietetics*, **4**, 369–73.
5. Goldstein, D. (1992) Beneficial health effects of modest weight loss. *International Journal of Obesity*, **16**, 397–15.
6. National Obesity Forum (2000) Guidelines on the Management of Adult Obesity. National Obesity Forum, Nottingham.
7. Harland, J., White, M., Drinkwater, C. *et al.* (1999) The Newcastle exercise project: a randomised controlled trial of methods to promote physical activity in primary care. *British Medical Journal*, **319**, 828–32.
8. Hauptman, J., Lucas, C., Boldrin, M.N. *et al.* (2000) Orlistat in the long term treatment of obesity in primary care settings. *Archives of Family Medicine*, **9**, 160–7.
9. Lean, M.E.J., Han, T.S. and Seidell, J.C. (1991) Impairment of health and quality of life in people with large waist circumference. *Lancet*, **351**, 853–6.
10. Sarvis, W.H.M. (1998) Physical activity in the treatment of obesity. Symposium on Obesity – the threat ahead, pp. 24–25.
11. Royal College of Physicians (1998) *Clinical Management of Overweight and Obese Patients with Particular Reference to the Use of Drugs*, RCP, London.

12. Hollander, P.A., Elbein, S.C., Hirsch, I.B. *et al.* (1998) Role of orlistat in the treatment of obese patients with type 2 diabetes. *Diabetes Care*, **21**, 1288–94.
13. Finer, N., Bloom, S.R., Frost, G.S. *et al.* (2000) Sibutramine is effective for weight loss and diabetic control in obesity with type 2 diabetes. *Diabetes, Obesity & Metabolism*, **2**, 105–12.
14. Jones, S.P., Smith, I.G., Kelly, F. and Gray, J.A. (1995) Long term weight loss with sibutramine. *International Journal of Obesity and Related Metabolic Disorders*, **19** (Suppl 2), 41.

15

Obesity and employment

Nerys Williams

Consultant Occupational Physician and former Honorary Consultant in Weight
Management, Birmingham Heartlands and Solihull NHS Trust, Birmingham, UK

15.1   Introduction

When the Human Resources director of a health club company was reported to have
sent an internal memo to staff relating to 'the impact of larger employees', despite
vigorous denials from the company, the press fed on the story with a frenzy. This
illustrated the sensitivity around weight as an employment and as a social issue.

Although obesity is recognized as a disease and is treated as such in the NHS, it is
likely that businesses will not directly be aware of its cost to their bottom line and
profits. They maybe aware of the toll of diabetes, heart disease and other complications
because these are commonly used categories on sickness absence recording systems but
the underlying and preventable cause, excess weight, is often over looked and not
appreciated. It is considered by many to be 'just a lifestyle issue' and a personal choice
to over indulge and not an area for employer involvement.

But the time has now come when obesity cannot be ignored, either at a public health
level or in the workplace. The epidemic will become more severe and will have a
growing impact on several aspects of work activity.

15.2   Obesity, health and work

The specialty of occupational health looks at the interaction between the worker and
the workplace from several different perspectives. The first is the effect of work on
health that is work as the cause of disease and illness. The second is the effect of health
on work – how a condition not caused by work, impacts on an individual's ability to do
their job effectively. This includes how a person does their job (e.g. related to their

Obesity and Diabetes, Second Edition   Edited by Anthony H. Barnett and Sudhesh Kumar
© 2009 John Wiley & Sons, Ltd

fitness) and how they can work safely (e.g. through the use of protective equipment). Third, occupational health looks at how people with health problems can be rehabilitated back into work and finally how the workplace can be used as a possible setting for health promotion and education activities through the provision of healthy food options and opportunities for exercise and for a positive environment which can support a diet and exercise weight management programme.

15.3   Effect of work on health

Relatively little research has been performed to see if specific jobs are actually obesogenic. Whilst anecdotally there seems to be over representation of people in catering and food trades attending NHS obesity clinics, studies have reported specific workplace activities and environments associated with excess weight gain [1]. Reported findings have differed across different studies, with some but not all suggesting that the risk of obesity may be increased in work environments that place high demands on workers yet give them low control over what they do and how they do it. The types of jobs which have these characteristics include production line work and work in certain types of call centres. Workers who work long hours have also been identified as being at risk of increased weight. This can occur in any industry but is frequently seen in offshore work and production facilities.

Box 15.1 Work conditions possibly associated with increased weight

High demand, low control jobs for example in call centres and on production lines

Jobs involving long hours

Shift work

Work stress

Obesity *per se* was also found to influence the acquisition of work related conditions and could:

1. Modify the risk of an individual developing a vibration induced injury. This was previously known as 'white finger' and is now called hand vibration syndrome (HAVS). It is one of the causes of secondary Raynaud's phenomenon and can be permanently disabling impacting on ability to work and undertake activities of daily living.

2. Act as a co-risk factor for the development of occupational asthma.

3. Modify a workers response to occupational stress and modify the risk of disease from occupational exposure to neurotoxins [1].

The relationship between body mass index (BMI) and work stress has also been investigated. [2] using cross sectional questionnaire data on 45 810 female and male

Finnish public sector workers. The researchers confirmed the association of high demand, low control jobs with BMI and an association between higher BMI and high effort-reward imbalance. In men who had lower job demands there was also an association with a higher BMI. Overall they reported a weak association between work stress and BMI.

15.4 Shift work

Associations between shift work and obesity have been well documented. Di Lorenzo *et al.* [3] reported on a cross sectional study of the metabolic effects of shift work in 319 glucose tolerant workers in the chemical industry in southern Italy. They found that shift workers had higher BMIs than day workers and that shift working was associated with BMI, independent of age and work duration. They also found that systolic blood pressure was also significantly higher but that it was influenced by BMI not shift work. Other studies have also shown obesity to be more prevalent in shift workers [4] and marked weight gain in shift working populations [5,6].

15.5 Work and response to treatment

Work and work organization may not only be a factor in causing obesity but certain aspects of work have also been reported to impact on individuals response to treatment by bariatric surgery. A retrospective study of 389 patients who had undergone Roux-en-Y gastric bypass surgery was undertaken [7]. The cohort contained a small number (eight) of shift workers. Weight loss post surgery was significantly lower in the shift workers than the non-shift workers at 3 months, (29.9% vs. 43.8% $p < 0.01$), at 6 months (46.4% vs. 61.3% ($p < 0.01$) and at 12 months (56.5% vs. 76.8% $p < 0.01$).

Although studies are rare, it is logical to assume that work can facilitate the development of obesity if it is sedentary by design (such as in offices or call centre work), if it removes the need for natural breaks and activity (e.g. by locating photocopiers and printers on desks rather than around the office so someone has to get up and move to use them) and if it provides opportunities for consumption of high calorie foods during working hours (e.g. through poor catering, the provision of free meals whilst on duty or the ready availability of food e.g. in confectionery manufacture). It may also facilitate weight gain through boredom or where the environment is such that eating is one of the few pleasures available (such as in offshore work).

15.6 Effect of health on work

The epidemic of obesity is impacting on the workplace and is becoming noticeable on an individual case basis in terms of sickness absence, ill health retirement, lack of fitness to work with poor performance and failure to pass medical standards. Yet few employers, or indeed occupational health physicians, are able to quantify its effects as often it is the comorbidities such as diabetes and coronary heart disease, which are the labels used to describe the health problem, rather than the underlying obesity.

15.7   Sickness absence and short-term disability

The links between sickness absence and obesity have been well described in the cohort of civil servants based in London in the Whitehall II study. Ferrie *et al.* [8] looked at the effect of BMI and changes in BMI from the age of 25 years as predictors of sickness absence. Data from 2564 women and 5853 men were analysed and compared to employers records of medically certified (>7 days) and self certified (1–7 days) spells of sickness absence. BMI was documented at baseline and then at a mean follow up period of 7.0 years later.

After adjustment for employment grade, health related behaviours and heath status, overweight (BMI = 25.0–29.9 kg/m^2 and obesity (BMI > 30 kg/m^2) were significant predictors of short and long absences in both sexes: rate ratios of (95% confidence intervals) ranged from 1.14 (1.05–1.21) to 1.51 (1.30–1.76) compared with a BMI of 21.0–22.9 kg/m^2.

The study also found that a BMI of 23.0–24.9 kg/m^2 predicted long-term absences in women and underweight (BMI < 21.0 kg/m^2 predicted short-term absences in men. Obesity at age 25 years predicted long-term absences and initial obesity, present at the start of the study, predicted short- and long-term absences in both men and women. Chronic obesity was a strong predictor of long absences in men, with a rate ratio of 2.61 (1.88–3.63). The authors concluded that the obesity epidemic might result in significant increases in sickness absence.

The finding of an association between BMI and sickness absence (short and particularly long term) was seen again in a Finnish study of Helsinki-based public sector employees and also found that working conditions had almost no effect on the association between BMI and short or long periods of sickness absence [9].

The independent effects of adiposity and body fat distribution and their relationship to sickness absence have been studied in the Belstress study in Belguim [10]. A cohort of 20 463 workers in 25 companies were identified and their sickness absence documented over the following year. The 75th percentile of the distribution of the total annual sickness days was used as a cut off to classify a high 1-year incidence rate of sick leave. BMI and waist circumference were measured to determine adiposity and distribution of body fat. The study found that central abdominal fatness (but not BMI) was an independent predictor of sickness absence for both sexes (both high incidence and long spells of absence).

Box 15.2 Obesity and sickness absence

Both overweight and obesity predict long- and short-term absence in male and females

Underweight predicts short-term absence in men

Central adiposity is an independent predictor of sickness absence in both sexes

15.8 Disability pensions

One of the consequences of extended sick leave is the award of a short-term pension or for retirement on health grounds. Terms of company and public sector retirement schemes vary but the impact of obesity on claims has proved to be of interest to employers and insurers. Arena *et al.* [11] studied employees of a financial services organization (so called 'white collar' workers) and found that after adjusting for multiple covariates, BMI was an independent predictor for short-term disability 'events'. It is likely that these correlate more with the United Kingdom and European concept of sickness absence given the differences in the United States and European social security schemes.

15.9 Is it reversible?

The clear links between high BMI and sickness absence should be a cause for concern of employers but are they reversible ? Serxner *et al.* [12] described the impact of a worksite health promotion campaign on short-term disability claims and found it to be cost effective in reducing days lost. However this is not comparable to the United Kingdom as in the United States all health care costs, including those of treatment, are borne by the employer and not the state health system. More hopeful data has been reported form the Swedish Obese Subjects study, which looked at sickness absence before and after bariatric surgery and conventional treatment [13]. They found that surgical treatment of obesity result in a reduction of sick leave and disability pensions, compared to controls, after the first year and particularly in subjects aged 47–60 years.

15.10 Accidents

Studies have looked at whether people who are obese and who have sleep apnoea have an increased risk of accidents, both occupational and on the roads. Teran-Santos *et al.* [14] conducted a case–control study of people with sleep apnoea and road traffic accidents. And found a strong association between sleep apnoea, as measured by the apnoea-hyponoea index, and the risk of traffic accidents. As compared to those without sleep apnoea, patients with an index of 10 or more had an odds ratio of 6.3 (95% confidence interval, 2.4–16.2) for having a traffic accident. This is highly relevant for occupations involving driving either full or part time. A sevenfold increase in risk of car accidents on patients with sleep apnoea has also been reported by Findley *et al.* [15] and Finkelstein *et al.* [16] have also reported an overall excess risks of all types of accident (traffic, falls, sporting) between BMI and the probability of sustaining an injury. The combination of obesity and high-risk occupations was found to be particularly detrimental. Increased accidents mean increased claims and costs. Ostbye *et al.* [17] found a linear relationship between BMI and claims with people with morbid obesity (BMI $> 40 \, \text{kg/m}^2$) having twice the number of claims of normal weight colleagues. There was an even stronger association with claims costs. The claims most strongly affected by BMI were to the lower extremity, wrist or hand and back.

Box 15.3 Accidents, claims, costs and obesity

Some studies suggest an association between obesity and all types of accident (road, sporting and falls)

A linear relationship has been reported between BMI and numbers of claims and an even stronger association with the cost of claims

If an obese person has sleep apnoea and daytime sleepiness then they are at more than twice the risk of occupational accidents

---

It is not just road traffic or sporting accidents that are influenced by obesity. If the individual has sleep apnoea then they are also at more than twice the risk of occupational accidents if they have both snoring and daytime sleepiness [18].

15.11   Fitness for work and ergonomics

Being overweight or obese can have other effects on ability to work and to work safely. Poor mobility due to weight, respiratory impairment or arthritis can inhibit the ability of an individual to evacuate a building in an emergency such as fire. It may be that because lifts cannot be used and the person cannot move down several flights of stairs that equipment in the form of an evacuation chair needs to be provided. Other individuals will need to be trained in its use with attendant risk of musculoskeletal injury in the rescuer.

The ability to give first aid requires mobility (to reach the casualty), flexibility (to bend to attend them on the floor), respiratory capacity (to provide mouth to mouth resuscitation) and physical stamina (to perform the necessary chest compressions). An overweight or obese person maybe unable to perform one or more of the above stages and may not be physically fit enough to be a first aider.

Personal protective equipment such as aprons protects not only the individual in the healthcare setting, also the patient through control of infection. Aprons are provided in a range of sizes but sometimes even the largest size is not adequate so healthcare staff wear them around their neck and not tied at the waist (because they do not fit around the waist), leading to a risk of transmission of infection. Respiratory masks worn to protect against inhalation of toxic chemicals and particles need to fit correctly. The obese face presents a challenge for adequate but even if the mask does fit, breathing against a filter requires enhanced respiratory capacity, which an obese person just may not have.

One of the most common areas where the impact of obesity is seen in the workplace is in ergonomic issues. In addition to the selection and fit of protective equipment as outlined above, chairs may need to be specially selected to withstand weight. Desks may need to be designed to allow someone with pronounced abdominal obesity get close enough to the desk and keyboard to use a computer safely and distances between desks and furniture in open plan offices may need to be increased to allow a large person to move around freely and without having to squeeze between furniture or bruise or injure themselves.

Uniforms may need to be specially ordered to ensure adequate fit, and in order to travel comfortably companies may need to purchase two adjoining airline seats, particularly for long-haul flights.

15.12 Medical standards

Relatively few occupations have medical standards but diving, work offshore, fire fighting and some jobs involving work on railways are a few that do. Standards are set, either to protect the individual against increased risk of ill health (e.g. diving where the risk of decompression illness is raised with raised BMI), or for the safety of others (e.g. emergency rescue crews). Obesity may impact on fitness to work purely because of increased size thus one of the requirement of offshore work is the ability to pass through the door of a helicopter wearing a survival suit – not easy if the individual is either very tall or very large.

Obesity due to a sedentary lifestyle and lack of physical fitness can mean a person does not meet the required standard. It may seem absurd that a train driver who sits all day in a cabin should have to meet a medical standard that considers obesity and physical fitness until you realize that it is essential that he or she is able to get in and out of the narrow cabin, up and down steps to and from the cabin at some stations and be able to run a quarter of mile to an emergency telephone to summon help.

Failure to meet a medical standard can mean loss of job, which has its own negative impact on health so a good proactive employer will ensure they take occupational health advice and plan a series of checks to identify individuals before they reach thresholds at which their employment is in danger. This allows the individual to make changes to their lifestyle, lose weight and continue at work.

15.13 Rehabilitation

Good employers have proactive rehabilitation programmes to help workers who are off work, either due to work or non-work-related health problems, to return to their jobs. Employees who are overweight and obese may experience gain in weight when off work and become fatigued when they return. Employers need to make sure they do not, despite good intentions, arrange work so employees become more inactive. Graded returns to physical jobs enable workers to get back to previous levels of fitness but may need to be undertaken over weeks rather than days. The Disability Discrimination Act 1995 requires employers to make reasonable adjustments to work places and work tasks for employees who have a 'physical or mental impairment' that affects one of more of seven domains of activities and if the condition is likely to last or has lasted for more than 12 months. There is considerable debate as to whether obesity *per se* is a condition covered by the Disability and Discrimination Act, but as it is a physical impairment, lasts more than 12 months and affects mobility, lifting, and so on, in the author's opinion it is likely to be covered; however, the definitive view can only be provided by an Employment Tribunal. Employers need to be careful that, whereas for other conditions, for example back pain, reasonable adjustments may mean reducing someone's activity; for obese patients this could lead to further weight gain and be against medical advice.

15.14   Stigma and discrimination

One topic worthy of inclusion is the stigma and discrimination around obesity, which may impact on employer's willingness to support staff at work. Little attention has so far been paid, in the United Kingdom at least, to the effect that the views of employers and practitioners in the healthcare system can have with regards to people with obesity. The workplace can be a hostile environment to people who are different but discrimination on grounds of gender, disability, religion and now age are all subject to discrimination legislation – not so obesity. Bullying, prejudice and discrimination have all been described in studies of obese workers, many of whom maybe depressed and have low self-esteem to start with.

Whilst little research has been undertaken in the United Kingdom, in the United States Professor Mark Roehling, from the Department of Management at Western Michigan University has concluded from his work that 'overall the evidence of consistent, significant discrimination against overweight employees is sobering' [19]. He found that overweight people were subject to discrimination in employment decisions based on body weight, they were stereotyped as emotionally impaired, socially handicapped and as possessing negative personality traits. The wages of mildly obese white women were 5.9% lower than standard weight counterparts and very obese women had wages 24.1% lower. Men only experienced penalties at the very highest weight levels.

Other studies have shown discrimination in recruitment and employee discharge (redundancy). Saporta and Halpern [20] investigated the effect of being overweight and of being thin in lawyers. By examining the salaries and personal measurements of respondents to the 1984 National Lawyer Survey, they found that overweight and thin male lawyers were paid less than normal weight individuals. The same was not found for women.

It has been long established that physical appearance is important to how people are treated. This attribution of special or better qualities due to appearance is known as the 'halo' effect of attractiveness, and even in professions unlikely to value physical appearance attractiveness ratings can predict future promotion. Weight is one of the most important determinants of attractiveness, but it is the ratio of height to weight which is thought to be most important [21]. A person's weight is thought to reflect many aspects of their character such as their motivation, willingness to work, ambition, their personal control and their discipline. This can influence employers' decisions regarding recruitment, promotion and salary.

The literature suggests that short people and unattractive people do not fare as well in the workplace as tall, attractive people. This comes from both laboratory experiments and field studies. Physical attractiveness has been found to affect interviewers' judgements when they assess curriculum vitae of potential managers [22].

The findings are stark: Roe and Eickwort [23] found in a survey of 81 employers (including human resources professionals) that 15.9% of employers held the view that obese applicants should be barred from employment and 43.9% believed that obesity was a valid medical reason for not employing a person. Studies have suggested that obese people are perceived to possess negative traits such as less conscientious (lazy) [24], lacking self-discipline and self control [25], less able to get on with customers and fellow workers [26].

An indication of the depth of prejudice against obese people which has been found is seen in the conclusions drawn by Kennedy and Homant [27] They found that that overweight job applicants were treated more harshly by employers when applying for work than ex-felons or individuals with a past history of mental ill health.

Compared to the US, relatively little research has been undertaken on the views of human resources practitioners. But a study published by *Personnel Today* [28] contains some worrying similarities with United States findings. In the survey of over 2000 human resources professionals, headline findings included:

- 93% said they would choose a 'normal' weight person over an obese applicant with the same qualifications and experience;

- 47% thought obesity negatively affected employee output;

- 30% thought obesity was a valid medical reason for not employing someone;

- 75% said their organization was doing little or nothing to tackle the issue and 69% said obesity was not discussed in their workplace;

- 11% thought employers could fairly dismiss someone because they were obese;

- 12% said obese people were unsuitable for client facing roles.

The literature review can be summarized as identifying significant discrimination against overweight and obese individuals at several stages of the employment process and beyond. Employers may feel they are justified in not recruiting obese people because of the ergonomic costs, raised sickness absence and greater healthcare costs. However, personal motivation, talent and skills can be overlooked when prejudice exists. The increased numbers of obese people both as employees and customers might have been expected to change attitudes and long-standing prejudices but this has yet to appear in studies. But this is more than just an issue that has significant implications for employment; it also affects self-esteem, which is pivotal to health behaviour changes.

Box 15.4 Obesity: Prejudice and discrimination

Studies have shown that obese people are less likely to be:

1. recruited

2. paid the same rates.

and are more likely to be:

1. selected for redundancy

2. perceived to be lazy and less able to get on with colleagues.

15.15 Health promotion

Workplaces are unique in that they have a captive population, many of whom are the individuals who do not ordinarily come into contact with their GP or practice nurse team and who have a reputation for late presentation of disease – notably young and middle aged men. Work can be a source of activity (not necessarily exercise) both in the job, in getting around at work and rarely, in the provision of actual facilities to exercise. Food is a feature of all workplaces either in canteens, snack bars or dispensing machines. In many workplaces there are occupational health professionals able to deliver consistent messages and support interested workers in learning more about diet, exercise and weight loss. But even in the absence of professional staff, workers can be included to set up their own competitions amongst staff with prizes awarded by management and a positive attitude towards participation.

Workplace weight reduction programmes have been shown to work either on their own or as part of a heart disease risk reduction programme) In some cases they have been reported to be more successful than weight clinics in the healthcare setting [29]. Health promotion activities can either be directed at the individual or at the whole working population but it is likely that the most effective interventions will be those, which remove the element of choice to make unhealthy decisions regarding food and nutrition by fundamentally changing the working environment. Work at the Mayo Clinic has looked at increased energy expenditure through the modification of common workplace activities, such as using a computer. By asking a worker to stand on a very slow treadmill and to work using a laptop they demonstrated an increase in energy consumption of 100 kcal/h. If used for 2–3 hours per day, and other components of energy balance remained constant, this would equate to a weight loss of 2–30 kg/year [30]. For workers who prefer to remain seated the Mayo Clinic has devised an office stepping device that can be sited under a normal desk and plugged into a PC for self-monitoring. The use of the device was found to lead to an increase in energy expenditure over and above just sitting in an office chair of 289 ± 102 kcal/hr ($p < 0.001$). The energy expenditure was greater for the obese (335 ± 99 kcal/hr) than for lean subjects (235 ± 80 kcal/hr $p = 0.03$). The increments in energy expenditure were similar to exercise-style walking. Researchers calculated that the use of the stepping device for 2 hours per day would result in loss of 20 kg/year if all other energy parameters remained the same [31].

Other studies looking at integrating exercise breaks into work routine have provided successful in improvements in body composition [32].

The effectiveness of conventional health promotion programmes, providing education on nutrition and exercise have been studied – Oberlinner *et al.* [33] reported on the BASF study which targeted all overweight and obese employees at a BASF site and put through a 9 month health promotion campaign and programme with a large prize draw for €10 000 for successful employees and their supporters; 2062 people took part and 658 reduced their weight, 440 having reduced their BMI by more than 2 points.

Specific occupational groups such as home workers and mobile staff present specific problems and challenges to the introduction of workplace schemes but it should not be assumed that single site factories and offices present less of a challenge. In today's' business environment staff maybe paid on productivity and time away, even for a good cause, which may have benefits for them and their employer, may not be welcomed by all staff or all employers. Guidance on how to introduce employee or workplace population-centred health promotion campaigns to prevent and reduce obesity is available, illustrated by case studies of campaigns undertaken across different size, industry sector, available budget and location [34].

In conclusion, obesity has many potential impacts on the workplace, many of which are currently unrecognized. If British businesses are to remain economically viable and profitable, as the obesity epidemic continues and gets worse, more effort will need to be devoted to helping people stop gaining weight and to support those who wish to lose weight. This not only has health benefits for the individual but also has economic and efficiency benefits, for the employer.

References

1. Schulte, P.A. *et al.* (2007) Work, obesity and occupational safety and health. *American Journal of Public Health*, **97**, 428–36.
2. Kouvonen, A., Kivimaki, M., Cox, S.J. *et al.* (2005) Relationship between work stress and body mass index among 45,810 female and male employees. *Psychosomatic Medicine*, **67**, 577–83.
3. Di Lorenzo, L. *et al.* (2003) Effect of shift work on body mass index: results of a study performed in 319 glucose tolerant men working in a Southern Italian industry. *International Journal of Obesity*, **27**, 1353–58.
4. Karlsson, B., Knuttsson, A. and Lindahl, B. (2001) Is there an association between shift work and having the metabolic syndrome ? Results from a population based study of 27485 people. *Journal of Occupational and Environmental Medicine*, **58**, 747–52.
5. Geliebter, A., Gluck, M.E., Tanowitz, M. *et al.* (2000) Work-shift period and weight change. *Nutrition*, **16**, 27–9.
6. Yamada, Y., Kameda, M., Noborisaka, Y., Suzuki, H., Honda, M. and Yamada, S. (2001) Comparisons of psychosomatic health and unhealthy behaviours between cleanroom workers in a 12 hour shift and those in an 8 hour shift. *Journal of Human Ergology (Tokyo)*, **1–2**, 399–403.

7. Ketchum, E.S. and Morton, J.M. (2007) Disappointing weight loss among shift workers after laparoscopic gastric bypass surgery. *Obesity Surgery*, **17**, 581–4.

8. Ferrie, J.E., Head, J., Shipley, M.J. *et al.* (2007) BMI, obesity and sickness absence in the Whitehall II study. *Obesity (Silver Spring)*, **15**, 1554–6.

9. Laaksonen, M., Phia, K. and Sarlio-Lahteenkorva, S. (2007) Relative weight and sickness absence. *Obesity (Silver Spring)*, **2**, 465–72.

10. Moreau, M., Valente, F., Mak, R. *et al.* (2004) Obesity, body fat distribution and incidence of sick leave in the Belgian workforce: the Belstress study. *International Journal of Obesity and Related Metabolic Disorders*, **28**, 574–82.

11. Arena, V.C., Padiyear, K.R., Burton, W.N. and Schwerha, K.J.J. (2006) The impact of body mass index on short term disability in the workplace. *Journal of Occupational and Environmental Medicine*, **48** (11), 1118–24.

12. Serxner, S., Gold, D., Anderson, D. and Williams, D. (2001) The impact of a worksite health promotion program on short term disability usage. *Journal of Occupational and Environmental Medicine/American College of Occupational and Environmental Medicine*, **43**, 25–9.

13. Narbro, K., Agren, G., Jonsson, E. *et al.* (1999) Sick leave and disability pension before and after treatment for obesity: a report from the Swedish Obese Subjects (SOS) study. *International Journal of Obesity and Related Metabolic Disorders*, **23**, 619–24.

14. Teran-Santos, J., Jimenez-Gomez, A. and Janson, C. (1999) The association between sleep apnoea and the risk of road traffic accidents. Cooperative Group Burgos-Santander. *New England Journal of Medicine*, **340**, 847–51.

15. Findley, L.J., Unverzagt, M.E. and Suratt, P.M. (1988) Automobile accidents involving patients with obstructive sleep apnoea. *American Review of Respiratory Disease*, **138**, 337–40.

16. Finkelstein E.A., Chen H., Prabhu M., Trogdon J.G. and Corso P.S. (2007) The relationship between obesity and injuries among US adults. *American Journal of Health Promotion*, **21** (5), 460–8.

17. Ostbye, T., Dement, J.M. and Krause, K.M. (2007) Obesity and workers' compensation: results from the Duke Health and Safety Surveillance System. *Archives of Internal Medicine*, **167**, 766–73.

18. Lindberg, E., Carter, N., Gislason, T. and Janson, C. (2001) Role of snoring and daytime sleepiness in occupational accidents. *American Journal of Respiratory and Critical Care Medicine*, **164**, 2031–5.

19. Roehling, M. (1999) Weight based Discrimination in employment: psychological and legal aspects. *Personnel Psychology*, **52**, 969–1016.

20. Saporta, I. and Halpern, J.J. (2002) Being different can hurt: effects of deviation from physical norms on lawyers' salaries. *Industrial Relations*, **41**, 442–66.

21. Patzer, G.L. (1985) *Physical Attractiveness Phenomena*, Plenum Press, New York.

22. Dipboye, R., Fromkin, H.L. and Willback, K. (1975) Relative importance of applicant sex, attractiveness and scholastic standing in evaluation of job applicants resumes. *Journal of Applied Psychology*, **60**, 39–43.

23. Roe, D.A. and Eickwort, K.R. (1976) Relationships between obesity and associated health factors with low employment among low- income women. *Journal of American Medical Women's Association*, **31**, 193–204.

24. Larkin, J.C. and Pines, H.A. (1979) No fat persons need apply: Experimental studies of the overweight stereotype and hiring preference. *Sociology of Work and Occupations*, **6**, 312–27.

25. Klesges, R.C., Klem, M.L., Hanson, C.L. *et al.* (1990) The effects of applicant's health status and qualifications on simulated hiring decisions'. *International Journal of Obesity*, **14**, 527–35.

26. Klassen, M.L., Jasper, C.R. and Harris, R.J. (1990) The role of physical appearance in managerial decisions. *Journal of Business and Psychology*, **8**, 181–98.

27. Kennedy, D.B. and Homant, R.J. (1984) Personnel managers and the stigmatised employee. *Journal of Employment Counselling*, **21**, 89–94.
28. Thomas, D. (2005 25 October) Fattism is the last bastion of employee discrimination. *Personnel Today*.
29. Winick, C., Rothacker, D.Q. and Norman, R.L. (2002) Four worksite weight loss programs with high-stress occupations using a meal replacement product. *Occupational Medicine*, **52**, 25–31.
30. Levine, J.A. and Miller, J.M. (2007) The energy expenditure of using a 'walk and work' desk for office workers with obesity. *British Journal of Sports Medicine*, **41**, 558–61.
31. McAlpine, D.A., Manohar, C.U., McCrady, S.K. *et al.* (2007) A workplace stepping device to promote workplace physical activity. *British Journal of Sports Medicine*, **41**, 903–7.
32. Lara, A., Yancey, A.K., Tapia-Conye, R. *et al.* (2008) Pausa para tu Salud: reduction of weight and waistlines by integrating exercise breaks into workplace organizational routine. *Preventing Chronic Disease*, **5**, A12.
33. Oberlinner, C., Lang, S., Germann, C. *et al.* (2007) Prevention of overweight and obesity in the workplace. BASF-health promotion campaign "trim down the pounds-losing weight without losing your mind". *Gesundheitswesen*, **69**, 385–92.
34. Williams, N. (2007) *Managing Obesity in the Workplace*, Radcliffe Medical Press, Oxford.

16
Obesity in different ethnic groups

Ponnusamy Saravanan, George Valsamakis and Sudhesh Kumar
Clinical Sciences Research Institute, Warwick Medical School, University of Warwick, Coventry, UK

16.1   Introduction – obesity and adiposity

Obesity is a strong risk factor for insulin resistance (IR), type 2 diabetes (T2D) and cardiovascular disease (CVD) [1,2]. Historically, excess body weight is expressed by body mass index (BMI). BMI is defined as body weight in kilograms divided by the square of height in metres (kg/m^2). Individuals with BMI between 25.0–30 kg/m^2 are classified as overweight, and $\geq$30.0 kg/m^2 as obese. These cut points were primarily derived by the evidence from the European populations and therefore raises the argument whether this is an appropriate tool to measure obesity in other ethnic populations [3]. BMI relies very much on body weight and therefore overestimates in individuals with higher muscle mass and underestimates in individuals with central obesity and lesser muscle mass. Hence, international organizations (World Health Organization, WHO) and other authors argue that BMI cut points should be defined according to the associated risks such as hypertension, T2D, CVD, and so on [4,5]. Interestingly, the first WHO consensus statement in 2000 argued the case for reducing the BMI cut points threshold to $\geq$23 kg/m^2 (over weight) and $\geq$25 kg/m^2 (obese) in Asians; a later one in 2004 suggested it should be the same as any other population ($\geq$25 kg/m^2 and $\geq$30 kg/m^2) as there is no added benefit [6]. To fuel the argument further, in a cross-sectional study comparing 4 different ethnic groups, Razak *et al.* showed the increased metabolic risk in non-Europeans appear approximately at six BMI points below the normal threshold [7].

Body fat is distributed in three major compartments: superficial subcutaneous, deep subcutaneous and visceral fat. Superficial subcutaneous fat is distributed both centrally

Obesity and Diabetes, Second Edition   Edited by Anthony H. Barnett and Sudhesh Kumar
© 2009 John Wiley & Sons, Ltd

as well as peripherally in the limbs. Deep subcutaneous fat and visceral fat are mainly centrally distributed [8–10]. Waist circumference is the best simple anthropometric measurement for central obesity and is sensitive to change. Several large epidemiological and intervention studies showed that central obesity correlates better with metabolic risk (such as T2D, hypertension and CVD) than BMI. While it is reasonably clear that limb fat, especially lower limb fat is protective against metabolic risk, there is ongoing debate about the relative adverse impact of central subcutaneous (both deep and superficial) and visceral fat [11,12]. Waist circumference (WC) alone does not take the limb fat in to consideration. To overcome this, some researchers use waist–hip ratio (WHR) while others use total body fat percentage and prefers the term 'adiposity' [13].

It has long been known that central obesity is distinctly different in different ethnic groups. For a given BMI, body fat percentage is higher in African–Americans but lower in Chinese, South Asians and Ethiopians [14]. Pima Indians have higher overall body fat while South Asians have higher central fat [15–17]. These factors resulted in international organizations introducing different cut points for WC to identify high risk patients in different ethnic population (Table 16.1) [18,19]. The prevalence of obesity, abdominal obesity and adiposity in different ethnic populations, especially the South Asians and their effects on metabolic risks will be discussed in details.

16.2 Prevalence of obesity and its relationship with metabolic risk in various ethnic sub-groups

Indoasians

Prevalence
There is no single study which included the various sub-populations in the Indian subcontinent to show the prevalence of obesity, abdominal obesity and adiposity (total body fat content in percentage). However, data from several single centre studies showed

Table 16.1 Guidelines for identifying high risk patients using waist circumference

Ethnic group	Waist circumference in cm (midway between lower end of ribs and top of the pelvis)	
	Male	Female
Europeans	$\geq$94	$\geq$80
South Asians	$\geq$90	$\geq$80
Chinese	$\geq$90	$\geq$80
Japanese	$\geq$90	$\geq$80
South and Central Americans	$\geq$90	$\geq$80
Africans (sub-Saharan)	$\geq$94	$\geq$80
Eastern Mediterranean	$\geq$94	$\geq$80
Middle East (Arab)	$\geq$94	$\geq$80

Modified with permission from Alberti *et al.* [19].

the prevalence is between 10 and 50%. Such wide variation is due to the sub-population studied and different cut points used for BMI, WC, WHR and total body fat percentage [13], reviewed in [20] (Table 16.2). Using the ATP III cut points for WC the presence of metabolic syndrome is surprisingly low in SAs [21,22]. Therefore it is preferable to use the revised consensus guidelines for WC and metabolic syndrome issued by the International Diabetes Federation (IDF) in 2004 for various ethnic populations [23] (Table 16.1). These data are mostly derived from cross sectional studies and therefore of limited value in asserting the causal relationship between obesity and metabolic risk.

Relationship between obesity and metabolic risk

SAs have higher mean glucose and insulin levels during oral glucose tolerant test, with resultant higher prevalence of T2D [24–28]. This, at least in part, appears to be due to higher central obesity and higher over all adiposity. Indians have more total body fat for a given BMI and is centrally distributed compared to white Caucasians and African–Americans [14,29]. This characteristic feature of high adiposity in South Asians was shown beautifully in a pictorial form, highlighting the limited usefulness of BMI in South Asians (Figure 16.1) [29]. In addition to the excess body fat, for a given amount of body fat (both total and central) Indians have higher IR than Caucasians [25,30]. The metabolic risk in Indians is characterized by dysglycaemia, higher insulin levels for a given glucose level, higher triglyceride levels, lower high density lipoprotein (HDL) levels, higher blood pressure, higher total cholesterol–HDL ratio but lower low density lipoprotein (LDL) levels. These associations between metabolic risk factors and central obesity appear to be stronger in South Asian women than in South Asian men [24]. A recent community-based study of 'apparently healthy' men in three geographical locations in India showed that overall adiposity is the most significant contributor to IR. This study also showed that the relative contribution of adiposity to IR is higher in urban population than rural population highlighting the potential possibility of differential activity of adipocytes as well as the important role of lifestyle and other environmental factors [13]. An elegant study by Chandalia *et al.* confirmed these findings in a study comparing South Asian and Caucasian men living in Texas, United States of America. They have showed that SA men have higher body fat (which is mainly subcutaneous rather than visceral) for a given BMI, higher subcutaneous adipocyte size, lower glucose disposal and lower adiponectin levels compared to Caucasians [31]. The higher incidence of IR, T2D and CVD in South Asians is therefore seem to be related to genetic, lifestyle, environmental and differential function of adipocytes. However, most of these studies are either cross-sectional or *in-vitro* studies. Prospective studies looking at the role of these risk factors on incident follow up of T2D and CVD are urgently needed.

Oriental Asians (Chinese and Japanese)

Prevalence

In a cross-sectional study, Chinese have lower BMI and lower WHR compared to South Indians and Malays living in Singapore [32]. However, the absolute prevalence of general or central obesity was not reported. Similar results were found by

Table 16.2 Prevalence of obesity in India

Study (year)	Centre	Age (years)	Population studied	Prevalence (%) Male	Prevalence (%) Female
Dhurandhar and Kulkarni (1992)	Bombay	31–50	$n = 1784$	10.7–53.1	–
Gopinath (1994)	Delhi	25–64	$n = 13\,414$	21.3	33.4
Gopalan (1998)	Nutrition Foundation of India	–	Upper strata	32.2	50
			Middle class	16.2	30.3
			Low socio-economic	7.0	27.8
			Poor urban slum	1.0	4.0
District Nutrition Profiles Survey (1998)	Food and Nutrition Board	–	Rural ($n = 142\,220$)	0.3	0.7
			Urban ($n = 35\,621$)	0.4	0.7
National Family Health Survey (1998–1999)	–	15–49	–	–	2.3
Zargar (2000)	Kashmir	>40	$n = 5083$	7.0	23.7
Mohan et al. (2001)	Chennai urban	>20	General obesity	22.8	31.8
			Abdominal obesity ($n = 1262$)	21.5	36.5
Deshmukh et al. (2006)	Rural Wardha	>18	General obesity	5.1	5.2
			Abdominal obesity ($n = 2700$)	7.6	8.7

Modified with permission from the review by Mohan and Deepa [20].

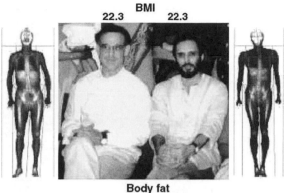

BMI
22.3   22.3

Body fat
9.1%   21.2%

Figure 16.1 Total body and central adiposity in South Asians and Caucasians. Legend: For an identical BMI, these two authors have wide variation in their total body adiposity measured by dual energy X-ray absorptiometry (DEXA) scan. Figure reproduced with permission from Yajnik and Yudkin [29]

Deurenberg-Yap *et al.* [33]. Interestingly, Chinese men had higher BMI and WHR compared to women while the Malayan and Indian women had higher BMI and WHR than their men counter parts. Over all Chinese men and women had significantly lower prevalence of obesity (BMI ≥ 30) and WHR (men ≥ 1.0 and women ≥0.85) using international criteria. Hence, the current recommendations are a WC of ≥90 cm in men and ≥80 cm in women should be used to identify individuals with higher metabolic risk. Studies of migrant Japanese–Americans living in the north-west of USA showed the prevalence of adiposity and central obesity are higher in second and third generation Japanese– Americans [34,35]. However, the absolute prevalence in comparison to native Japanese is not known. In an attempt to provide population wide cut points for generalized and central obesity, the Japanese society for obesity conducted a large cross-sectional study of more than 1100 individuals. Nearly 34% of men and 25% of women were found obese using a BMI cut point of ≥25 [36]. The authors also conclude a WC of ≥85 in men and ≥90 in women predicts metabolic risk. However, this is debated and re-analysis of this data suggested WC of ≥90 cm in men and ≥80 cm in women should be used, which are the same as South Asians and Chinese, until more data is available [37].

Relationship between obesity and metabolic risk
Though Chinese are shorter and lighter, with higher HDL levels, lower fasting insulin levels, lower glucose intolerance and lower triglyceride levels, the relationship between obesity and the metabolic risk factors are similar in Chinese compared to Indians and Malays [32,38]. For a given BMI Chinese men and women had higher prevalence of hypertension compared to American whites and non-Hispanic whites but not with American Blacks. This increased risk appears to get worse when the BMI ≥23 kg/m^2 [39]. In a study comparing four ethnic groups, Razak *et al.* beautifully demonstrated that among the various metabolic factors, blood pressure seem to

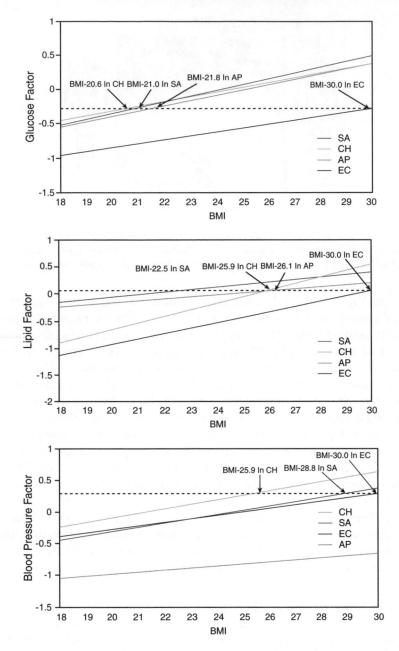

Figure 16.2 (a–c) Relationship between BMI and metabolic risk factors in various ethnic subgroups (a) BMI and glycaemia (b) BMI and lipids (c) BMI and blood pressure. CH, Chinese; SA, South Asians; EC, Europeans; AP, Aboriginals. Figure adapted and reproduced with permission from Razak *et al.* [7]

increase much earlier than glucose levels and lipid parameters with increasing BMI (Figure 16.2) [7]. The migrant Japanese–American studies showed that visceral adiposity correlates better with insulin resistance [40]. The prevalence of visceral obesity and its contribution to insulin resistance in migrant Japanese–American are higher compared to Caucasians. The prevalence of T2D in migrant Japanese-Americans are two- to fourfold higher compared to non-migrants and is approximately two- to threefold higher compared to white Caucasians [41–43]. These studies highlight the significance of environmental influences on the development of metabolic risk.

Afro-origin groups

Similar to South Asians, people of African and Afro-Caribbean decent also have distinct but different anthropometric characteristics and metabolic risk factors. Over all they have higher BMI, but tend to have less visceral adiposity than Caucasians at a given level of WHR. Indeed, BMI seem to be a better marker of obesity, especially in black women [44,45]. However, the overall evidence base for differences in the association of BMI, WC and total body adiposity with morbidity is limited in this ethnic group. People from this ethnic minority group have high incidence of T2D (two- to threefold), higher blood pressure (three- to fourfold), hyperuricaemia but lower triglyceride levels and higher HDL levels compared to Caucasians [46–49]. Studies comparing native and migrant black populations reveal adoption of a western lifestyle contributes to higher blood pressure as well as to higher mortality related to metabolic disorders [50,51]. This increased clustering of metabolic risk factors translates into higher incidence of stroke and end-stage renal failure but lower incidence of coronary heart disease (CHD) [52,53]. While the higher salt and lower potassium intake seems to contribute to the excess mortality from stroke, lower fibrinogen level in addition to the protective lipid profile (lower triglycerides and higher HDL) may in part explain the reduced risk of CHD [55,54].

Mexican–Americans (Hispanics)

Obesity is common among Mexican–Americans and 30% of women aged above 60 have a BMI $\geq$30 kg/m^2. Mexican–American women had higher central obesity (measured by skinfold thickness and WHR) than non-Hispanic white women. Similarly, Mexican–American males had higher central obesity than non-Hispanic white males, but differences in WHR disappeared after adjusting for BMI suggesting the higher amount of subcutaneous fat (higher skinfold thickness) in this population [56]. Compared to non-Hispanic whites, there is a three- to fivefold increased risk of T2D in Hispanics living in the USA. The prevalence of diabetes increases with age in Mexican Americans, and one in four over the age of 60 years have T2D [57–60]. Resistance to insulin-mediated glucose uptake appears to be a primary pathophysiological abnormality predisposing to T2D. This higher insulin resistance has been documented in older Hispanic women [61] and also appears to be present even in Mexican–American children. They have higher fasting plasma insulin, triglycerides, systolic blood pressure levels, lower HDL-cholesterol levels and a greater prevalence of multiple adverse risk factors compared with non-Hispanic white children [62]. These apparent ethnic differences were greater among boys than among girls, perhaps because of differences in adiposity [63]. The presence of higher metabolic risk factors in children including adiposity suggests the potential influence of genetic factors in this ethnic sub-group.

American Indians

Pima Indians have been extensively studied as they have an exceptionally high prevalence rate for T2D. They are very prone to obesity and are more insulin resistant compared to Caucasians of the same BMI [64]. Data from the Strong Heart Study indicated a propensity to high insulin concentrations, high WHR and dyslipidaemia characterized by elevated triglycerides, low HDL and small dense LDL particles. It showed that plasma insulin concentrations were a significant correlate in men, triglycerides were significant in women and HDL had a strong inverse correlation in both men and women [65]. The Atherosclerosis Risk in Communities study suggests that rates of CHD in American Indians may exceed those of other US populations and it is almost two fold higher in American Indian men and women than Caucasians. T2D is the strongest determinant of CVD in this ethnic group, contributing to 56% of the events in men and 78% of the events in women. Despite the higher incidence of CVD, the total and LDL cholesterol levels lower than the US average [66,67]. Hypertension is common in American Indian communities except for South/North Dakota and its prevalence is greater than in the general US population [68].

In a small study, Gautier *et al.* showed that Pima Indians have similar amounts of visceral fat compared to age, sex and BMI matched Caucasians but are less sensitive to the metabolic action of insulin and secrete more insulin. The difference in metabolic parameters and the higher risk of dysglycaemia in Pima Indians compared to Caucasians, despite controlling for obesity, suggests that unique genetic factors contribute to insulin resistance and hyperinsulinaemia in Pima Indians [69]. Intriguingly, visceral adipose tissue is not highly correlated with insulin resistance in Pima Indians.

Potential mechanisms of increased metabolic risk in ethnic groups

Several attempts have been made to identify the pathophysiological reasons for distinct anthropometric and metabolic characteristics in different ethnic groups. Over the last few decades it is also evident that the natural history of diabetes in these ethnic groups behaves differently, resulting in sub-classification of diabetes. In addition, it is now well recognized that development of complications due to diabetes is different in different populations – for example people of African and Afro-Caribbean decent develop more strokes, while people with origins from Indian subcontinent develop more heart disease and kidney disease [70]. Despite these advances in our understanding, the precise mechanisms of: the difference in body fat distribution, translation of adiposity into metabolic risk, effects of migration, relative contribution of individual risk factors to CVD and pharmacogenetics of common drugs in different ethnic population is far from certain.

Thrifty genotype hypothesis

Nearly half a century ago, the 'thrifty genotype hypothesis' was proposed by Neel in an attempt to explain the widespread prevalence of IR and T2D in modern society. He suggested that despite its association with conditions detrimental to health and survival today, it must have provided a survival advantage to the human species during evolution for it to have such a high frequency within present day populations [71]. Neel argued that hyperinsulinaemia conferred a survival advantage to humans when cycles of feast and famine were common, as it provides a mechanism by which mankind could take maximal advantage of such a pattern of food supply in times of plenty. Wendorf and Goldfine further added to this hypothesis that the presence of selective IR in muscle not only contributes to hyperinsulinaemia but also helps the excess energy available is preferentially stored in the liver and fat [72]. While this would not be detrimental to health in a feast-famine environment, in an environment of persistent calorie excess, these characteristics would predispose to obesity, T2D and the metabolic syndrome.

This hypothesis provides a plausible basis for the high prevalence of T2D in the Pima Indians, Nauruans and Australian Aborigines. The central feature of this hypothesis is the existence of hyperinsulinaemia. The case for hyperinsulinaemia as the primary defect in T2D was further supported by numerous studies. Ethnic variability in plasma insulin responses was shown in Pima Indians, Micronesians and Polynesians, Australian Aborigines, Asian Indians, Chinese and Creoles. Hyperinsulinaemia is a characteristic feature of populations with a high prevalence of T2D such as American Indians, Micronesian Nauruans and Polynesians, Mexican–Americans, Australian Aborigines, Asian Indians and Americans. It is unclear whether the thrifty genotype ever occurred in the ancestors of developed European populations with frequencies of a magnitude similar to those now seen in the above populations. If it was common at some time in the past, then it may well have been selected against until the gene(s) reached a relative low potency and constant population frequency, consistent with the currently observed pattern of disease onset in middle and older age, following completion of the reproductive phase. While the existence of the thrifty genotype has not been proven, the concept provides a reasonable explanation of the phenomenon of epidemic levels of T2D in certain ethnic groups.

Thrifty phenotype hypothesis

Some investigators have questioned the existence of a genetic component to the metabolic syndrome and suggest that IR, T2D and the metabolic syndrome seen in adulthood are the result of an adverse intrauterine and neonatal environment and therefore manifestations of a 'thrifty phenotype'. Barker *et al.* showed that with increasing birth weight and weight at one year, the death rate from heart disease fell while no similar trend could be shown in non-circulatory illness [73]. Further studies on this cohort of men looking specifically for the presence of metabolic syndrome (2-hour glucose ≥ 7.8 mmol/l, systolic BP ≥ 160 and triglycerides ≥ 1.4 mmol/l) showed that it reduces progressively from 30 to 6% as birth weight rose from <2.5 to >4.1 kg. Based on these findings, Barker proposed that the abnormalities that form the metabolic syndrome coexist because they share a common origin in the form of a suboptimal environment in early life. Data from developing countries that are undergoing rapid westernization, as well as data from migrants moved from their native environment to 'food affluent' environments, supports this hypothesis further. For example adults living in their native environment such as rural Africa and the highlands of Papua New Guinea have one of the lowest prevalence of T2D (less than 1%) [74,75]. In contrast, the indigenous population living in North American and western Pacific societies have the highest prevalence of T2D (up to one third of the adult population) found in the world [74,76]. The hypothesis that the disease is the outcome of reduced early growth is consistent with these geographic variations. If growth restraint during fetal life and infancy results in impaired growth and function of beta-cells, a sudden change to relative over nutrition during childhood and adulthood could explain the high diabetes rate in the Nauruan islanders. This population suffered severe nutritional deficiency during the Second World War. Thereafter, they became affluent from phosphate mining, and diabetes on the island became epidemic. A similar situation was shown in the Ethiopian Jews transported to Israel, among whom a high prevalence of diabetes was observed [77]. Thus, it seems, poor nutrition in fetal and early infant life is detrimental to the mechanisms maintaining carbohydrate tolerance. Two longitudinal studies, both from India, confirmed the critical role of the 'intrauterine environment'. These studies confirmed that lower birth weight, especially when associated with accelerated early childhood growth, results in higher metabolic risk [78,79]. Further analysis of one of the cohorts suggests that maternal micronutrient levels and their potential epigenetic regulation of DNA might be contributing to the increased metabolic risk of the offspring [80], a concept supported by animal studies [81]. These findings are fascinating and worth careful consideration and replication in carefully designed prospective studies.

The common soil hypothesis

This hypothesis was initially proposed by Stern from many observations that although atherosclerosis is often considered to be a complication of diabetes, they both share many of the genetic and environmental antecedents [82]. This will explain the increased risk of atherosclerosis and CVD in patients with impaired glucose tolerance. Therefore both should be considered as consequences of the metabolic syndrome that is spring from a 'common soil'. There is, in fact, a large body of evidence to suggest this may indeed be the case. However, this hypothesis alone does not explain the higher incidence of CVD in patients with diabetes and the presence of CVD in patients without diabetes.

The adipose tissue overflow hypothesis

In an attempt to explain the differences in body fat distribution in different ethnicity, Snidermann and colleagues recently hypothesized that the primary adipose tissue compartment is superficial subcutaneous adipose tissue and is less well developed in South Asians compared to white Caucasians [83]. Because of the limited capacity of the superficial subcutaneous adipose tissue to expand, the excess energy is stored as adipose tissue in the deep subcutaneous and visceral compartment; both of them are centrally distributed and known to be more metabolically active. This would explain why at a similar BMI, higher central adiposity and adverse atherogenic lipoprotein profile are more pronounced in South Asians compared to white Caucasians. However, testing this hypothesis needs carefully characterized, large cohort studies that are followed for a long period, preferably from intrauterine life along side with complex pathophysiological studies on IR, beta cell dysfunction and adipocyte biology.

Points to learn from migration studies

Increased metabolic and cardiovascular risk in migrant South Asians compared to other ethnic groups has been observed as early as the 1950s [84–91]. This is also true for ethnic sub-populations such as Punjabis, Gujaratis, Sikhs, Bangladeshis, and so on [92]. This excess is remarkably consistent in South Asian populations living outside India, even if the migration occurred many generations earlier, suggesting the critical role of genetic factors [27,28,93]. However, the stepwise increase in the prevalence of the metabolic risk in rural, urban migrants inside India and migrants outside India suggest the vital role of gene–environment interaction [13,94]. While affluence is associated with higher obesity in the individuals migrating inside the country, it has the opposite effect on the individuals who migrated outside the country. Excess food (especially high calorie fast foods) and lack of awareness about the impact of healthy life style on obesity seem to be the common denominators in both of these migrant populations. It is therefore clear that the increased cardiovascular risks are likely due to increasing prevalence of obesity from these lifestyle and dietary changes in addition to the genetic predisposition. These migrant studies also highlight the contribution of 'non-traditional risk factors' to the increased cardiovascular risk [95].

16.3 Conclusion

There is a significant variation in the pattern of obesity, complications of diabetes, including blood pressure and cardiovascular disease, amongst the various ethnic groups in the world. Indians have more central fat distribution and higher incidence of CHD than any other ethnic group. People of African origin seem to have higher non-esterified fatty acids, more likely to be insulinopenic, more likely to develop high blood pressure and suffer from stroke. European men are taller, heavier and are at lower risk for T2D. Chinese are shorter and lighter with lower triglyceride and 2 hour glucose levels and at higher risk of developing T2D and hypertension. While different stages of epidemiological transition may explain part of this variance, the diversity of gene–environment interactions is the factor that contributes most to this variability. Ethnic differences are also relevant in assessing CHD risk. Models that assume an 'average' HDL cholesterol concentration rather than a measured value are not appropriate in a multi-ethnic setting as they underestimate risk in groups such as Indo-Asians who tend to have low HDL levels. From a practical point of view, these differences must be borne in mind when carrying out studies involving the metabolic syndrome across different ethnic groups and when assessing the risk of complications including CHD in ethnic minority groups.

Prevention and control of metabolic diseases should be a high priority for any nation and obesity management should form an important part of its strategy. Prevention of obesity, diabetes and cardiovascular diseases can be classified as primary prevention – by providing better health for prenatal women; secondary – by providing education on healthy living for children, adolescents and adults; and tertiary – by early detection of these conditions with aggressive risk reduction strategies. Though the prevalence of obesity is lower in South Asia than in Europe the health risks associated with obesity occur at a lower BMI in Asian populations [96,97]. Therefore efforts to initiate these prevention strategies should be implemented at an early stage, recognizing ethnic differences in susceptibility to complications. Prevention strategies can also be implemented by two mechanisms: nationwide strategies targeting the whole population and selective and targeted strategies targeting the high risk groups. While the nation-wide strategies need policies involving governments, targeting high risk groups can be implemented in appropriate settings at local and regional level (e.g. schools, primary care venues, community and religious centres). This will not only allow easy access for these high risk groups but also provide more opportunities to engage them as well as to develop tailor-made strategies according to the local need. Such targeted prevention aiming to: prevent weight gain in overweight individuals and to reduce the number of people with weight-related disorders who are already obese or those with biological markers associated with excess adiposity who are not yet obese, will make huge difference to the individuals affected as well as the nation as a whole.

References

1. McKeigue, P.M., Shah, B. and Marmot, M.G. (1991) Relation of central obesity and insulin resistance with high diabetes prevalence and cardiovascular risk in South Asians. *Lancet*, **337** (8738), 382–6.
2. Shelgikar, K.M., Hockaday, T.D. and Yajnik, C.S. (1991) Central rather than generalized obesity is related to hyperglycaemia in Asian Indian subjects. *Diabetic Medicine*, **8** (8), 712–7.
3. World Health Organization (1998) Obesity: Preventing and Managing the Global Epidemic – Report on a WHO consultation on obesity. WHO/NUT/NCD/98. 1; Geneva.
4. World Health Organization (2002) Report of a WHO expert consultation on appropriate BMI for Asian populations and its implications for policy and intervention strategies, WHO Consultation, Geneva.

5. Stevens, J. (2003) Ethnic-specific revisions of body mass index cut-offs to define overweight and obesity in Asians are not warranted. *International Journal of Obesity and Related Metabolic Disorders*, **27** (11), 1297–9.

6. WHO (2004) Appropriate body-mass index for Asian populations and its implications for policy and intervention strategies. *Lancet* **363** (9403), 157–63.

7. Razak, F., Anand, S.S., Shannon, H. *et al.* (2007) Defining obesity cut points in a multiethnic population. *Circulation*, **115** (16), 2111–8.

8. Markman, B. and Barton, F.E., Jr (1987) Anatomy of the subcutaneous tissue of the trunk and lower extremity. *Plastic and Reconstructive Surgery*, **80** (2), 248–54.

9. Johnson, D., Dixon, A.K. and Abrahams, P.H. (1996) The abdominal subcutaneous tissue: computed tomographic, magnetic resonance, and anatomical observations. *Clinical Anatomy (New York, NY)*, **9** (1), 19–24.

10. Deschenes, D., Couture, P., Dupont, P. and Tchernof, A. (2003) Subdivision of the subcutaneous adipose tissue compartment and lipid-lipoprotein levels in women. *Obesity Research*, **11** (3), 469–76.

11. Lebovitz, H.E. and Banerji, M.A. (2005) Point: visceral adiposity is causally related to insulin resistance. *Diabetes Care*, **28** (9), 2322–5.

12. Miles, J.M. and Jensen, M.D. (2005) Counterpoint: visceral adiposity is not causally related to insulin resistance. *Diabetes Care*, **28** (9), 2326–8.

13. Yajnik, C.S., Joglekar, C.V., Lubree, H.G. *et al.* (2008) Adiposity, inflammation and hyperglycaemia in rural and urban Indian men: Coronary Risk of Insulin Sensitivity in Indian Subjects (CRISIS) Study. *Diabetologia*, **51** (1), 39–46.

14. Deurenberg, P., Yap, M. and van Staveren, W.A. (1998) Body mass index and percent body fat: a meta analysis among different ethnic groups. *International Journal of Obesity and Related Metabolic Disorders*, **22** (12), 1164–71.

15. Knowler, W.C., Pettitt, D.J., Savage, P.J. and Bennett, P.H. (1981) Diabetes incidence in Pima Indians: contributions of obesity and parental diabetes. *American Journal of Epidemiology*, **113** (2), 144–56.

16. Cappuccio, F.P., Cook, D.G., Atkinson, R.W. and Strazzullo, P. (1997) Prevalence, detection, and management of cardiovascular risk factors in different ethnic groups in south London. *Heart (British Cardiac Society)*, **78** (6), 555–63.

17. Balarajan, R. (1991) Ethnic differences in mortality from ischaemic heart disease and cerebrovascular disease in England and Wales. *British Medical Journal (Clinical Research Ed)*, **302** (6776), 560–4.

18. The IDF consensus worldwide definition of the metabolic syndrome. Last accessed on 10th June at www.idf.org/webdata/docs/MetS_def_update2006.pdf (2006).

19. Alberti, K.G., Zimmet, P. and Shaw, J. (2007) International Diabetes Federation: a consensus on type 2 diabetes prevention. *Diabetic Medicine*, **24** (5), 451–63.

20. Mohan, V. and Deepa, R. (2006) Obesity and abdominal obesity in Asian Indians. *Indian Journal of Medical Research*, **123** (5), 593–6.

21. Tan, C.E., Ma, S., Wai, D. *et al.* (2004) Can we apply the National Cholesterol Education Program Adult Treatment Panel definition of the metabolic syndrome to Asians? *Diabetes Care*, **27** (5), 1182–6.

22. Snehalatha, C., Viswanathan, V. and Ramachandran, A. (2003) Cutoff values for normal anthropometric variables in Asian Indian adults. *Diabetes Care*, **26** (5), 1380–4.

23. Alberti, K.G., Zimmet, P. and Shaw, J. (2005) The metabolic syndrome – a new worldwide definition. *Lancet*, **366** (9491), 1059–62.

24. McKeigue, P.M., Pierpoint, T., Ferrie, J.E. and Marmot, M.G. (1992) Relationship of glucose intolerance and hyperinsulinaemia to body fat pattern in south Asians and Europeans. *Diabetologia*, **35** (8), 785–91.

25. Chandalia, M., Abate, N., Garg, A. *et al.* (1999) Relationship between generalized and upper body obesity to insulin resistance in Asian Indian men. *Journal of Clinical Endocrinology and Metabolism*, **84** (7), 2329–35.

26. Simmons, D., Williams, D.R. and Powell, M.J. (1991) The Coventry Diabetes Study: prevalence of diabetes and impaired glucose tolerance in Europids and Asians. *Quarterly Journal of Medicine*, **81** (296), 1021–30.

27. Ramachandran, A., Snehalatha, C., Dharmaraj, D. and Viswanathan, M. (1992) Prevalence of glucose intolerance in Asian Indians. Urban–rural difference and significance of upper body adiposity. *Diabetes Care*, **15** (10), 1348–55.

28. Cappuccio, F.P. (1997) Ethnicity and cardiovascular risk: variations in people of African ancestry and South Asian origin. *Journal of Human Hypertension*, **11** (9), 571–6.

29. Yajnik, C.S. and Yudkin, J.S. (2004) The Y-Y paradox. *Lancet*, **363** (9403), 163.

30. Ramachandran, A., Snehalatha, C., Viswanathan, V. *et al.* (1997) Risk of noninsulin dependent diabetes mellitus conferred by obesity and central adiposity in different ethnic groups: a comparative analysis between Asian Indians. Mexican Americans and Whites. *Diabetes Research and Clinical Practice*, **36** (2), 121–5.

31. Chandalia, M., Lin, P., Seenivasan, T. *et al.* (2007) Insulin resistance and body fat distribution in South Asian men compared to Caucasian men. *PLoS One*, **2** (8), e812.

32. Hughes, K., Aw, T.C., Kuperan, P. and Choo, M. (1997) Central obesity, insulin resistance, syndrome X, lipoprotein(a), and cardiovascular risk in Indians, Malays, and Chinese in Singapore. *Journal of Epidemiology and Community Health*, **51** (4), 394–9.

33. Deurenberg-Yap, M., Chew, S.K., Lin, V.F. *et al.* (2001) Relationships between indices of obesity and its co-morbidities in multi-ethnic Singapore. *International Journal of Obesity and Related Metabolic Disorders*, **25** (10), 1554–62.

34. Bergstrom, R.W., Newell-Morris, L.L., Leonetti, D.L. *et al.* (1990) Association of elevated fasting C-peptide level and increased intra-abdominal fat distribution with development of NIDDM in Japanese-American men. *Diabetes*, **39** (1), 104–11.

35. Fujimoto, W.Y., Bergstrom, R.W., Boyko, E.J. *et al.* (1994) Diabetes and diabetes risk factors in second- and third-generation Japanese Americans in Seattle, Washington. *Diabetes Research and Clinical Practice*, **24** (Suppl), S43–S52

36. The Examination Committee of Criteria for 'Obesity Disease' in Japan (2002) New criteria for 'obesity disease' in Japan. *Circulation Journal*, **66** (11) 987–92.

37. Alberti, K.G., Zimmet, P. and Shaw, J. (2006) Metabolic syndrome–a new world-wide definition. A Consensus Statement from the International Diabetes Federation. *Diabetic Medicine*, **23** (5), 469–80.

38. Patel, S., Unwin, N., Bhopal, R. *et al.* (1999) A comparison of proxy measures of abdominal obesity in Chinese, European and South Asian adults. *Diabetic Medicine*, **16** (10), 853–60.

39. Ko, G.T., Chan, J.C., Cockram, C.S. and Woo, J. (1999) Prediction of hypertension, diabetes, dyslipidaemia or albuminuria using simple anthropometric indexes in Hong Kong Chinese. *International Journal of Obesity and Related Metabolic Disorders*, **23** (11), 1136–42.

40. Fujimoto, W.Y. (1992) The growing prevalence of non-insulin-dependent diabetes in migrant Asian populations and its implications for Asia. *Diabetes Research and Clinical Practice*, **15** (2), 167–83.

41. Fujimoto, W.Y., Leonetti, D.L., Kinyoun, J.L. *et al.* (1987) Prevalence of diabetes mellitus and impaired glucose tolerance among second-generation Japanese-American men. *Diabetes*, **36** (6), 721–9.

42. Burchfiel, C.M., Curb, J.D., Rodriguez, B.L. *et al.* (1995) Incidence and predictors of diabetes in Japanese-American men. The Honolulu Heart Program. *Annals of Epidemiology*, **5** (1), 33–43.

43. Edwards, K.L., Burchfiel, C.M., Sharp, D.S. *et al.* (1998) Factors of the insulin resistance syndrome in nondiabetic and diabetic elderly Japanese-American men. *American Journal of Epidemiology*, **147** (5), 441–7.

44. Kaufman, J.S., Durazo-Arvizu, R.A., Rotimi, C.N. *et al.* (1996) Obesity and hypertension prevalence in populations of African origin. The Investigators of the International Collaborative Study on Hypertension in Blacks. *Epidemiology*, **7** (4), 398–405.

45. Luke, A., Durazo-Arvizu, R., Rotimi, C. *et al.* (1997) Relation between body mass index and body fat in black population samples from Nigeria, Jamaica, and the United States. *American Journal of Epidemiology*, **145** (7), 620–8.

46. Chaturvedi, N., McKeigue, P.M. and Marmot, M.G. (1993) Resting and ambulatory blood pressure differences in Afro-Caribbeans and Europeans. *Hypertension*, **22** (1), 90–6.

47. Chaturvedi, N., McKeigue, P.M. and Marmot, M.G. (1994) Relationship of glucose intolerance to coronary risk in Afro-Caribbeans compared with Europeans. *Diabetologia*, **37** (8), 765–72.

48. Cooper, R., Rotimi, C., Ataman, S. *et al.* (1997) The prevalence of hypertension in seven populations of west African origin. *American Journal of Public Health*, **87** (2), 160–8.

49. Miller, G.J., Kirkwood, B.R., Beckles, G.L. *et al.* (1988) Adult male all-cause, cardiovascular and cerebrovascular mortality in relation to ethnic group, systolic blood pressure and blood glucose concentration in Trinidad, West Indies. *International Journal of Epidemiology*, **17** (1), 62–9.

50. Kaufman, J.S., Rotimi, C.N., Brieger, W.R. *et al.* (1996) The mortality risk associated with hypertension: preliminary results of a prospective study in rural Nigeria. *Journal of Human Hypertension*, **10** (7), 461–4.

51. Poulter, N.R., Khaw, K.T., Hopwood, B.E. *et al.* (1990) The Kenyan Luo migration study: observations on the initiation of a rise in blood pressure. *British Medical Journal (Clinical Research Ed)*, **300** (6730), 967–72.

52. Raleigh, V.S. (1997) Diabetes and hypertension in Britain's ethnic minorities: implications for the future of renal services. *British Medical Journal (Clinical Research Ed)*, **314** (7075), 209–13.

53. Schmidt, M.I., Duncan, B.B., Watson, R.L. *et al.* (1996) A metabolic syndrome in whites and African-Americans. The Atherosclerosis Risk in Communities baseline study. *Diabetes Care*, **19** (5), 414–8.

54. Cruickshank, J.K., Cooper, J., Burnett, M. *et al.* (1991) Ethnic differences in fasting plasma C-peptide and insulin in relation to glucose tolerance and blood pressure. *Lancet*, **338** (8771), 842–7.

55. Cook, D.G., Cappuccio, F.P., Atkinson, R.W. *et al.* (2001) Ethnic differences in fibrinogen levels: the role of environmental factors and the beta-fibrinogen gene. *American Journal of Epidemiology*, **153** (8), 799–806.

56. Haffner, S.M., Stern, M.P., Hazuda, H.P. *et al.* (1986) Upper body and centralized adiposity in Mexican Americans and non-Hispanic whites: relationship to body mass index and other behavioural and demographic variables. *International Journal of Obesity*, **10** (6), 493–502.

57. Diehl, A.K. and Stern, M.P. (1989) Special health problems of Mexican-Americans: obesity, gallbladder disease, diabetes mellitus, and cardiovascular disease. *Advances in Internal Medicine*, **34**, 73–96.

58. Gardner, L.I., Jr, Stern, M.P., Haffner, S.M. *et al.* (1984) Prevalence of diabetes in Mexican Americans. Relationship to percent of gene pool derived from native American sources. *Diabetes*, **33** (1), 86–92.

59. Stern, M.P., Rosenthal, M., Haffner, S.M. *et al.* (1984) Sex difference in the effects of sociocultural status on diabetes and cardiovascular risk factors in Mexican Americans. The San Antonio Heart Study. *American Journal of Epidemiology*, **120** (6), 834–51.

60. Flegal, K.M., Ezzati, T.M., Harris, M.I. *et al.* (1991) Prevalence of diabetes in Mexican Americans, Cubans, and Puerto Ricans from the Hispanic Health and Nutrition Examination Survey, 1982–1984. *Diabetes Care*, **14** (7), 628–38.

61. Aguirre, M.A., Jones, C.N., Pei, D. *et al.* (1997) Ethnic differences in insulin resistance and its consequences in older Mexican American and non-Hispanic white women. *Journals of Gerontology. Series A, Biological Sciences and Medical Sciences*, **52** (1), M56–M60.

62. Batey, L.S., Goff, D.C., Jr. Tortolero, S.R. *et al.* (1997) Summary measures of the insulin resistance syndrome are adverse among Mexican-American versus non-Hispanic white children: the Corpus Christi Child Heart Study. *Circulation*, **96** (12), 4319–25.

63. Haffner, S.M., Stern, M.P., Hazuda, H.P. *et al.* (1986) Upper body and centralized adiposity in Mexican Americans and non-Hispanic whites: relationship to body mass index and other behavioral and demographic variables. *International Journal of Obesity*, **10** (6), 493–502.

64. Nagulesparan, M., Savage, P.J., Knowler, W.C. *et al.* (1982) Increased in vivo insulin resistance in nondiabetic Pima Indians compared with Caucasians. *Diabetes*, **31** (11), 952–6.

65. Howard, B.V., Lee, E.T., Cowan, L.D. *et al.* (1999) Rising tide of cardiovascular disease in American Indians. The Strong Heart Study. *Circulation*, **99** (18), 2389–95.

66. Haffner, S.M., Stern, M.P., Hazuda, H.P. *et al.* (1986) The role of behavioral variables and fat patterning in explaining ethnic differences in serum lipids and lipoproteins. *American Journal of Epidemiology*, **123** (5), 830–9.

67. Chambless, L.E., Heiss, G., Folsom, A.R. *et al.* (1997) Association of coronary heart disease incidence with carotid arterial wall thickness and major risk factors: the Atherosclerosis Risk in Communities (ARIC) Study, 1987–1993. *American Journal of Epidemiology*, **146** (6), 483–94.

68. Howard, B.V., Lee, E.T., Yeh, J.L. *et al.* (1996) Hypertension in adult American Indians. The Strong Heart Study. *Hypertension*, **28** (2), 256–64.

69. Gautier, J.F., Milner, M.R., Elam, E. *et al.* (1999) Visceral adipose tissue is not increased in Pima Indians compared with equally obese Caucasians and is not related to insulin action or secretion. *Diabetologia*, **42** (1), 28–34.

70. Bellary, S., O'Hare, J.P., Raymond, N.T. *et al.* (2008) Enhanced diabetes care to patients of south Asian ethnic origin (the United Kingdom Asian Diabetes Study): a cluster randomised controlled trial. *Lancet*, **371** (9626), 1769–76.

71. Neel, J.V. (1962) Diabetes mellitus: a 'thrifty' genotype rendered detrimental by 'progress'? *American Journal of Human Genetics*, **14**, 353–62.

72. Wendorf, M. and Goldfine, I.D. (1991) Archaeology of NIDDM. Excavation of the 'thrifty' genotype. *Diabetes*, **40** (2), 161–5.

73. Barker, D.J., Hales, C.N., Fall, C.H. *et al.* (1993) Type 2 (non-insulin-dependent) diabetes mellitus, hypertension and hyperlipidaemia (syndrome X): relation to reduced fetal growth. *Diabetologia*, **36** (1), 62–7.

74. King, H., Heywood, P., Zimmet, P. *et al.* (1984) Glucose tolerance in a highland population in Papua New Guinea. *Diabetes Research (Edinburgh, Lothian)*, **1** (1), 45–51.

75. McLarty, D.G., Swai, A.B., Kitange, H.M. *et al.* (1989) Prevalence of diabetes and impaired glucose tolerance in rural Tanzania. *Lancet*, **1** (8643), 871–5.

76. Knowler, W.C., Bennett, P.H., Hamman, R.F. and Miller, M. (1978) Diabetes incidence and prevalence in Pima Indians: a 19-fold greater incidence than in Rochester, Minnesota. *American Journal of Epidemiology*, **108** (6), 497–505.

77. Cohen, M.P., Stern, E., Rusecki, Y. and Zeidler, A. (1988) High prevalence of diabetes in young adult Ethiopian immigrants to Israel. *Diabetes*, **37** (6), 824–8.

78. Bhargava, S.K., Sachdev, H.S., Fall, C.H.D. *et al.* (2004) Relation of serial changes in childhood body-mass index to impaired glucose tolerance in young adulthood. *New England Journal of Medicine*, **350** (9), 865–75.

79. Joglekar, C.V., Fall, C.H., Deshpande, V.U. *et al.* (2007) Newborn size, infant and childhood growth, and body composition and cardiovascular disease risk factors at the age of 6 years: the Pune Maternal Nutrition Study. *International Journal of Obesity (London)*, **31** (10), 1534–44.

80. Yajnik, C.S., Deshpande, S.S., Jackson, A.A. *et al.* (2008) Vitamin B(12) and folate concentrations during pregnancy and insulin resistance in the offspring: the Pune Maternal Nutrition Study. *Diabetologia*, **51** (1), 29–38.

81. Sinclair, K.D., Allegrucci, C., Singh, R. *et al.* (2007) DNA methylation, insulin resistance, and blood pressure in offspring determined by maternal periconceptional B vitamin and methionine status. *Proceedings of the National Academy of Sciences of the United States of America*, **104** (49), 19351–6.

82. Stern, M.P. (1995) Diabetes and cardiovascular disease. The 'common soil' hypothesis. *Diabetes*, **44** (4), 369–74.

83. Sniderman, A.D., Bhopal, R., Prabhakaran, D. *et al.* (2007) Why might South Asians be so susceptible to central obesity and its atherogenic consequences? The adipose tissue overflow hypothesis. *International Journal of Epidemiology*, **36** (1), 220–5.

84. Danaraj, T.J., Acker, M.S., Danaraj, W. *et al.* (1959) Ethnic group differences in coronary heart disease in Singapore: an analysis of necropsy records. *American Heart Journal*, **58**, 516–26.

85. Adelstein, A.M. (1963) Some aspects of cardiovascular mortality in South Africa. *British Journal of Preventive & Social Medicine*, **17**, 29–40.

86. Tuomilehto, J., Ram, P., Eseroma, R. *et al.* (1984) Cardiovascular diseases and diabetes mellitus in Fiji: analysis of mortality, morbidity and risk factors. *Bulletin of the World Health Organization*, **62** (1), 133–43.

87. Ramachandran, A., Jali, M.V., Mohan, V. *et al.* (1988) High prevalence of diabetes in an urban population in south India. *British Medical Journal (Clinical Research Ed)*, **297** (6648), 587–90.

88. McKeigue, P.M., Miller, G.J. and Marmot, M.G. (1989) Coronary heart disease in south Asians overseas: a review. *Journal of Clinical Epidemiology*, **42** (7), 597–609.

89. Snehalatha, C., Ramachandran, A., Vijay, V. and Viswanathan, M. (1994) Differences in plasma insulin responses in urban and rural Indians: a study in southern-Indians. *Diabetic Medicine*, **11** (5), 445–8.

90. McKeigue, P.M. (1996) Metabolic consequences of obesity and body fat pattern: lessons from migrant studies. *Ciba Foundation Symposium*, **201**, 54–64.

91. Cappuccio, F.P., Cook, D.G., Atkinson, R.W. and Strazzullo, P. (1997) Prevalence, detection, and management of cardiovascular risk factors in different ethnic groups in south London. *Heart (British Cardiac Society)*, **78** (6), 555–63.

92. Bhatnagar, D., Anand, I.S., Durrington, P.N. *et al.* (1995) Coronary risk factors in people from the Indian subcontinent living in west London and their siblings in India. *Lancet*, **345** (8947), 405–9.

93. McKeigue, P.M., Marmot, M.G., Adelstein, A.M. *et al.* (1985) Diet and risk factors for coronary heart disease in Asians in northwest London. *Lancet*, **2** (8464), 1086–90.

94. Misra, A., Khurana, L., Vikram, N.K. *et al.* (2007) Metabolic syndrome in children: current issues and South Asian perspective. *Nutrition*, **23** (11–12), 895–910.

95. Bhopal, R., Unwin, N., White, M. *et al.* (1999) Heterogeneity of coronary heart disease risk factors in Indian, Pakistani, Bangladeshi, and European origin populations: cross sectional study. *British Medical Journal (Clinical Research Ed)*, **319** (7204), 215–20.

96. Deurenberg-Yap, M., Yian, T.B., Kai, C.S. *et al.* (1999) Manifestation of cardiovascular risk factors at low levels of body mass index and waist-to-hip ratio in Singaporean Chinese. *Asia Pacific Journal of Clinical Nutrition*, **8** (3), 177–83.

97. Inoue, S., Zimmet, P., Caterson, I. *et al.* (2000) The Asia Pacific Perspective: Redefining Obesity and its Treatment. WHO, IOTF, IASO, Hong Kong.

Index

Obesity and Diabetes, Second Edition   Edited by Anthony H. Barnett and Sudhesh Kumar
© 2009 John Wiley & Sons, Ltd